AF904406

Thoracic Anesthesia Procedures

Thoracic Anesthesia Procedures

Edited by

Alan D. Kaye, MD, PhD, DABA, DABPM, DABIPP, FASA
Vice-Chancellor of Academic Affairs, Chief Academic Officer, and Provost
Tenured Professor of Anesthesiology, Pharmacology, Toxicology, and Neurosciences
LSU School of Medicine
Shreveport, LA, USA

Richard D. Urman, MD, MBA, FASA
Associate Professor
Department of Anesthesiology
Perioperative and Pain Medicine
Brigham and Women's Hospital
Boston, MA, USA

OXFORD
UNIVERSITY PRESS

OXFORD
UNIVERSITY PRESS

Oxford University Press is a department of the University of Oxford. It furthers the University's objective of excellence in research, scholarship, and education by publishing worldwide. Oxford is a registered trade mark of Oxford University Press in the UK and certain other countries.

Published in the United States of America by Oxford University Press
198 Madison Avenue, New York, NY 10016, United States of America.

© Oxford University Press 2021

All rights reserved. No part of this publication may be reproduced, stored in a retrieval system, or transmitted, in any form or by any means, without the prior permission in writing of Oxford University Press, or as expressly permitted by law, by license, or under terms agreed with the appropriate reproduction rights organization. Inquiries concerning reproduction outside the scope of the above should be sent to the Rights Department, Oxford University Press, at the address above.

You must not circulate this work in any other form
and you must impose this same condition on any acquirer.

Library of Congress Cataloging-in-Publication Data
Names: Kaye, Alan D., editor. | Urman, Richard D., editor.
Title: Thoracic anesthesia procedures / Alan D. Kaye and Richard D. Urman.
Description: New York, NY : Oxford University Press, [2021] |
Includes bibliographical references and index.
Identifiers: LCCN 2020047807 (print) | LCCN 2020047808 (ebook) |
ISBN 9780197506127 (paperback) | ISBN 9780197506141 (epub) |
ISBN 9780197506158 (online)
Subjects: MESH: Thoracic Surgical Procedures | Anesthesia
Classification: LCC RD536 (print) | LCC RD536 (ebook) |
NLM WF 980 | DDC 617.9/6754—dc23
LC record available at https://lccn.loc.gov/2020047807
LC ebook record available at https://lccn.loc.gov/2020047808

DOI: 10.1093/med/9780197506127.001.0001

This material is not intended to be, and should not be considered, a substitute for medical or other professional advice. Treatment for the conditions described in this material is highly dependent on the individual circumstances. And, while this material is designed to offer accurate information with respect to the subject matter covered and to be current as of the time it was written, research and knowledge about medical and health issues is constantly evolving and dose schedules for medications are being revised continually, with new side effects recognized and accounted for regularly. Readers must therefore always check the product information and clinical procedures with the most up-to-date published product information and data sheets provided by the manufacturers and the most recent codes of conduct and safety regulation. The publisher and the authors make no representations or warranties to readers, express or implied, as to the accuracy or completeness of this material. Without limiting the foregoing, the publisher and the authors make no representations or warranties as to the accuracy or efficacy of the drug dosages mentioned in the material. The authors and the publisher do not accept, and expressly disclaim, any responsibility for any liability, loss, or risk that may be claimed or incurred as a consequence of the use and/or application of any of the contents of this material.

1 3 5 7 9 8 6 4 2

Printed by Marquis, Canada

To my wife Dr. Kim Kaye and my children, Aaron and Rachel Kaye, for being the best family a man could ask for in his life.

To my mother Florence Feldman who made me the man I am today.

Thank you to all my patients that I have had the honor to take care of over the past 30 plus years.

I am grateful to my mentors, friends, brother Adam, sister Sheree, and other family members for your support throughout my life.

—Alan D. Kaye, MD, PhD, DABA, DABPM, DABIPP, FASA

To my patients who inspired me to write this book to help other practitioners improve their care

To my mentors for their encouragement and support

To my students and trainees so that they can use this guide to better prepare to take care of their patients

To my family: my wife Dr. Zina Matlyuk-Urman, MD, my daughters Abigail and Isabelle who make it all possible and worth it, every day.

And finally, to my parents, Tanya and Dennis Urman.

—Richard D. Urman, MD, MBA, FASA

Contents

Foreword

Historically, injury or disease within the chest was considered in most instances to be fatal. It would take hundreds of years to understand human anatomy and physiology for doctors and scientists to develop surgical techniques to provide surgeons and anesthesiologists the understanding and skills to work in a small space to treat diseases of the thorax.

Today, technological advances have paved the way for miraculous cures for infection, anatomical disorders, vascular abnormalities, malignant tumors, benign masses, and other thorax pathologies. These treatments promote healing for a wide variety of clinical conditions, and the evoluation of anesthesia techniques has allowed for less postoperative pain and improved outcomes.

We hope that our book, Thoracic Anesthesia Procedures, provides an inspiration for lessons in thorax surgery and anesthesia for medical students, residents, fellows, and attending staff. We have worked methodically to recruit experts from numerous medical fields and professional disciplines. The result is an easy to read and very visual book sharing expertise and knowledge in the field of thoracic surgery. We welcome your comments and hope you enjoy our book focused on thoracic disease and treatment.

Contributors

Harendra Arora, MD, FASA, MBA
Professor
Department of Anesthesiology
University of North Carolina School of Medicine
Chapel Hill, NC, USA

Alexandra L. Belfar, MD
Assistant Professor
Department of Anesthesiology
Michael E. DeBakey Veterans Affairs Medical Center
Department of Anesthesiology
Baylor College of Medicine
Houston, TX, USA

Joseph Capone, DO
Resident
Department of Anesthesiology
Advocate Illinois Masonic Medical Center
Chicago, IL, USA

Indranil Chakraborty, MBBS, MD, DNB
Professor
Department of Anesthesiology
College of Medicine, University of Arkansas for Medical Sciences
Little Rock, AR, USA

Xiangdong Chen, MD, PhD
Chairman and Professor
Department of Anesthesiology
Tongji Medical College Wuhan Union Hospital
Huazhong University of Science & Technology
Wuhan, China

Daniel Demos, MD
Assistant Professor of Surgery
Division of Thoracic and Cardiac Surgery
Department of Surgery
University of Florida College of Medicine
Gainesville, FL, USA

Yi Deng, MD
Assistant Professor of Cardiothoracic Anesthesiology and Critical Care Medicine
Associate Director of Cardiothoracic Anesthesiology at Ben Taub Hospital
Department of Anesthesiology
Baylor College of Medicine
Houston, TX, USA

Tricia Desvarieux, MD
Assistant Professor of Anesthesiology and Critical Care Medicine
Department of Anesthesiology and Critical Care Medicine
George Washington University School of Medicine & Health Sciences
Washington, DC, USA

Kevin Duong, MD
Resident Physician
Department of Anesthesiology
Baylor College of Medicine
Houston, TX, USA

Zipei Feng, MD, PhD
Resident Physician
Department of Otolaryngology
Baylor College of Medicine
Houston, TX, USA

Loren Francis, MD
Cardiothoracic Anesthesiologist
Department of Anesthesia and Perioperative Medicine
Medical University of South Carolina
Charleston, SC, USA

Parker D. Freels, MD
Physician
Department of Radiology
University of Florida College of Medicine
Jacksonville, FL, USA

Giuseppe Giurattabocchetta, MD
Department of Anesthesiology
University of Florida College of Medicine
Jacksonville, FL, USA

Thimothy Graham, MD
Department of Radiology
University of Florida College of Medicine
Jacksonville, FL, USA

Priya Gupta, MD
Associate Professor
Department of Anesthesiology
College of Medicine, University of Arkansas for Medical Sciences
Little Rock, AR, USA

Gary R. Haynes, MD, MS, PhD, FASA
Professor and the Merryl and Sam Israel Chair in Anesthesiology
Department of Anesthesiology
Tulane University School of Medicine
New Orleans, LA, USA

Phi Ho, MD
Resident Physician
Department of Anesthesiology
Baylor College of Medicine
Houston, TX, USA

Jose C. Humanez, MD
Assistant Professor
Department of Anesthesiology
University of Florida College of Medicine
Jacksonville, FL, USA

George M. Jeha
Medical Student
Louisiana State University Health Sciences Center
New Orleans, LA, USA

William Johnson, MD
Resident Physician
Department of Anesthesiology
Baylor College of Medicine
Houston, TX, USA

Tyler Kabes, MD
Resident Physician
Department of Anesthesiology
University of Florida College of Medicine
Gainesville, FL, USA

Alan D. Kaye, MD, PhD, DABA, DABPM, DABIPP, FASA
Vice-Chancellor of Academic Affairs, Chief Academic Officer, and Provost
Tenured Professor of Anesthesiology, Pharmacology, Toxicology, and Neurosciences
LSU School of Medicine
Shreveport, LA, USA

W. Kirk Fowler, MD
Physician
Department of Anesthesiology
University of Florida College of Medicine
Gainesville, FL, USA

Neeraj Kumar, MD
Assistant Professor
Department of Anesthesiology
College of Medicine, University of Arkansas for Medical Sciences
Little Rock, AR, USA

Henry Liu, MD, MS, FASA
Professor of Anesthesiology
Department of Anesthesiology and Perioperative Medicine
Penn State Milton S. Hershey Medical Center
Hershey, PA, USA

Brian P. McClure, MD
Assistant Professor
Department of Anesthesiology
Tulane University School of Medicine
New Orleans, LA

Edward McGough, MD
Associate Professor of Anesthesia
Divisions of Critical Care Medicine and Cardiac Anesthesia
Program Director
Cardiothoracic Anesthesia Fellowship
Department of Anesthesiology
University of Florida College of Medicine
Gainesville, FL, USA

Jared McKinnon, MD
Assistance Professor
Department of Anesthesiology and Perioperative Medicine
Medical University of South Carolina
Charleston, SC, USA

Travis Meyer, MD
Physician
Department of Radiology
University of Florida Health, Clinical Center
Jacksonville, FL, USA

Paul Mongan, MD
Professor
Department of Anesthesiology
University of Florida College of Medicine
Jacksonville, FL, USA

Juan C. Mora, MD
Assistant Professor of Anesthesiology
Department of Anesthesiology
University of Florida College of Medicine
Gainesville, FL, USA

Melissa Nikolaidis, MD
Assistant Professor of Anesthesiology
Department of Anesthesiology
Director of Cardiothoracic Anesthesiology at Ben Taub Hospital
Baylor College of Medicine
Houston, TX, USA

Geoffrey D. Panjeton, MD
Fellow
Department of Anesthesiology
University of Florida College of Medicine
Gainesville, FL, USA

Hess Panjeton, MD
Northside Anesthesiology Consultants
Atlanta, GA, USA

Kishan Patel, MD
Physician
Department of Anesthesiology
University of Florida College of Medicine
Jacksonville, FL, USA

Tiffany D. Perry

Raymond Pla, MD
Assistant Professor of Medicine
Department of Anesthesiology and Critical Care
George Washington University School of Medicine
Washington, DC, USA

Rene Przkora, MD, PhD
Professor of Anesthesiology and Chief, Pain Medicine Division
Department of Anesthesiology
University of Florida College of Medicine
Gainesville, FL, USA

Jordan S. Renschler
Medical Student
Louisiana State University Health Sciences Center
New Orleans, LA, USA

Nahel Saied, MD
Professor of Anesthesiology and Critical Care
University of Arkansas for Medical Sciences
Little Rock, AR, USA

Saurin Shah, MD
Department of Anesthesiology
University of Florida College of Medicine
Jacksonville, FL, USA

Geetha Shanmugam, MD
Assistant Professor of Medicine
Department of Anesthesiology and Critical Care
George Washington University School of Medicine
Washington, DC, USA

Kevin Sidoran, MD
Resident Physician
Department of Anesthesiology and Critical Care
George Washington University Hospital
Washington, DC, USA

Alan Smeltz, MD
Assistant Professor
Department of Anesthesiology
University of North Carolina School of Medicine
Chapel Hill, NC, USA

Hanan Tafesse, MD
Anesthesia Resident
Department of Anesthesiology
The George Washington University Hospital
Washington, DC, USA

Antony Tharian, MD
Program Director
Department of Anesthesiology
Advocate Illinois Masonic Medical Center
Chicago, IL, USA

Richard D. Urman, MD, MBA, FASA
Associate Professor
Department of Anesthesiology
Perioperative and Pain Medicine
Brigham and Women's Hospital
Boston, MA, USA

Jeffrey D. White, MD
Clinical Associate
Department of Anesthesiology
University of Florida College of Medicine
Gainesville, FL, USA

Justin W. Wilson, MD
Associate Professor of Anesthesiology and Director
Division of Cardiothoracic Anesthesiology
Department of Anesthesiology
University of Texas Health Science Center at San Antonio
San Antonio, TX, USA

Lacey Wood, DO
Resident
Department of Anesthesiology
Advocate Illinois Masonic Medical Center
Chicago, IL, USA

Mengjie Wu, MD
Resident Physician
Department of Anesthesiology
UT Houston
Houston, TX, USA

Gregory C. Wynn, MD
Associate Professor
Department of Radiology
University of Florida College of Medicine
Jacksonville, FL, USA

Zhongyuan Xia, MD, PhD
Professor and Chairman
Department of Anesthesiology
Renmin Hospital of Wuhan University,
Hubei General Hospital
Wuhan, China

Manxu Zhao, MD, MS
Director
Department of Anesthesiology
Cedar Sinai Medical Center
Los Angeles, CA, USA

1

Normal Respiratory Physiology

Basic Concepts for the Clinician

Jordan S. Renschler, George M. Jeha, and Alan D. Kaye

Physiological and Anatomical Consideration of Patient Positioning

Introduction

Patient positioning should optimize exposure for surgery while minimizing potential harm to the patient. Concerns for patient positioning include interfering with respiration or circulation, compressing peripheral nerves of skin, and causing musculoskeletal discomfort. Factors that should be considered when choosing optimal patient positioning include procedure length, the surgeon's preference, the type of anesthesia administered, and patient specific risk factors, including age and weight.[1]

Supine

Supine is the most used surgical position and poses the lowest risk to patient[2] (Figure 1.1). In the supine position the patient is placed on their back with the spinal column in alignment and legs extended parallel to the bed. Changing a person from upright to the supine position results in a fall of about 0.8 to 1 L in functional residual capacity (FRC).[2,3] After induction of anesthesia, the FRC decreases another 0.4 to 0.5 L due to relaxation of the intercostal muscles and diaphragm. This drop in FRC contributes to small airway collapse and a decrease in oxygenation.

Lateral Decubitus: Closed Chest

The lateral decubitus position is often used in surgeries of the hip, retroperitoneum, and thorax (Figure 1.2). To achieve this position, patients are anesthetized supine then turned so the nonoperative side is in contact with the bed. The shoulders and hips should be turned simultaneously to prevent torsion of the spine and great vessels. The lower leg is flexed at hip, and the upper leg is completely extended. There is a decrease in FRC and total volumes of both lungs due to the patient being in a supine position. In lateral decubitus, the dependent

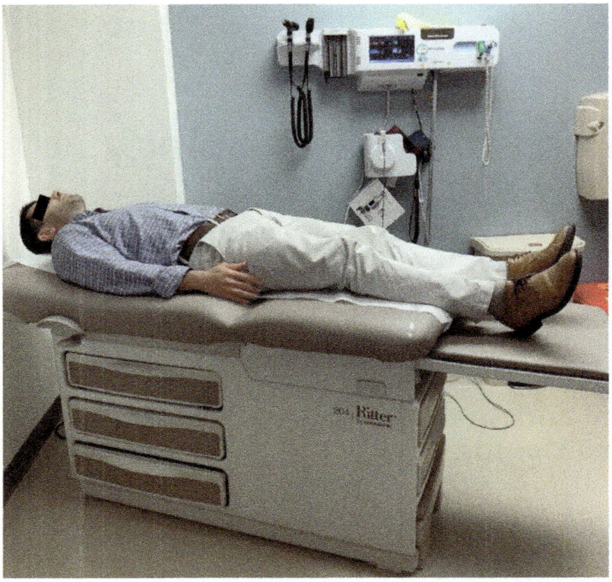

Figure 1.1 Supine position.

lung is better perfused due to gravity but has a decreased compliance to the increased intra-abdominal pressure and pressure from the mediastinum.[2] This leads to better ventilation of the poorly perfused, nondependent lung. These alterations result in significant ventilation-perfusion mismatch.

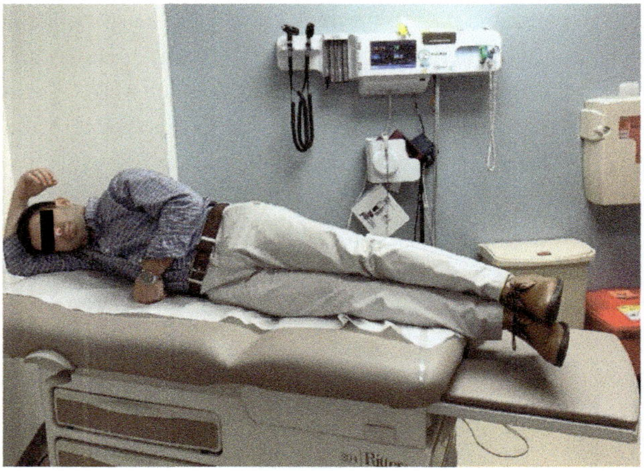

Figure 1.2 Lateral decubitus position.

Open Chest

Opening the chest in lateral decubitus poses additional physiologic effects. Opening a large section of the thoracic cavity removes some constraint of the chest wall on the nondependent lung. This increases ventilation of the lung, which worsens the ventilation-perfusion mismatch.[4] Because the intact hemithorax is generating negative pressures, the mediastinum can shift toward the closed section, changing hemodynamics in a potentially dangerous way. The closed hemithorax can also pull air from the open hemithorax, resulting in paradoxical breathing.[5]

Lung Isolation Techniques

Introduction

Lung isolation may be desired in surgery to optimize surgical access. By collapsing a single lung, the surgeon has greater access to the thorax and prevents puncturing the lung. Single-lung ventilation can also prevent contamination of healthy lung tissue by a diseased lung in cases of severe infection or bleeding. This section discusses methods of lung isolation including double-lumen tubes and bronchial blockers.

Anatomical Landmarks

The trachea is the entrance to the respiratory system and is kept patent by C-shaped cartilaginous rings. These rings maintain the structure of the trachea and are incomplete on the posterior aspect of the trachea. The trachea splits into the right and left mainstem bronchus at the carina (Figure 1.3). Notice the right bronchus lies in a more vertical plane and is typically shorter and wider. The right bronchus supplies the right lung, which has three lobes—the superior, middle, and inferior lobes—whereas the left lung consists of only the superior and

(A) (B)

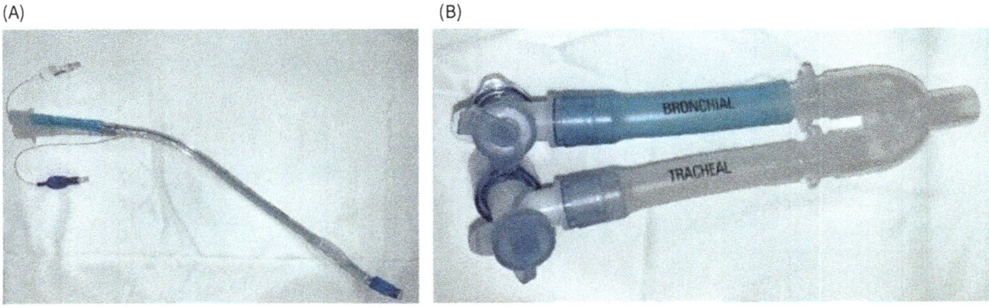

Figure 1.3 The trachea splits into the right and left mainstem bronchus at the carina.

inferior lobes and is supplied by the left bronchus. Each lobe is supplied by a secondary bronchus, coming from the respective mainstem bronchus. Secondary bronchi split further into bronchioles.

Double-Lumen Tubes

Double-lumen tubes are the main method of anatomical and physiologic lung isolation in most thoracic surgery cases. Double-lumen tubes are composed of two unequal length endotracheal tubes molded together. The longer tube has a blue cuff and is designed to sit in the primary bronchus, while the shorter tube has a clear cuff and is placed in the trachea (Figure 1.4). By inflating the tracheal cuff and deflating the bronchial cuff, ventilation of both lungs is achieved. Lung isolation is achieved when the bronchial cuff is inflated.[6]

- Double-lumen tubes come in right and left models. Adult double-lumen tubes are available in different sizes: 25 Fr, 28 Fr, 32 Fr, 35 Fr, 37 Fr, 39 Fr, and 41 Fr. 39 Fr and 41 Fr are commonly used in adult males, and 35 Fr and 37 Fr are used for adult females.[7] Size choice should prevent trauma or ischemia to the airway from a tube too large, but it must be large enough to adequately isolate the lung when inflated. The tubes should pass without resistance during insertion. Smaller tubes are more likely to be displaced and are more difficult to suction and ventilate through. Double-lumen tubes are also commercially available

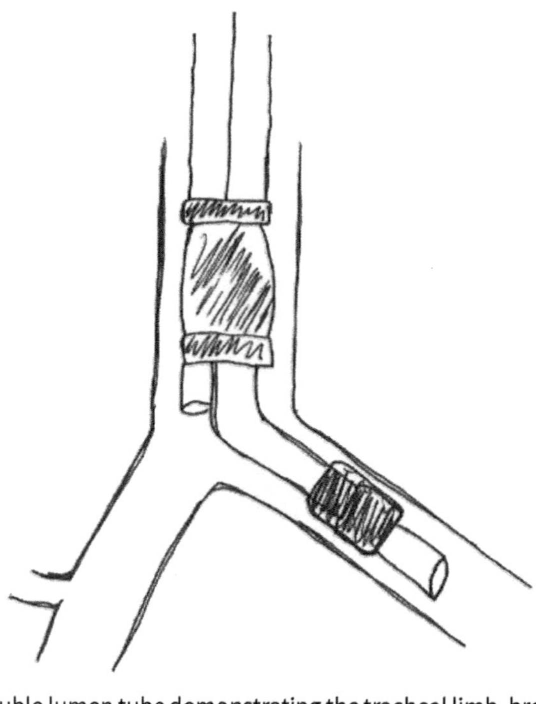

Figure 1.4 A 39 Fr double lumen tube demonstrating the tracheal limb, bronchial limb, oropharyngeal curve, tracheal cuff, and bronchial cuff (A). An enlarged image displaying the bronchial and tracheal limbs (B).

for patients with tracheostomy and are shorter and curved between the intratracheal and extratracheal components.

- Components of double-lumen tube package:
  - Double-lumen tube
  - Adaptor for ventilation of both ports
  - Extension for each port
  - Stylet
  - Suction catheter
  - Apparatus to deliver continuous positive pressure airway to the nonventilated lung (variable depending on manufacturer)
- Additional equipment:
  - Laryngoscope blade
  - Fiberoptic bronchoscope
  - Stethoscope
  - Hemostat to clamp the tube extension on the nonventilated side
- Blind placement[7]:
  - *Preparation*: Prior to the case, prepare and assemble the supplies to prevent delays later. Lubricate the stylet and place it into the double-lumen tube. Connect the adaptor to both port extension.
  - *Intubating the patient*: Visualize the vocal cords by direct laryngoscopy. Advance the double-lumen tube with the bronchial tip oriented so the concave curve faces anteriorly through the vocal cords until the bronchial cuff passes the cords. Rotate the tube 90° to the left when using a left-sided tube or to the right if using a right-side tube. Then advance the tube until there is resistance, while having another clinician remove the stylet. Attach the adaptor/extension piece. Following adequate positioning, inflate the tracheal cuff. Confirm both lungs are being ventilated by visualized chest rise and auscultation. Next verify ventilation from the bronchial lumen by inflating the bronchial cuff 1 mL at a time until leak stops. Stop gas flow through the tracheal lumen, then open the tracheal sealing cap to air. Clamp off gas flow through the bronchial lumen to confirm isolation of the other lung through the tracheal lumen. Connect the double-lumen tube to the ventilator circuit using the connector provided in the packaging. End-tidal carbon dioxide (CO_2) confirms placement in the trachea. Oxygenate the patient fully with a fraction of inspired oxygen of 100%.
  - *Confirmation of placement*: Confirm correct placement of the tube using a fiberoptic bronchoscope through the endotracheal lumen (gold standard), by auscultation, and/or with lung ultrasound.
  - *Relative contraindications*: Placement of a double-lumen tube is difficult due to the larger size and design; therefore, relative contraindications include a difficult airway, limited jaw mobility, a tracheal constriction, and a pre-existing trachea or stoma. In these cases, a single lumen tube with a bronchial blocker is an advisable alternative.
- Considerations:
  - Left-sided double-lumen tubes have a higher margin of safety because the left primary bronchus is longer than the right.
  - The proximity of the right-upper lobe bronchus to the carina poses an additional challenge in placing a right-sided double-lumen tube.[8]

- Reviewing prior lung imaging may aid in locating the right upper lobe position relative to the right primary bronchus.

Bronchial Blocker

Bronchial blockers are another method used for selective ventilation of an individual lung. The blocker is a catheter with a balloon at the tip that is inflated to occlude the lung of the bronchus it is placed in. Open-tipped bronchial blockers offer the ability to apply continuous positive pressure and to suction the airway, making them more useful than the alternative close-tipped bronchial blockers.[6] The smallest size is a 2 French, which may be used in a 3.5 or 4.0 mm endotracheal tube. Proper placement of bronchial blockers is especially difficult in smaller children. To assure proper placement of the bronchial blocker, one must visualize key anatomical structures during placement. Fiberoptic bronchoscopy is a reliable method to confirm proper placement of the bronchial blocker.

Advantages of bronchial blockers compared to double-lumen tubes include bronchial blockers utility in airway trauma, ability to be placed through an existing endotracheal tube, and ability to selectively block a lung lobe.[9,10] Disadvantages include being especially difficult to place, particularly in the right upper lobe, as well as being more likely to be dislodged.

- Placement of bronchial blocker
  - *Preparation*: Prior to intubation, verify that the bronchial blocker attached to the fiberoptic scope fits through the endotracheal tube.
  - *Intubation*: Using a single-lumen tube, intubate the trachea. Confirm endotracheal tube intubation with end-tidal CO_2 and auscultation. Fully ventilate the patient with a fraction of inspired oxygen of 100% prior to placing the bronchial blocker.
  - *Placement of the bronchial blocker*: Attach the blocker to the very distal tip of the fiberoptic bronchoscope using the loop/lariat of the blocker. Advance the attached bronchial blocker into the endotracheal tube. Use the fiberoptic bronchoscope to visualize the airway, guiding the blocker into the selected primary bronchus. Place the bronchial blocker by releasing the loop/lariat that connect the blocker to the fiberoptic bronchoscope. Withdraw the bronchoscope to slightly above the carina and visualize the primary bronchi. While observing from this view, inflate the balloon with air or saline as instructed by the manufacturer. Remove the fiberoptic bronchoscope and auscultate to confirm positioning of blocker. Confirm that peak airway pressures are appropriate and not excessive.
- Risks: Bronchial blockers may cause local trauma to the tracheal mucosa during placement. Additionally, using a bronchial blocker or overinflation of the balloon that is too large can damage the mucosa of the airway. If the bronchial block is inflated within the trachea ventilation of both lungs is blocked.

Bronchoscopy

Bronchoscopy allows for visualization of the airways and has utility in diagnostic and therapeutic procedures. There are two main types of bronchoscopes, rigid and flexible. The rigid bronchoscope is a metal tube with a beveled tip. The flexible bronchoscope has several variations. Traditionally, they have a long flexible tube encircling a fiberoptic system with a light source. The handle of the scope has an eyepiece, control lever for tip movement, suction button, and access to the suction channel.[11] Indications for rigid and flexible bronchoscopes overlap, but flexible bronchoscopes are preferred in confirmation of double-lumen tube and bronchial blocker placement.[12]

Indications for Bronchoscopy	
Diagnostic	*Therapeutic*
Tracheoesophageal fistula, hemoptysis management, chronic cough, stridor, nodal staging of lung cancer, hilar lymphadenopathy tracheomalacia, posttransplant surveillance, pulmonary infiltrates	Lung resection, hemoptysis management, foreign body removal, airway dilatation and stent placement, lavage, tumor debulking, thermoplasty for asthma[13]

When using a double-lumen tube or bronchial blocker, fiberoptic bronchoscopy is a reliable method to confirm tube placement and lung isolation.[14] Auscultation is less reliable for determining adequate ventilation of the selected lung. Mispositioning of the double-lumen tube can result in hypoventilation, hypoxia, atelectasis, and respiratory collapse.[15]

When using fiberoptic bronchoscopy to confirm the position of a blindly inserted tube, it is advanced through the tracheal lumen to confirm[11]:

- The bronchial portion is in the correct bronchus.
- The bronchial cuff does not cover the carina.
- The bronchial rings are anterior and longitudinal fibers are posterior.

When advancing the bronchoscope through the endobronchial lumen:

- For left-sided tubes, visualize the origins of the left upper and lower bronchi to assure the endobronchial tip is not occluding a bronchi.
- For the right-sided tube, because of the alternate size and angle, ensure the alignment between the opening of the endobronchial lumen and the opening of the right upper lobe bronchus is optimal. Visualize the middle and lower bronchus as patent and ventilated.

Bronchoscopy may be used to aid in placing the double-lumen tube by placing the bronchoscope through the bronchial lumen and positioning the double-lumen tube over the scope.

- *Complications*: Potential complications of bronchoscopy include laryngospasm, bronchospasm, hypoxemia, mucosal damage resulting in bleeding, pneumothorax, cardiac arrhythmias, and exacerbation of hypoxia. The benefits of bronchoscopy must outweigh the risks.

Pulmonary Function Changes During Thoracic Anesthesia

Introduction

During thoracic anesthesia, a significant reduction in pulmonary function occurs, with a decrease of up to 50% in forced expiratory volume in 1 second (FEV1), forced vital capacity, and FRC.[16] Anesthetic agents themselves, particularly the volatile anesthetics, lead to hypercarbia and hypoxia. Depression of reflexes, increased secretions, changes in hemodynamics, and alterations in rib cage movement during thoracic anesthesia further alter pulmonary function. These alterations lead to a high risk of hypoxia and atelectasis, resulting in respiratory complications comprising most perioperative causes of morbidity and mortality.

Lung Mechanics and Pulmonary Function

The lungs' primary function is to maintain oxygenation and remove CO_2 from the blood, thus allowing for respiration at the cellular level to occur. Arterial CO_2 is detected by chemoreceptors of the carotid body and medulla and is the primary driver of respiration. Patent alveoli and capillaries within the lung are the site of gas diffusion. Alveolar ventilation (Va) refers to the gas exchange occurring between the alveoli and external environment, while perfusion (Q) is the blood flow the lung receives. Perfusion of the lung tissue is heavily dependent on gravity, so patient positioning alters which areas of the lung are most perfused.[17] Different methods of thoracic anesthesia and positioning of the patient alter Va and Q. Thoracic anesthesia causes a dose-dependent decrease in minute ventilation, or the total volume the lung receives in 1 minute.[18] The additional decrease in FRC and FEV1 leads to alveolar collapse and an increase of shunting within the lungs. Some of this loss of lung function can be overcome with positive end-expiratory pressure and alveolar recruitment maneuvers, improving overall patient outcomes. Mechanical ventilation improves the Va/Q ratio by increasing the volume of air the lung receives and limiting atelectasis.[19]

Predictive Postoperative Pulmonary Lung Function

FEV1 and the diffusion capacity of CO_2 are quantitative preoperative assessment values of thoracic anesthesia patients undergoing partial lung resection. FEV1 is a measure of the respiratory mechanics whereas diffusing capacity for CO_2 (DLCO) measures the lung parenchymal function. Reduction in FEV1 and DLCO are associated with increased respiratory morbidity and mortality rates.[20] In the setting of a normal FEV1, DLCO should still be measured because of its utility in predicting morbidity in patients with no airflow limitations.[21,22]

Forced Expiratory Volume in 1 Second

ppoFEV1% = preoperative FEV1% × (1 – %functional lung tissue removed/100)

A predicted postoperative FEV1 percentage (ppoFEV1%) above 40% is low risk for postoperative respiratory complication, while less than 30% is considered high risk.[23] Following the surgery, the remaining lung will compensate and eventually FEV1 will increase slightly.[24]

Diffusion Capacity of CO_2

ppoDLCO = preoperative DLCO × (1 – %functional lung tissue removed/100)

Diffusion capacity is a measure of gases ability to cross the alveolar-capillary membranes. A predicted postoperative DLCO percentage (ppoDLCO) less than 40% is correlated with increased postoperative cardiopulmonary complications.[21] DLCO is the strongest predictor for morbidity and mortality after lung resection and predicts cardiopulmonary complications in the setting of a normal FEV1. The DLCO value has also been associated with postoperative quality of life and long-term survival.[22] Guidelines recommend DLCO measurement prior to lung resection in all cases.

One-Lung Ventilation

Introduction

In most circumstances, the lungs of patients undergoing mechanical ventilation are inflated and deflated in unison. In some instances, however, it is beneficial to mechanically separate the two lungs to ventilate only one lung while the other is deflated. This is termed one-lung ventilation (OLV). OLV is commonly used to provide exposure to the surgical field during thoracic surgery or to anatomically isolate one lung from pathologic processes related to the other lung.

Indications for One-Lung Ventilation

OLV is routinely utilized to enhance exposure of the surgical field in a variety of surgical procedures, including:

- Pulmonary resection (including pneumonectomy, lobectomy, and wedge resection).
- Video-assisted thoracoscopic surgery (including wedge resection, biopsy, and pleurodesis).

- Mediastinal surgery.
- Esophageal surgery.
- Thoracic vascular surgery.
- Thoracic spine surgery.
- Minimally invasive cardiac valve surgery.

The nonsurgical indications for OLV include[6]:

- Protective isolation of one lung from pathologic processes occurring in the contralateral lung, such as:
  - Pulmonary hemorrhage.
  - Infection or purulent secretions.
- Control of ventilation in circumstances such as:
  - Tracheobronchial trauma.
  - Broncho-pleural or broncho-cutaneous fistula.

Methods of Lung Separation

There are three methods used to isolate a lung:

1. *Single-lumen endobronchial tube*: The single-lumen endobronchial tube differs from normal endotracheal tube in that the former has a smaller external diameter, smaller external cuff, and longer length. The single-lumen endobronchial tube is utilized far less frequently than the double-lumen endobronchial tube for achieving lung isolation but may be useful in emergency situations in select patients with abnormal tracheobronchial anatomy or in cases involving small children.[8,9] Placement of a single-lumen endobronchial tube within the right or left mainstem bronchus allows for ventilation of only the intubated lung, while the contralateral lung is allowed to spontaneously collapse.
2. *Double-lumen endobronchial tube*: Since its introduction in the 1930s, the double-lumen endobronchial tube has been the most commonly utilized method of lung isolation. Its design consists of two separate lumens: a bronchial lumen and a tracheal lumen. This allows for isolation, selective ventilation, and intermittent suctioning of either lung.[6,8,9]
3. *Endobronchial blockers*: Endobronchial blockers are inflatable balloon-tipped stylets which may be placed within the mainstem bronchus, resulting in collapse of lung distal to the blocker.[9,25,26]

Physiology

By inhibiting the ventilation of one lung, single-lung ventilation alters normal respiratory physiology. Disruption of normal respiratory physiology is often followed by the development of hypoxemia. Hypoxemia in the context of one lung ventilation may be attributable to several factors, including reduced oxygen stores, lung compression, dissociation of oxygen from hemoglobin, and matching of ventilation and perfusion.[8,27,28]

- *Reduced oxygen stores*: Because one lung is collapsed during OLV, the FRC is reduced. Accordingly, there is a decrease in the body's stores of oxygen. Additionally, the disease process at play within the thorax may contribute to decreased oxygen stores.
- *Lung compression*: Compression of the ventilated lung may contribute to hypoxemia. During OLV, the ventilated lung may be compressed by the weight of the mediastinum. After diaphragmatic paralysis, the weights of the abdominal contents may also contribute to compression of the ventilated lung.[6,28,29]
- *Oxygen dissociation from hemoglobin*: During OLV, the absence of ventilation to one lung reduces the surface area available for gas exchange by approximately one half, leading to a reduction in arterial partial pressure of oxygen and increased CO_2 levels. The result is more rapid dissociation of oxygen from hemoglobin. This phenomenon is known as the Bohr effect.[8,28,30]
- *Ventilation and perfusion matching*: Under normal circumstances, ventilation and perfusion are anatomically well-matched. However, during OLV, ventilation is interrupted to one of the lungs while its perfusion remains unaffected. This wasted perfusion leads to the development of a right-to-left intrapulmonary shunt and relative hypoxemia. In practice, however, the shunt fraction is actually lower than expected. The reasons for this are as follows[6,8]:
  - Manipulation of the nonventilated lung leads to partial obstruction of its blood supply.
  - By positioning the patient in the lateral position, gravity causes an increase in perfusion to the ventilated lung.
  - Blood flow to hypoxic and poorly ventilated regions of the lung is diverted to more ventilated segments via the mechanism of hypoxic pulmonary vasoconstriction.

Optimum Driving Pressure

Driving pressure (ΔP) is calculated as the difference between airway pressure at the end of inspiration (plateau pressure, P_{plat}) and positive end-expiratory airway pressure (PEEP). Two pressures comprise the driving pressure: the transpulmonary pressure (ΔP_L) and the pressure applied to the chest wall (ΔP_{cw}). By rearranging the standard respiratory compliance (C_{RS}) equation, it is demonstrated that driving pressure equals the tidal volume (VT) divided by C_{RS}. Consequently, driving pressure can be interpreted as the tidal volume corrected for the patient's C_{RS} and thus related to global lung strain. When adjusting the tidal volume, driving pressure may be used as a safety limit to minimize lung strain in intubated patients. Although optimal driving pressure is the subject of ongoing research, it is currently generally accepted that safe driving pressures lie between 14 and 18 cm H_2O.[31–33]

$$\Delta P = P_{plat} - PEEP$$

$$C_{RS} = \frac{VT}{Pplat - PEEP} = \frac{VT}{\Delta P}$$

$$\Delta P = \frac{VT}{CRS}$$

Optimum Positive End-Expiratory Airway Pressure

PEEP is defined as the positive pressure remaining within the airways at the end of exhalation. During mechanical ventilation, extrinsic PEEP may be utilized to keep open atelectatic lung tissue, thereby increasing oxygenation and minimizing ventilation-perfusion mismatches. However, if PEEP is too high, this may lead to increased plateau pressure and subsequent barotrauma. It is generally recommended that PEEP of 5 to 10 cm H_2O should be applied to patients undergoing OLV with low tidal volumes.[34,35] It is important to use caution while ventilating patients with obstructive airways disease, as these patients have relatively higher levels of intrinsic PEEP, which makes the effects of extrinsic PEEP less predictable. Intrinsic PEEP is a complication of mechanical ventilation that arises when the lungs are not evacuated completely, leading to entrapment of air at the end of expiration. If this process is repeated with each respiratory cycle, the result is a pathologic increase in plateau pressure.[34,36] Factors that predispose to generation of intrinsic PEEP include:

- Airway inflammation and mucus plugs leading to dynamic airway obstruction.
- Increased lung compliance (e.g., patients with obstructive airways disease).
- Ventilator settings with high tidal volumes or inappropriately short expiratory times.
- Resistance of artificial airways such as the double-lumen tube.

Physiological Impact of Fluid Management: Restricted vs Goal Target

The goal of perioperative and intraoperative fluid management is the maintenance of central euvolemia as well as electrolyte and tissue homeostasis. While there is uncertainty surrounding the optimal composition and volume of intraoperative fluid therapy, it is known that adequate maintenance of intravascular volume status is important for improving postsurgical outcomes. Factors that may predispose to imbalances in intravascular volume status during the perioperative period include[37]:

- Dehydration as a result of preoperative fasting.
- Use of mechanical bowel preparation.
- Ongoing disease processes causing inflammation and interstitial edema and subsequent volume losses.
- Ongoing bleeding during surgery.
- Insensible perspiration during surgery.
- Prolonged operating times.
- Anesthetic-mediated vasodilation.

Maintenance of euvolemia is ideal, as both hypovolemia and hypervolemia leading to tissue edema are associated with undesirable effects:

Consequences of Hypovolemia	Consequences of Tissue Edema
Decreased blood pressure	Pulmonary edema
Low cardiac output	Decreased gastrointestinal motility
Impaired tissue perfusion	Impaired clotting
Shock	Impaired wound healing
Multiorgan failure	Wound dehiscence

Hypoxic Pulmonary Vasoconstriction: Physiology and Anesthesia Impact

Introduction

Within systemic circulation, hypoxia causes arteries to dilate to meet the metabolic demands of surrounding tissues. In contrast, intrapulmonary arteries constrict in response to hypoxia. This unique homeostatic mechanism, known as hypoxic pulmonary vasoconstriction, allows for the diversion of blood flow from oxygen-poor areas of the lung to better-oxygenated areas of the lungs, thus optimizing oxygen uptake during diseased states such as pneumonia, atelectasis, or acute respiratory distress syndrome.

Physiology

The mechanism of hypoxic pulmonary vasoconstriction involves specialized pulmonary arterial smooth muscle and endothelial cells (oxygen-sensing cells) that are sensitive to small changes in oxygen levels. During states of hypoxia, pulmonary artery vasoconstriction is largely mediated via inhibition of potassium channels, which depolarizes the smooth muscle cells and leads to subsequent calcium channel activation. The increased levels of calcium within the cytosol trigger hypoxic pulmonary vasoconstriction.[27,38,39]

Impact on Anesthesia

When performing OLV, the isolation of one lung leaves the other lung with minimal ventilation. This wasted ventilation creates a right-to-left intrapulmonary shunt, which predisposes to the development of systemic hypoxemia. However, during one-lung anesthesia, this shunt is minimized due to the diversion of blood to more ventilated segments via the mechanism of hypoxic pulmonary vasoconstriction.[27,38,39] Should this mechanism become impaired, the patient is more prone to develop systemic hypoxemia. While an adequate understanding of hypoxic pulmonary vasoconstriction is important for anesthesiologists, strategies for optimizing this physiologic phenomenon in intubated patients undergoing surgical procedures should be the subject of future clinical trials.

References

1. Hagan K, Gottumukkala V. Surgical positioning: physiology and perioperative implications. In: DE Longnecker, SC Mackey, MF Newman, WS Sandberg, WM Zapol, eds. *Anesthesiology*. 3rd ed. New York, NY McGraw-Hill Education:316–325.
2. Armstrong M, Moore RA. *Anatomy, patient positioning. StatPearls*. http://www.ncbi.nlm.nih.gov/pubmed/30020692. Published 2020. Accessed February 11, 2020.
3. Mezidi M, Guerin C. Effects of patient positioning on respiratory mechanics in mechanically ventilated ICU patients. *Ann Transl Med*. 2018;6(19):10. doi:10.21037/19858
4. McLean SR, Lohser J. Physiology of the lateral decubitus position, open chest, and one-lung ventilation. In: PD Slinger, RS Blank, J Campos, J Lohser, K McRae, eds. *Principles and Practice of Anesthesia for Thoracic Surgery*. Cham, Switzerland: Springer International; 2019:93–105. doi:10.1007/978-3-030-00859-8_5
5. Positioning in thoracic surgery. *Open Anesthesia*. https://www.openanesthesia.org/positioning_in_thoracic_surgery/. Published 2020. Accessed February 29, 2020.
6. Mehrotra M, Jain A. Single lung ventilation. *StatPearls*. http://www.ncbi.nlm.nih.gov/pubmed/30855898. Published 2019. Accessed February 29, 2020.
7. Bora V, Arthur ME. Double lumen endobronchial tubes. *StatPearls*. http://www.ncbi.nlm.nih.gov/pubmed/30570987. Published 2019. Accessed February 11, 2020.
8. Purohit A, Bhargava S, Mangal V, Parashar VK. Lung isolation, one-lung ventilation and hypoxaemia during lung isolation. *Indian J Anaesth*. 2015;59(9):606–617. doi:10.4103/0019-5049.165855
9. Narayanaswamy M, McRae K, Slinger P, et al. Choosing a lung isolation device for thoracic surgery: a randomized trial of three bronchial blockers versus double-lumen tubes. *Anesth Analg*. 2009;108(4):1097–1101. doi:10.1213/ane.0b013e3181999339
10. Neustein SM. The use of bronchial blockers for providing one-lung ventilation. *J Cardiothorac Vasc Anesth*. 2009;23(6):860–868. doi:10.1053/j.jvca.2009.05.014
11. Hertz MI, Gustafson P. Bronchoscopy. In: JH Abrams, P Druck, FB Cerra, eds. *Surgical Critical Care*. 2nd ed. Boca Raton, FL: CRC/Taylor and Francis; 2005:905–914.
12. Arndt GA, Buchika S, Kranner PW, DeLessio ST. Wire-guided endobronchial blockade in a patient with a limited mouth opening. *Can J Anaesth*. 1999;46(1):87–89. doi:10.1007/BF03012521
13. Galway U, Zura A, Khanna S, Wang M, Turan A, Ruetzler K. Anesthetic considerations for bronchoscopic procedures: a narrative review based on the Cleveland clinic experience. *J Thorac Dis*. 2019;11(7):3156–3170. doi:10.21037/jtd.2019.07.29
14. Klein U, Karzai W, Bloos F, et al. Role of fiberoptic bronchoscopy in conjunction with the use of double-lumen tubes for thoracic anesthesia. *Anesthesiology*. 1998;88(2):346–350. doi:10.1097/00000542-199802000-00012
15. Kabadayi S, Bellamy MC. Bronchoscopy in critical care. *BJA Educ*. 2017;17(2):48–56. doi:10.1093/bjaed/mkw040
16. Bigler DR. Lung function changes during anesthesia and thoracic surgery. *Ugeskr Laeger*. 2003;165(3):232–235.
17. Lohser J, Ishikawa S. Physiology of the lateral decubitus position, open chest and one-lung ventilation. In: PD Slinger, RS Blank, J Campos, J Lohser, K McRae, eds. *Principles and Practice of Anesthesia for Thoracic Surgery*. Cham, Switzerland: Springer; 1995:71–82. doi:10.1007/978-1-4419-0184-2_5
18. Saraswat V. Effects of anaesthesia techniques and drugs on pulmonary function. *Indian J Anaesth*. 2015;59(9):557–564. doi:10.4103/0019-5049.165850

19. Blank RS, Colquhoun DA, Durieux ME, et al. Management of one-lung ventilation: impact of tidal volume on complications after thoracic surgery. *Anesthesiology.* 2016;124(6):1286–1295. doi:10.1097/ALN.0000000000001100
20. Ponce MC, Sharma S. Pulmonary function tests. *StatPearls.* http://www.ncbi.nlm.nih.gov/pubmed/29493964. Published 2020. Accessed February 29, 2020.
21. Liptay MJ, Basu S, Hoaglin MC, et al. Diffusion lung capacity for carbon monoxide (DLCO) is an independent prognostic factor for long-term survival after curative lung resection for cancer. *J Surg Oncol.* 2009;100(8):703–707. doi:10.1002/jso.21407
22. Ferguson MK, Dignam JJ, Siddique J, Vigneswaran WT, Celauro AD. Diffusing capacity predicts long-term survival after lung resection for cancer. *Eur J Cardiothorac Surg.* 2012;41(5):e81–e86. doi:10.1093/ejcts/ezs049
23. Brunelli A, Kim AW, Berger KI, Addrizzo-Harris DJ. ACCP. *Chest.* 2013;143(5):e166S–e190S. doi:10.1378/chest.12-2395
24. Handy JR, Asaph JW, Skokan L, et al. What happens to patients undergoing lung cancer surgery? Outcomes and quality of life before and after surgery. *Chest.* 2002;122(1):21–30. doi:10.1378/chest.122.1.21
25. Inoue H, Shohtsu A, Ogawa J, Koide S, Kawada S. Endotracheal tube with movable blocker to prevent aspiration of intratracheal bleeding. *Ann Thorac Surg.* 1984;37(6):497–499. doi:10.1016/s0003-4975(10)61140-x
26. Dumans-Nizard V, Liu N, Laloë P-A, Fischler M. A comparison of the deflecting-tip bronchial blocker with a wire-guided blocker or left-sided double-lumen tube. *J Cardiothorac Vasc Anesth.* 2009;23(4):501–505. doi:10.1053/j.jvca.2009.02.002
27. Evans AM. Hypoxic pulmonary vasoconstriction. *Essays Biochem.* 2007;43:61–76. doi:10.1042/BSE0430061
28. Brinkman JE, Sharma S. *Physiology, respiratory drive. StatPearls.* https://www.ncbi.nlm.nih.gov/books/NBK482414/. Published 2020. Accessed on February 3, 2020.
29. Mortola JP. How to breathe? Respiratory mechanics and breathing pattern. *Respir Physiol Neurobiol.* 2019;261:48–54. doi:10.1016/j.resp.2018.12.005
30. Tyuma I. The Bohr effect and the Haldane effect in human hemoglobin. *Jpn J Physiol.* 1984;34(2):205–216. doi:10.2170/jjphysiol.34.205
31. Williams EC, Motta-Ribeiro GC, Melo MFV. Driving pressure and transpulmonary pressure: how do we guide safe mechanical ventilation? *Anesthesiology.* 2019;131(1):155–163. doi:10.1097/ALN.0000000000002731
32. Amato MBP, Meade MO, Slutsky AS, et al. Driving pressure and survival in the acute respiratory distress syndrome. *N Engl J Med.* 2014;372(8):747–755. doi:10.1056/NEJMsa1410639
33. Neto AS, Hemmes SNT, Barbas CSV, et al. Association between driving pressure and development of postoperative pulmonary complications in patients undergoing mechanical ventilation for general anaesthesia: a meta-analysis of individual patient data. *Lancet Respir Med.* 2016;4(4):272–280. doi:10.1016/S2213-2600(16)00057-6
34. Mora Carpio AL, Mora JI. *Positive end-expiratory pressure (PEEP). StatPearls.* https://www.ncbi.nlm.nih.gov/books/NBK441904/. Published 2020. Accessed on February 15, 2020.
35. Motta-Ribeiro GC, Hashimoto S, Winkler T, et al. Deterioration of regional lung strain and inflammation during early lung injury. *Am J Respir Crit Care Med.* 2018;198(7):891–902. doi:10.1164/rccm.201710-2038OC
36. Blankman P, Hasan D, Erik GJ, Gommers D. Detection of "best" positive end-expiratory pressure derived from electrical impedance tomography parameters during a decremental positive end-expiratory pressure trial. *Crit Care.* 2014;18(3):R95. doi:10.1186/cc13866
37. Jacob M, Chappell D, Hofmann-Kiefer K, Conzen P, Rehm M. A rational approach to perioperative fluid management. *Anesthesiology.* 2008;109(4):723–740. doi:10.1097/ALN.0b013e3181863117
38. Dunham-Snary KJ, Wu D, Sykes EA, et al. Hypoxic pulmonary vasoconstriction: from molecular mechanisms to medicine. *Chest.* 2017;151(1):181–192. doi:10.1016/j.chest.2016.09.001
39. Khan M, Sharma S. Physiology, pulmonary vasoconstriction. *StatPearls.* https://www.ncbi.nlm.nih.gov/books/NBK499962/. Published 2020. Accessed on January 27, 2020.

2

Thoracic Radiology

Thoracic Anesthesia Procedures

Parker D. Freels, Gregory C. Wynn, Travis Meyer, and Giuseppe Giuratrabocchetta

Introduction

Despite the more recent introduction of advanced cross-sectional imaging techniques, the chest radiograph remains one of the most commonly performed radiologic studies and is routinely utilized in preprocedural planning and postoperative follow-up. It is often the first diagnostic study ordered for a patient and frequently dictates the course of treatment. However, it is also one of the most difficult examinations to interpret. The evaluation of a three-dimensional object (the thorax) is limited by a two-dimensional display. Various densities (e.g., air, fat, fluid, soft tissue, calcium, and metal) attenuate X-ray beams differently as they pass through a patient, and these differing tissues may be projected over a single point in the image. The delineation of intrathoracic structures becomes difficult as areas of interest are superimposed on one another, potentially masking pathology. An optimal exam is one in which the patient is able to stand erect and follow respiratory and positioning commands delivered by the radiologic technologist. Obtaining both posterior-to-anterior and lateral views yields a more complete examination to include improved visualization of normal regional anatomy and better localization of thoracic pathology (Figure 2.1). Often determined by a patient's clinical condition, an anterior-to-posterior projection radiograph is regularly performed instead, but optimal localization of anatomy and support devices is limited without a lateral view. For example, in the intensive care setting, multiple support lines, tubes, and instruments can interfere with adequate visualization of adjacent structures (Figure 2.2), and having a thorough understanding of normal anatomy and the radiographic appearance of these support devices is necessary for discovering intrathoracic pathology.

Several other imaging modalities are available and useful for evaluation of the chest. In computed tomography (CT), an X-ray beam is emitted from an X-ray tube in a helical pattern around a patient as he or she moves through the CT machine. This yields data with spiral geometry, capable of generating very high resolution multiplanar images and exquisite detail of the patient's anatomy. Additionally, the administration of oral and intravenous contrast during the CT study provides improved detail of vascular and alimentary tract structures. Although limited by poor transmission through air-/gas-containing anatomy, ultrasound imaging carries the advantages of relatively low cost, portability, speed, and high diagnostic

(A) (B)

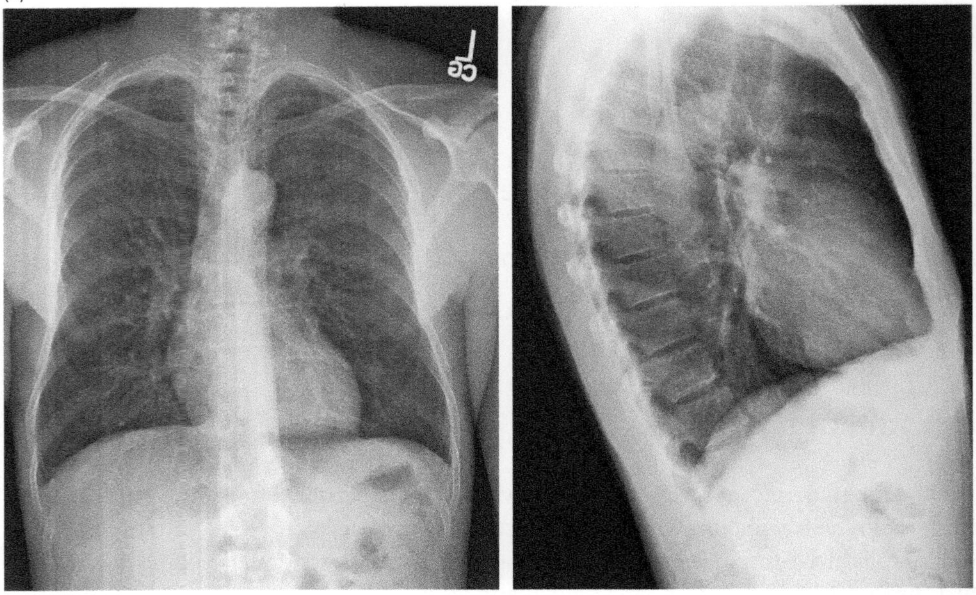

Figure 2.1 Normal chest X-ray. (A) The posteroanterial view demonstrates intact osseous structures, midline trachea, well-aerated lungs, pulmonary vascular markings extending out to the periphery, hemidiaphragms forming sharp costophrenic angles bilaterally, and a cardiac silhouette of normal size. (B) The lateral view shows the more perceptible inferior thoracic spine relative to its super portion, a dense hilum, the arch and descending portion of the aorta, and a clear anterior mediastinum.

sensitivity and accuracy in image-guided procedures. Fluoroscopy also provides both anatomic and functional information about a patient's respiratory and gastrointestinal systems.

Nonetheless, the risks associated with these diagnostic tools should be considered in conjunction with the benefit they can provide. Each modality should be selected with careful consideration when deciding which study to order for an individual patient. Radiation dose, contrast side effects, cost, and ability to answer the clinical question are concerns the provider should address before ordering a study. Consultation with a radiologist is recommended if, when attempting to answer a clinical question, uncertainty regarding the most efficacious diagnostic imaging path arises.

Airways and Lungs

Anatomy of the Trachea and Bronchopulmonary System

The trachea bridges the larynx and bronchi as it moves inferiorly to its bifurcation at the carina. Membranous tissue and anywhere from 14 to 19 C-shaped semicircular rings of cartilage form the anterior portion of the trachea, while its posterior portion is composed of smooth muscle and mucus-producing goblet cells. The elasticity of the muscular posterior portion allows for tracheal compliance during swallowing as the esophagus expands against

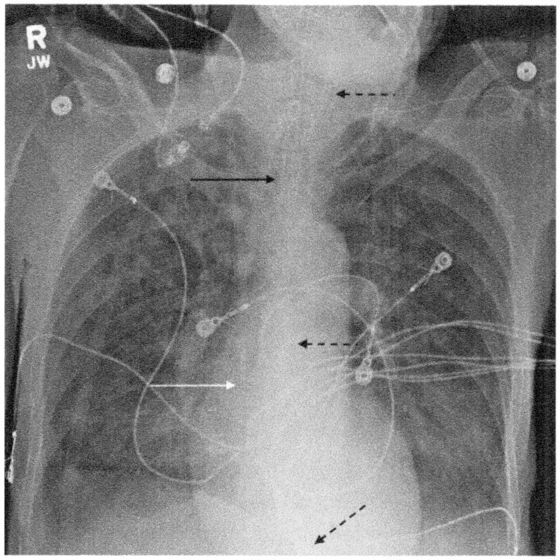

Figure 2.2 Chest X-ray in the intensive care unit. Common support lines and tubes in the critical care setting can be difficult to perceive on a radiograph, but it is imperative to confirm their location. The endotracheal tube should terminate 4 to 6 cm superior to the carina (solid black arrow). Enteric tubes should course subdiaphragmatically (dashed black arrows). Jugular, subclavian, and peripherally inserted central catheter lines should all terminate at the cavoatrial junction (solid white arrow).

the more anteriorly located trachea.[1] The trachea continues to divide into the right and left mainstem bronchi.

Beyond the mainstem bronchi, the airways are referred to as the bronchus intermedius on the right and divide into segments within the lobes of the lungs as they branch more peripherally. The right upper lobe bronchus branches into apical, anterior, and posterior segmental bronchi, and the right middle lobe bronchus divides into a medial and lateral segmental bronchi. The right lower lobe bronchus branches into a superior segment and multiple basilar segments including anterior, medial, lateral, and posterior portions. The left lung shares space with the heart in the left chest and, therefore, is smaller in size with one less lobe relative to the right lung. The lingula, analogous to the right middle lobe, is a tongue-shaped process projecting from the most anterior portion of the left upper lobe. The left upper lobe bronchus branches into apical, anterior, and posterior segmental bronchi as well as superior and inferior lingular segmental bronchi. The left lower lobe bronchus gives rise to a superior segmental bronchus, and similar to the right lower lobe, multiple segmental bronchi, which aerate the anterior, medial, lateral, and posterior basilar segments.

Atelectasis

Atelectasis results when a portion or whole lung is not aerated and collapses, leading to an abnormally dense or opaque region of the respective lung tissue on imaging. There is also associated volume loss involving the same region as the atelectatic lung. If the volume loss is great

(A) (B)

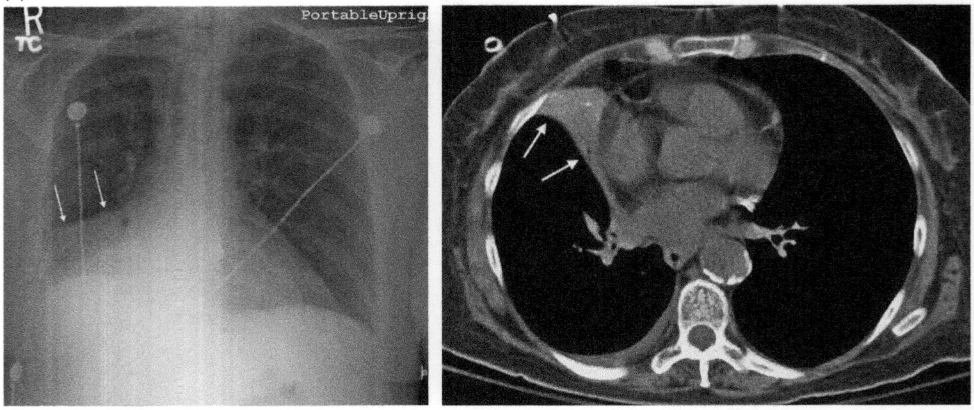

Figure 2.3 Atelectasis. (A) The frontal view of the chest depicts a well-defined linear opacity in the right lung base with a similar radiographic density as the neighboring heart (white arrows). The border between the two is not well-delineated, suggesting a more anterior location of the lung pathology. This is an example of the silhouette sign, and these findings support a right middle lobe location of the opacity as the right middle lobe is situated more anteriorly in the chest than the right lower lobe. (B) A computed tomography image was obtained in the same patient that validates the opacity's location in the right middle lobe of the lung (white arrows). There is also a subtle shift of the heart toward the opacity, indicating the process is causing volume loss. These findings are consistent with a subsegmental form of right middle lobe atelectasis.

enough, a compensatory shift in mobile structures of the chest toward the collapsed lung will occur (including the trachea, heart, and hemidiaphragm) (Figure 2.3)[2]. Atelectasis can be easily identified on a chest X-ray, but the type of atelectasis may be better classified on CT.

There are five types of atelectasis. First, obstructive atelectasis develops from proximal occlusion of an airway leading to distal collapse of the corresponding lung ventilated by that airway. Common causes include bronchogenic carcinoma, foreign object, mucous plug, and endotracheal (ET) tube. The right mainstem bronchus is commonly and preferentially intubated due to its shallower angle relative to the left mainstem bronchus. When this occurs, the left lung is not adequately aerated and complete collapse of the left lung may occur (Figure 2.4). Retracting the ET tube so that its tip terminates at the targeted level of 4 to 6 cm superior to the carina can quickly reverse this phenomenon. Compressive atelectasis originates within the lung parenchyma adjacent to a mass, abscess, or bullae, while passive atelectasis is caused by extrinsic mass effect upon the lung from a pleural or extrapleural process, usually a pleural effusion or pneumothorax. Most commonly found in premature infants with underdeveloped lungs, adhesive atelectasis develops from surfactant deficiency causing inadequate lung expansion. Finally, cicatricial atelectasis results from fibrotic changes following radiation therapy and tuberculosis infection. It is important to consider a patient's history in conjunction with the imaging findings when deciphering the etiology of the detected atelectasis. Recognizing the acute development of atelectasis on imaging (e.g., mucous plugging) and providing the appropriate treatment can lead to a prompt resolution of related symptoms.

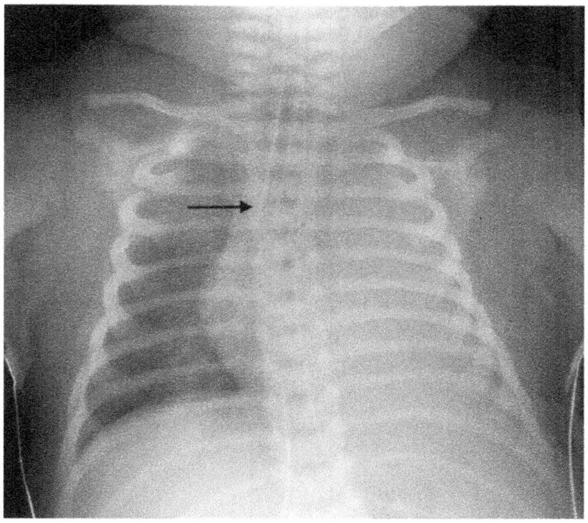

Figure 2.4 Right mainstem bronchus intubation. Due to its relatively shallow angle of origin compared to the left bronchus, the right mainstem bronchus is commonly and preferentially intubated (black arrow). This restricts ventilation to the contralateral lung and promotes its collapse. In a neonate, like the one depicted in this image, mere millimeters of change in the position of the endotracheal tube can make drastic differences in the quality of pulmonary aeration. After intubation, a chest X-ray should be performed to confirm proper placement of the endotracheal tube 4 to 6 cm superior the carina in adults and 1 to 2 cm superior the carina in pediatric patients.

Pneumonia

In general, pneumonia develops from consolidation of the lung or part of the lung by inflammatory exudate which fills the alveoli or pulmonary interstitium. This is usually due to the body's response to an infectious organism, and on a chest X-ray, the diseased lung will demonstrate increased density or opacification (Figure 2.5). Chest radiography remains the gold standard for the diagnosis of pneumonia, but proof of pneumonia on a chest X-ray may be delayed anywhere from 24 to 72 hours relative to the onset of typical symptoms of fever and productive cough.[6] Compared to the more well-defined linear appearance of atelectasis, pneumonia tends to have more indistinct margins. If the airways remain patent and the surrounding lung parenchyma is consolidated, air bronchograms may be visualized as the lucent air-filled bronchi are accentuated by the adjacent opaque exudate. Although they are a nonspecific finding, air bronchograms help support the diagnosis of pneumonia in the appropriate clinical setting.

Other key findings on a chest radiograph can help localize a pneumonia within the chest. If two objects of very similar radiographic density border one another, the boundary between the structures is not radiographically defined. However, if their densities significantly differ, their interface is well visualized. This phenomenon, known as the silhouette sign, is useful in localizing disease with knowledge of which anatomical structures abut each other. Of course, an orthogonal projection further assists in pinpointing a pneumonia's location, but a patient's condition may limit the acquisition of this projection. If the lateral view is available, follow the thoracic spine inferiorly, which should gradually appear darker as one approaches

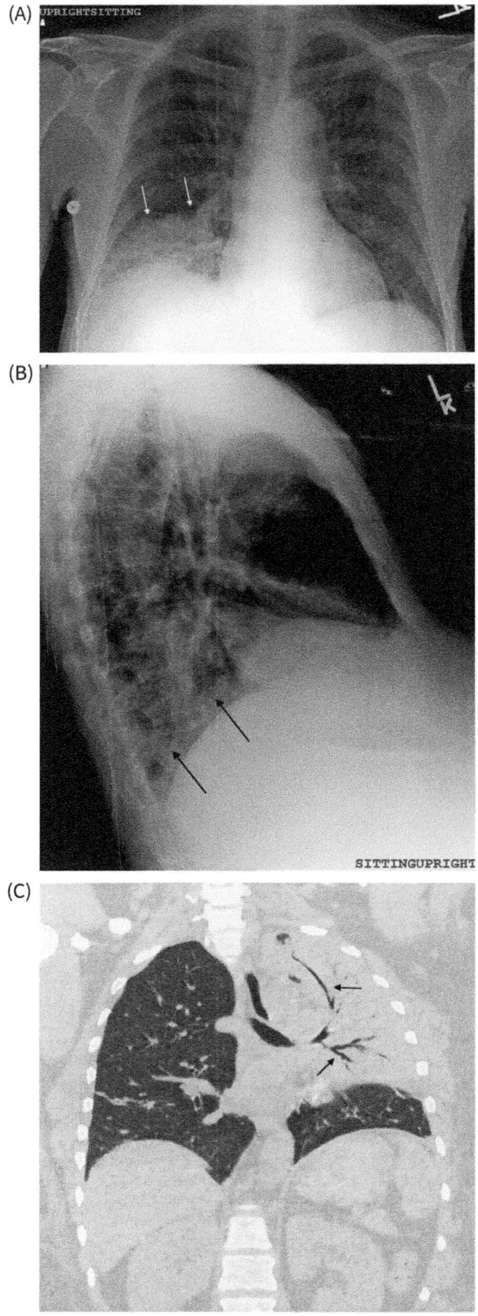

Figure 2.5 Pneumonia. (A) The anteroposterior view shows increased consolidation within the right lung base with indistinct margins (white arrows), which is compatible with an airspace disease like pneumonia. The right heart border is well visualized and not silhouetted by the opacity, indicating a more posterior location. (B) The right lower lobe pneumonia absorbs some of the X-rays traversing the chest, making the lower thoracic spine appear more dense and white on a lateral radiograph (black arrows). This is called the spine sign and helps localize the opacity within the posterior portion of the right lower lobe of the lung. (C) Black, branching, air bronchograms with distinct margins are seen on this computed tomography coronal image of the chest in a different patient with left upper lobe pneumonia (black arrows). As surrounding airspaces continue to fill with inflammatory exudate, the airways will remain patent. When these findings are seen on imaging, it helps support the diagnosis of pneumonia.

the diaphragm. The spine sign is useful in confirming diseases that increase the density of the lower lobe, such as pneumonia. Accurately localizing the pneumonia can provide diagnostic clues for the etiology of the disease and direct the course of treatment. For example, abnormal opacity within the right middle lobe or lower lobes in a patient who is intubated suggests aspiration pneumonia.

Different patterns of pneumonia are largely determined by the anatomic structures involved, the causative microorganism, and the timeline of the disease. Although these patterns are not specific to any one organism, they help establish a diagnosis to guide proper treatment for a patient. In the case of classic lobar pneumonia due to infection by *Streptococcus pneumoniae*, the infection will homogeneously opacify most of a lobe of the lung normally resulting in the silhouette sign and air bronchograms. Patients may develop an adjacent pleural effusion. Segmental pneumonia is typically caused by staphylococcal species, tends to be multifocal, and causes volume loss if bronchi are filled with exudate (lack of air bronchograms). In mycoplasma and pneumocystis infection, a fine reticular pattern of interstitial pneumonia is caused by inflammation of the bronchial walls and alveolar septa. In younger pediatric patients, communications between alveoli, known as pores of Kohn and canals of Lambert, have not developed, limiting the spread of infection and resulting in the round pneumonia seen on chest radiographs.[7] Finally, cavitary pneumonia is a hallmark of postprimary *Mycobacterium tuberculosis*, which classically leads to localized necrosis within the upper lobes.

Pulmonary Edema

As fluid accumulates in the lungs due to physiologic pressure differences, findings of pulmonary edema develop on imaging. The causes of pulmonary edema may be either cardiogenic in origin or noncardiogenic, and the associated patterns on imaging overlap between the etiologies. Clinical history is crucial in establishing the cause, which, in turn, assists in determining the correct treatment. Cardiogenic pulmonary edema is commonly related to a history of congestive heart failure, with cardiomegaly, pleural effusions, and the radiograph finding of Kerley B lines (prominent interstitial septae) (Figure 2.6A). In contrast, a chest X-ray in a patient with noncardiogenic pulmonary edema is often absent of the above findings, and instead displays an "winged" appearance with a perihilar distribution of indistinct opacities with ill-defined margins (Figure 2.6B). However, in both cardiogenic and noncardiogenic pulmonary edema alike, both lungs are usually affected. If recognized and treated appropriately with oxygen supplementation, intravenous diuretics, and adequate blood pressure control, pulmonary edema generally resolves within 48 hours. Patients should receive repeat imaging until resolution is confirmed.[8]

Chronic Obstructive Pulmonary Disease

Emphysema is a specific entity within the category of chronic obstructive pulmonary disease and is defined as destruction of the alveoli with permanent dilation of the airways distal to the terminal bronchioles. It is caused by multiple risk factors including environmental exposure, genetics, and, most commonly, tobacco smoking. Hundreds of millions of individuals worldwide are affected by the disease, which leads to significant morbidity

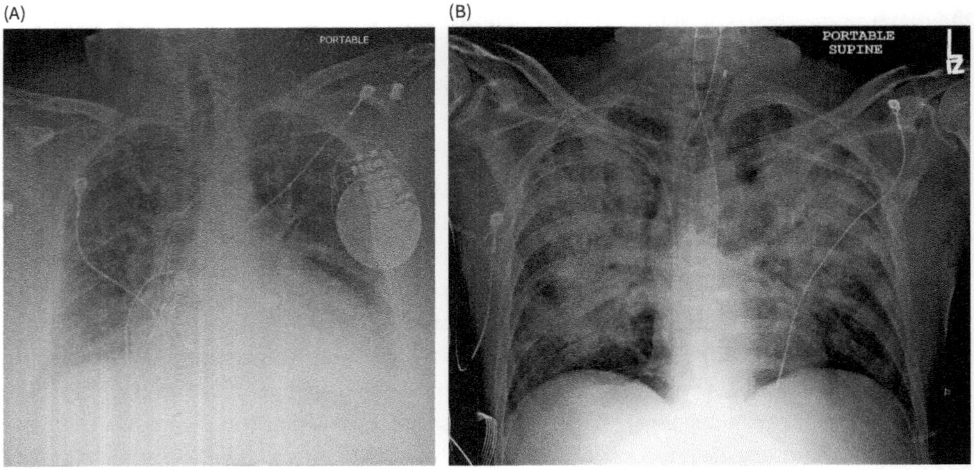

Figure 2.6 Pulmonary edema. (A) This anteroposterior projection demonstrates cardiomegaly and a diffuse, fine, reticular pattern of increased density extending to the periphery and fissures. These findings are suggestive of congestive heart failure causing retrograde fluid overload within the pulmonary circulation. There is also mild blunting of the left costophrenic angle, consistent with a small left pleural effusion. (B) Noncardiogenic pulmonary edema is typically caused by inflammatory changes, malignancy, or volume overload, which leads to increased capillary permeability. Compared to the cardiogenic variety, this type of pulmonary edema shows a perihilar, indistinct pattern of air space density that spares the periphery of the lung (winged appearance). The heart appears normal in size and the pulmonary capillary wedge pressure is typically within normal limits.

and mortality.[4] Flattening of the diaphragm from hyperinflation, increased lucency with decreased visibility of the vascular markings, and prominent central pulmonary arteries related to secondary pulmonary arterial hypertension are typical features seen on chest X-ray in a patient with chronic obstructive pulmonary disease. Of note, if more than eight to nine ribs are seen projected over the lungs on a chest X-ray in the frontal view in a patient with known risk factors for lung disease, it is indicative of hyperinflation possibly related to an underlying obstructive lung disease.

The greater anatomical detail inherent to CT allows for better visualization of the previously mentioned features in addition to identifying areas of air trapping and bullae that result from destruction of alveoli (Figure 2.7). These anatomical deficits should be closely correlated with a patient's pulmonary function during preoperative planning, especially in the setting of thoracic surgery when a single lung is often ventilated to operate on the contralateral lung. Preoperative X-rays are not required in patients with emphysema. However, they are beneficial in optimizing a patient to treat reversible conditions like pneumonia. They can also help in understanding the risk of general anesthesia administration in a patient with chronic obstructive pulmonary disease (i.e., help reduce the risk of a pneumothorax in a patient with pre-existing bullous disease).[5] Still yet, if a patient's pulmonary function is poor and their emphysematous disease is too advanced, they may not be a surgical candidate. Preoperative imaging is influential in the decision-making process of whether or not to place a patient with severe emphysematous disease under general anesthesia.

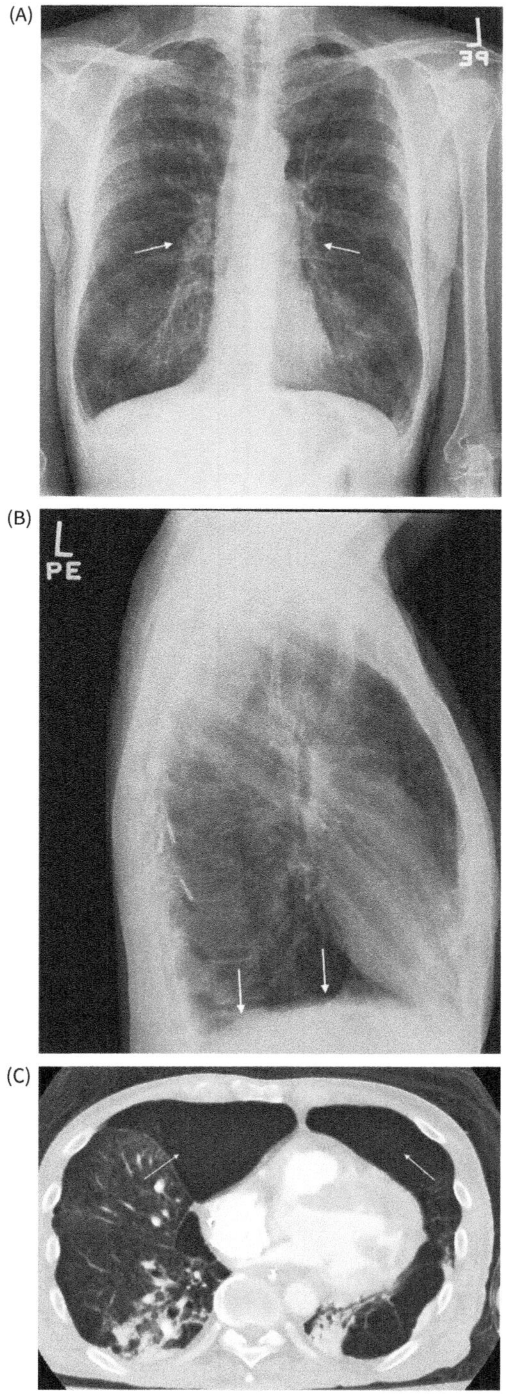

Figure 2.7 Chronic obstructive pulmonary disease. (A) The lungs appear hyperinflated with decreased vascular markings. Additionally, the prominent pulmonary arteries (solid white arrows) are indicative of underlying pulmonary hypertension. (B) There is also associated flattening of the diaphragms (solid white arrows) due to increased intrathoracic pressure. (C) An axial computed tomography slice in a different patient displays advanced destructive changes of chronic obstructive pulmonary disease, where normal lung parenchyma is replaced by thin walled and air filled bullae (solid white arrows).

Asthma

Asthma is a very common disease, and the diagnosis is typically made clinically and not by radiologic means. A chest radiograph obtained during an acute asthmatic attack may display pulmonary hyperinflation with flattening of the diaphragms and peribronchial thickening. However, these findings are nonspecific and not always present in a patient with asthma. During an acute asthma attack, prompt treatment with bronchodilators, steroids, and in the case of severe respiratory distress, intubation should not be interrupted by imaging.[3] However, imaging studies may be beneficial in determining the source of the patient's exacerbation or disease complication. For example, in the setting of fever, pneumonia should be suspected and can be confirmed by a chest X-ray once the patient has been clinically stabilized.

Lung Cancer

Malignancy within the chest is largely categorized by both the anatomical structures involved and by the cell type. The mediastinum is arbitrarily divided into anterior, middle, and posterior compartments, and certain classes of neoplasms are known to commonly arise from a specific compartment. Lymphoma, substernal thyroid neoplasms, thymomas, and teratomas (the prototypical *T*s) classically originate within the anterior mediastinum. Lymphadenopathy from metastatic disease is more prevalent within the middle mediastinum, and neurogenic or nerve sheath tumors are normally found within the posterior mediastinum. However, the borders between compartments are not well defined, and there is often overlap in the distribution of these malignancies.

Cancer within the lung is broadly divided into two categories: small cell carcinoma and nonsmall cell carcinoma. Small cell carcinoma has a neurosecretory component, tends to be more centrally located, and is typically more aggressive in its behavior (metastasis often occurs prior to the cancer's discovery). Squamous cell carcinoma is found more centrally and is the most common histological type to appear as a cavitary lesion on imaging, and it very often will be the source of airway obstruction leading to pneumonitis or atelectasis (Figure 2.8). Finally, adenocarcinoma is generally located peripherally, and it is the slowest growing of the three types described here. In contrast, metastatic neoplasms will usually present as multiple scattered nodules within the lungs and are not amenable to surgery, but they may require a tissue sample to determine the cell type.

Arguably the most important question to answer regarding a nodule within the lung is its malignant potential. Generally speaking, incidental solitary pulmonary nodules less than 4 mm in a low-risk patient are benign and do not require follow-up. According to the Fleischner criteria, nodules larger than this in high-risk patients (i.e., smokers between the ages of 55 and 74) require closer imaging follow-up.[9]

Pleura

Pneumothorax

The inner visceral layer and outer parietal layer of the pleura are tightly adhered to each other by constant negative pressure. However, when air enters the pleural space and increases

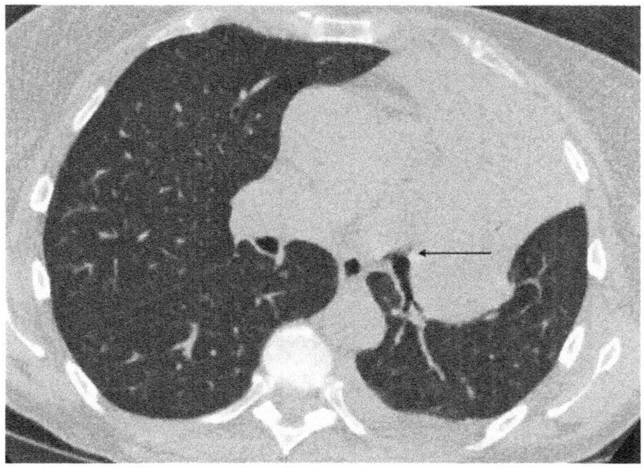

Figure 2.8 Lung cancer. This axial computed tomography slice shows a lung mass within the upper lobe of the left lung, which is causing obstruction of the left upper bronchus (solid black arrow). Impeding ventilation to the portion of the lung distal to this mass results in obstructive atelectasis and collapse of the corresponding lung. A tissue biopsy later confirmed squamous cell carcinoma in this patient.

pressure to a level higher than the intra-alveolar pressure within the lungs, the lung collapses and a pneumothorax results. The etiology of pneumothorax is variable, with chest trauma being the most common cause, but it can also be spontaneous (related to underlying parenchymal disease) or iatrogenic from positive pressure mechanical ventilation or procedures. A postprocedure chest X-ray is useful for confirming where a tube or line terminates, but it is also necessary to exclude a pneumothorax following its placement. CT is more sensitive than X-ray for the diagnosis of pneumothorax, but clinical urgency, availability, and cost precludes patients from receiving a postprocedure CT rather than a chest radiograph.[2]

On a chest X-ray, identification of the dense white visceral pleural line with absence of lung markings more peripherally is the radiologic criteria for diagnosis of pneumothorax (Figure 2.9). Skin folds and the medial border of the scapula may be confused for the visceral pleura. Additionally, air-filled lung bullae or pneumatocysts can mimic a pneumothorax radiographically. Therefore, the *lack* of lung markings is not always an indicator of a pneumothorax, so careful attention should be used identifying the visceral pleural edge to confirm the diagnosis.

In critically ill patients, performing an upright chest X-ray is often not possible and portable supine anteroposterior radiographs are usually obtained. As a result, the typical apical collection of air within the pleural space seen on an erect radiograph may not be identified. In this scenario, lateral decubitus chest X-ray, performed with the suspected side of the pneumothorax in the nondependent position, may be required for complete evaluation.

Suspicion of a tension pneumothorax is raised in the setting of trauma when breath sounds are not heard on auscultation. If intrapleural pressure is great enough, hemodynamic instability can result from compression of vital structures like the inferior vena cava, compromising venous return to the heart. Treatment of a tension pneumothorax requires emergent needle decompression of the pneumothorax. This should not be delayed by imaging, but if a preprocedure radiograph was obtained, displacement of mobile structures in the chest (the heart and mediastinum) away from the side of the pneumothorax would be visible.

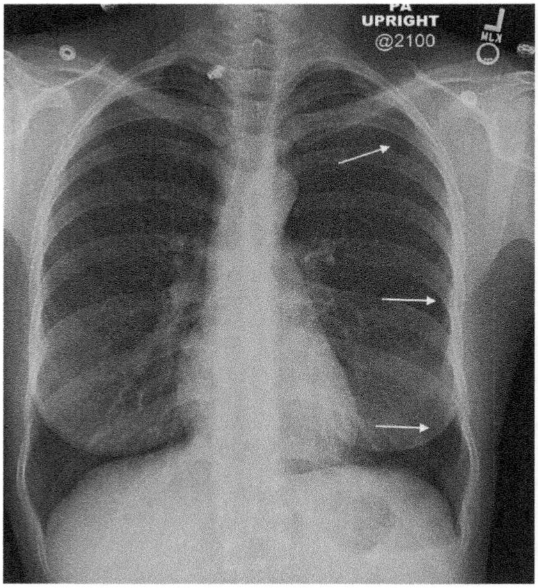

Figure 2.9 Pneumothorax. In a patient with chest pain and shortness of breath, a chest radiograph was obtained and depicts a left pneumothorax. When air enters the pleural space, the visceral and parietal layers separate. As pressure increases in the pleural space, the lung collapses, and the visceral layer is identified on a chest X-ray as a thin radiopaque line matching the contour of the lung (solid white arrows). Additionally, radiolucent air within the pleural space is visualized instead of the lung markings normally seen in the peripheral zones of the chest.

Pleural Effusion

Fluid can also fill the space between the visceral and parietal layers of the pleura. Under normal physiologic conditions, pulmonary capillary beds in the parietal pleura produce a few hundred milliliters of pleural fluid per day, which is then resorbed by the visceral pleura and lymphatics. A pleural effusion results if more fluid is produced than is resorbed. Pleural effusions are classified as either transudative (from increased intravascular hydrostatic pressure or decreased osmotic pressure) or exudative (due to inflammatory changes). This characterization of a pleural effusion is confirmed by sampling and analyzing the fluid as determined by Light's criteria.[10] Imaging is beneficial in confirming the presence or resolution of a pleural effusion (Figure 2.10). Conventional radiography and CT are useful in detecting a pleural effusion, but ultrasonography is a particularly valuable tool in a patient with respiratory compromise who requires imaged guided pleurocentesis.

Vasculature

Thoracic Vascular Anatomy

The vascular system within the chest is complex, consisting of both a systemic and pulmonary circulation that meet within the heart. Cardiac anatomy will not be discussed in this

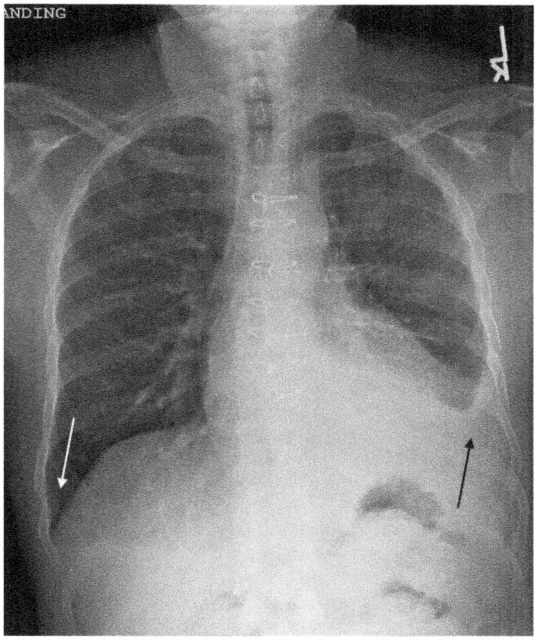

Figure 2.10 Pleural effusion. This posteroanterior chest X-ray shows fluid in the inferior portion of the left pleural space (solid black arrow), which blunts the left costophrenic angle and forms a U-shaped meniscus. The right costophrenic angle is well visualized and sharp (solid white arrow). The meniscal sign results from adhesive forces of the pleural fluid acting against the elastic recoil of the lung indicative of a left pleural effusion. Additionally, postoperative changes from a median sternotomy, coronary artery bypass grafting, and cholecystectomy are incidentally seen.

chapter, but other components of thoracic vasculature will briefly be reviewed as well as a few commonly encountered radiologic abnormalities of the thoracic vasculature.[11]

As the aorta arises from the left ventricle, the left and right main coronary arteries are the first branches of this large vessel's root. The aorta then courses superiorly, posteriorly, and to the left as the ascending thoracic aorta, aortic arch, and descending thoracic aorta before it enters the abdomen through the diaphragmatic aortic hiatus. In most individuals, the aortic arch gives rise to the innominate artery (branching into the right subclavian artery and right common carotid artery), the left common carotid artery, and the left subclavian artery. The subclavian arteries continue to branch into the bilateral vertebral arteries, thyrocervical trunks, internal mammary arteries (commonly used as an autograft during coronary artery bypass grafting), and the costocervical trunks. As the aortic arch transitions to the descending thoracic aorta distal to the subclavian branches, it extends further into a parietal and visceral system. The parietal branches include posterior intercostal, subcostal, and superior phrenic arteries. The visceral branches include pericardial, mediastinal, esophageal, and bronchial arteries. In comparison to the pulmonary arteries (whose primary role is gas exchange), the bronchial arteries are the main delivery method of nutrients to the lung parenchyma.

The inferior vena cava receives deoxygenated blood from organs inferior to the diaphragm and enters the right atrium inferiorly like the superior vena cava (SVC) does superiorly. The valveless SVC is formed as the right and left brachiocephalic veins converge and, apart from the heart and lungs, receives deoxygenated blood from structures superior to the diaphragm. The azygos–hemiazygos venous system demonstrates considerable anatomical variability and forms a collateral system between the inferior vena cava and SVC as it drains the thoracoabdominal walls, mediastinal structures, and the posterior thorax.

In the pulmonary arterial system, the right and left pulmonary arteries originate from the right ventricle via the pulmonary artery trunk and course peripherally until their branches terminate and deliver deoxygenated blood to capillaries at the level of the alveolar walls. After gas exchange has occurred, the pulmonary venous system carries oxygenated blood back to the heart as left and right superior and inferior pulmonary veins drain into the left atrium.[12]

Thoracic Aortic Aneurysm

When a vessel exceeds 50% of its original size, an aneurysm has developed. If that abnormal dilation contains all three layers of a vessel wall (the intima, media, and adventitia), it is considered a true aneurysm. A pseudoaneurysm occurs when fewer than three layers are involved. Atherosclerosis is the most common etiology leading to an aneurysm, which can be further exacerbated by the presence of hypertension.

A thoracic aortic aneurysm is normally discovered incidentally, as most patients are asymptomatic. In the chest, the ascending aorta is normally less than 3.5 cm in maximal diameter, and the descending aorta typically measures less than 3 cm. Although radiography may reveal abnormal aortic enlargement, contrast-enhanced CT is the standard for diagnosis of a thoracic aortic aneurysm, which is defined as dilation (either fusiform or saccular in shape) greater than 4 cm. If the thoracic aorta exceeds 5 cm in diameter or grows at a rate of greater than 1 cm/year, surgical intervention is recommended.[2]

Thoracic Aortic Dissection

In a patient with chest pain radiating to the back and a history of trauma, atherosclerosis, and less commonly, connective tissue disorder or untreated syphilis, a provider should consider thoracic aortic dissection in the differential diagnosis. Especially in the setting of a deceleration type traumatic injury, disruption of the medial layer occurs at sites where the aorta is fixed (the heart, ligamentum arteriosum, etc.). Once an aortic dissection occurs, lethal consequences can rapidly develop if the dissection causes aortic rupture or involves the region of the root or valve.

Conventional radiography may display what is typically described as a “widened mediastinum,” but a chest X-ray is not sufficient to confirm a diagnosis. Contrast-enhanced CT is more sensitive and specific for thoracic aortic dissection. It confirms the presence of an intimal flap causing a filling defect within the vessel lumen, which is indicative of the development of a true lumen and false lumen (Figure 2.11). Coincident myocardial infarction may also occur with an ascending aortic dissection as blood flow through the coronary vessels branching from the aortic root is compromised. In general, an ascending aortic dissection

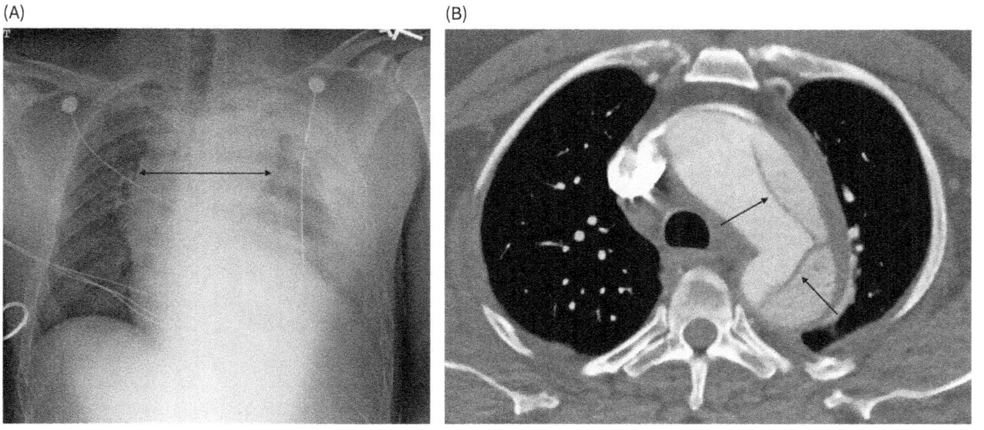

Figure 2.11 Thoracic aortic dissection. (A) A widened mediastinum is demonstrated on this chest radiograph (double black arrow), which is often considered characteristic of a thoracic aortic dissection. However, this sign is infrequently seen on a chest X-ray. (B) This axial computed tomography slice in a different patient demonstrates the presence of an intimal flap within the thoracic aorta (solid black arrows). This is consistent with a Stanford type B dissection as it involves the descending aortic arch. The false lumen is created after blood dissects further into the media layer of the vessel, and the true lumen is usually smaller in size relative to the false lumen.

(Stanford type A) requires surgical treatment, while a descending aortic dissection (Stanford type B) can be treated medically with blood pressure modification.

Pulmonary Embolism

In a patient presenting with pleuritic chest pain and/or dyspnea with a history of recent surgery, cancer, or reduced mobility, consider the diagnosis of pulmonary embolism (PE). Most emboli develop from thrombi in the deep venous system of the pelvis or lower extremities and migrate to the pulmonary circulation. As mentioned previously, the lungs receive a dual blood supply from both the pulmonary and bronchial arterial system. Pulmonary infarction is rare but can occur if the embolism is large enough to restrict flow to the lung parenchyma distal to the obstruction. Increased pulmonary arterial pressure may also develop, leading to right heart failure in a matter of minutes to hours.

A chest X-ray has low sensitivity in the diagnosis of PE, but it may show a wedge-shaped peripheral opacity (Hampton's hump) due to infarction, localized lucency due to hypovolemia distal to the PE (Westermark sign) or engorged pulmonary artery (knuckle sign). Especially in patients whose kidney function is poor and who cannot tolerate contrast administration, a ventilation–perfusion scan may be performed to rule out a PE. However, CT pulmonary angiography has become the standard for the diagnosis of PE.[2] A PE is seen as a filling defect within the lumen of the contrast enhanced pulmonary vasculature (Figure 2.12). Depending on the severity of the embolus and the patient's symptoms, prompt treatment with anticoagulation or thrombolytics should be administered to prevent a devastating outcome.

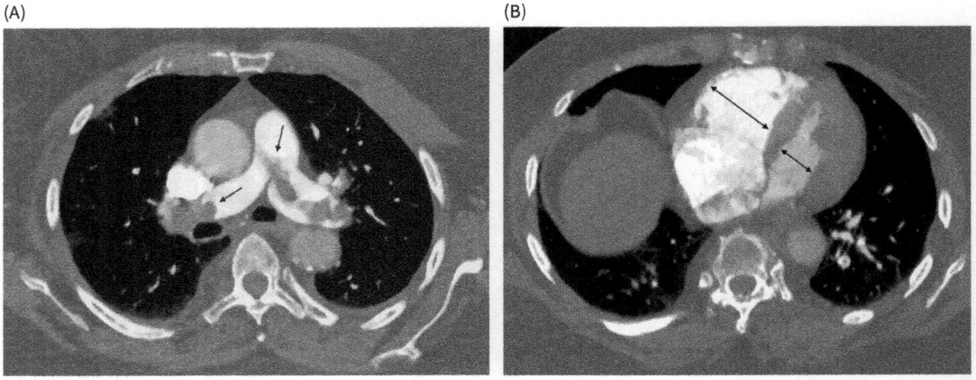

Figure 2.12 Pulmonary embolism. (A) An axial slice of a computed tomography angiography study depicts both partial and complete filling defects within contrast-enhanced pulmonary arteries (solid black arrows). (B) More inferiorly in the same study, the dimension of the right ventricle relative to the left ventricle is increased (double black arrows). These findings are consistent with large pulmonary emboli causing right heart strain.

Esophagus

Anatomy of the Esophagus

The esophagus functions to move ingested material from the inferior pharynx to the stomach. Voluntary action of skeletal muscle superiorly helps propagate food or fluid through the esophagus where a combination of involuntary contraction and relaxation of sphincters advances a bolus into the stomach. The esophagus is positioned between the trachea anteriorly and vertebral bodies posteriorly and courses inferiorly through its diaphragmatic hiatus until it terminates at the gastroesophageal junction. Even under direct visualization, the tracheal and esophageal relationship can appear complex and confusing. Equipment may be mistakenly positioned in the wrong structure during ET tube or enteric tube placement. Radiography should follow these procedures to confirm the correct placement of an ET tube terminating superior to the carina and enteric tube coursing subdiaphragmatically (Figure 2.13).

Hiatal Hernia

Hiatal hernias are classified as either sliding type (most common) or paraesophageal. In the sliding type, the gastroesophageal junction resides above the diaphragm. In contrast, the gastroesophageal junction remains infradiaphragmatic and within the diaphragm in a paraesophageal type, with a portion of the stomach migrating superiorly through the diaphragmatic hiatus to lie adjacent to the esophagus (Figure 2.14). Hiatal hernias are also usually found incidentally, and many patients are asymptomatic. Nevertheless, patients may

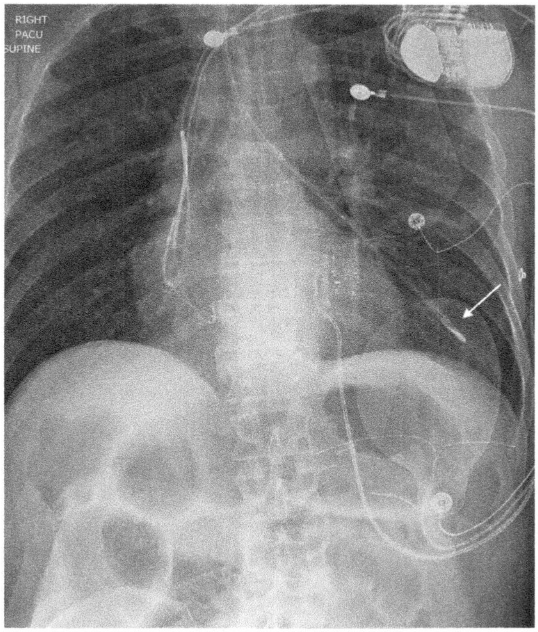

Figure 2.13 Incorrect enteric tube placement. An enteric tube should course subdiaphragmatically into the region of the stomach or more distally into the small intestine. After placement of the tube, its location should be confirmed with a radiograph. In this patient, the enteric tube was inadvertently placed within the left bronchus/lung (solid white arrow), requiring positional readjustment.

(A) (B)

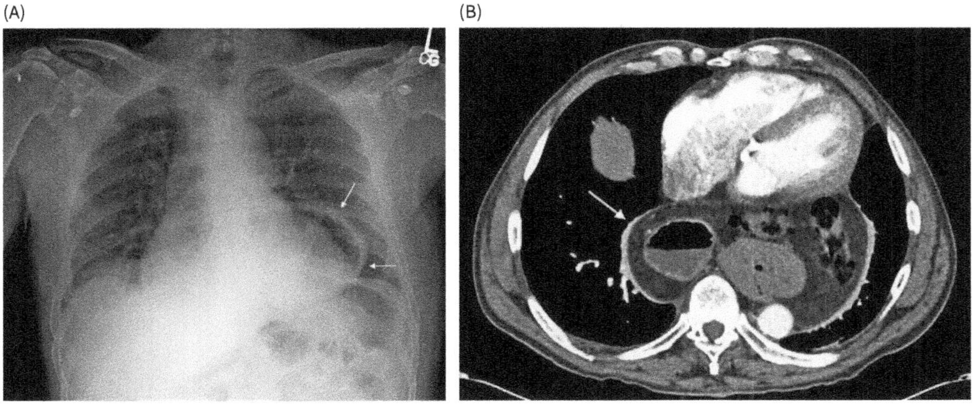

Figure 2.14 Hiatal hernia. (A) A retrocardiac opacity with internal lucency and air fluid levels is seen on this chest X-ray (solid white arrows). (B) The axial computed tomography scan confirms the presence of a large hernia containing both stomach and bowel extending superiorly within the thorax above the diaphragm and behind the heart (solid white arrow).

complain of gastroesophageal reflux type pain as gastric acid more easily flows retrograde into the esophagus.

Esophageal Cancer

The esophagus lacks a serosal border and is rich in a lymphatic network, which contributes to a poor prognosis for patients with esophageal cancer as many will have metastatic disease at the time of diagnosis. The major histological types include squamous cell carcinoma and adenocarcinomas. Patients with a history of extended tobacco or alcohol use are at an increased risk of developing squamous cell carcinoma of the esophagus. In esophageal adenocarcinoma, metaplastic transformation of the normal esophageal squamous epithelium to a columnar type promotes the development of premalignant Barrett esophagus. Eventually, with repetitive insult of chronic gastroesophageal reflux, histological transformation occurs and malignant neoplastic disease develops. As it progresses, patients will often complain of increasing dysphagia and odynophagia, initially with solid foods and eventually with liquids. A barium esophagram is typically the study of choice in the initial evaluation of patients with these types of symptoms (Figure 2.15), but confirmation will require endoscopic direct visualization and tissue sampling.

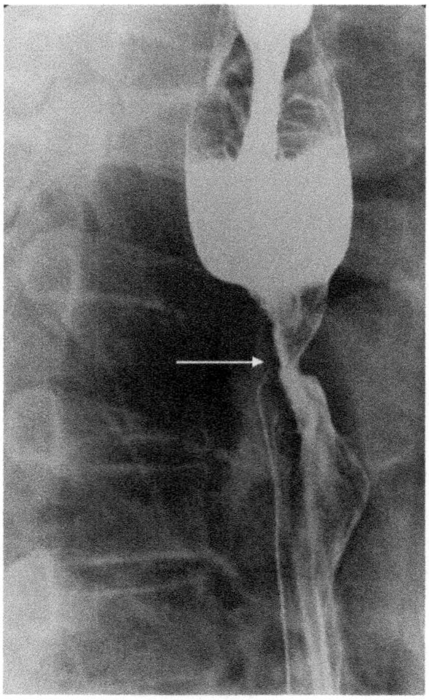

Figure 2.15 Esophageal carcinoma. This fluoroscopic barium swallow study reveals an irregular contour of the esophageal lumen. There is evidence of annular constriction (solid white arrow) leading to proximal esophageal dilation and obstruction of esophageal contents. These findings are concerning for esophageal carcinoma, and this was later confirmed under direct visualization and tissue sampling with endoscopy.

Summary

The descriptive information presented above serves as a foundation for understanding common thoracic pathology and its associated radiologic manifestations. Perioperative diagnostic imaging provides insight into a patient's unique thoracic anatomy, potential underlying pathology and, therefore, vital information for operative planning. This knowledge should be well understood and communicated by all providers to optimize perioperative patient care.

References

1. Kamel KS, Lau G, Stringer, MD. In vivo and in vitro morphometry of the human trachea. *Clin Anat.* 2009;22(5):571–579.
2. Herring W. *Learning Radiology: Recognizing The Basics.* 3rd ed. New York: Elsevier; 2016.
3. Pollart SM, Compton RM, Elward KS. *Am Fam Physician.* 2011;84(1):40–47.
4. Kemp SV, Polkey MI, Shah PL. The epidemiology, etiology, clinical features, and natural history of emphysema. *Thorac Surg Clin.* 2009;19(2):149–158. doi:10.1016/j.thorsurg.2009.03.003
5. Lumb A, Biercamp C. Chronic obstructive pulmonary disease and anaesthesia. *Cont Ed Anaesth Crit Care Pain.* 2014;14(1):1–5.
6. Bartlett JG, Dowell SF, Mandell LA, et al. Practice guidelines for the management of community-acquired pneumonia in adults. *Clin Infect Dis.* 2000;31:347–382.
7. Bramson RT, Griscom NT, Cleveland RH. Interpretation of chest radiographs in infants with cough and fever. *Radiology.* 2005;236(1):22–29.
8. Purvey M, Allen G. Managing acute pulmonary oedema. *Austr Prescrib.* 2017;40(2):59–63. doi:10.18773/austprescr.2017.012
9. MacMahon H, Naidich DP, Goo JM, et al. Guidelines for management of incidental pulmonary nodules detected on CT Images: from the Fleischner Society 2017. *Radiology.* 2017;284(1):228–243.
10. Light RW. Clinical practice: pleural effusion. *N Engl J Med.* 2002;346(25):1971–1977.
11. Patel AA. Thoracic vascular anatomy: a brief review. *J Vasc Interv Radiol.* 2014;13(2):P318–P321.
12. Kandathil A, Chamarthy M. Pulmonary vascular anatomy & anatomical variants. *Cardiovasc Diagn Ther.* 2018;8(3):201–207. doi:10.21037/cdt.2018.01.04.

3
Physiology of One-Lung Ventilation

Geetha Shanmugam and Raymond Pla

Introduction

Anesthesia for most thoracic surgical procedures involves one-lung ventilation (OLV), with the patient in the lateral decubitus position for optimal surgical access. OLV, achieved with a double-lumen tube or bronchial blocker, selectively inhibits ventilation of one lung while perfusion of that lung continues. The result is a right-to-left intrapulmonary shunt, with deoxygenated systemic blood returning to the circulation without pulmonic oxygenation. The prevention of sustained hypoxemia from selective lung ventilation requires an in-depth understanding of one-lung physiology.

The Ventilation/Perfusion Relationship

Ventilation involves the entry and exit of air from the lungs, while perfusion involves the flow of blood through alveolar pulmonary capillaries. Both are necessary for the diffusion of oxygen into and carbon dioxide out of the bloodstream. Under physiologic conditions, ventilation and perfusion are matched for optimal gas exchange. However, neither ventilation nor perfusion is uniformly distributed throughout the lung.

Perfusion varies across a gravitational gradient, with more dependent areas better perfused. Perfusion is influenced by a complex interaction of pulmonary artery pressure, alveolar pressure, and pulmonary venous pressure. This relationship was originally described by West and Dollery who described three distinct zones of the lung.[1] (See Figure 3.1.)

Zone 1 is the least dependent zone of the lung, in which alveolar pressure is equal to atmospheric pressure and pulmonary artery pressure is subatmospheric but greater than pulmonary venous pressure ($P_{alv} > P_{art} > P_v$). Because alveolar pressure is greatest, pulmonary vascular collapse occurs, and perfusion is absent in Zone 1. Alveolar ventilation without perfusion is termed "dead space." Although generally small under normal physiologic conditions, the size of Zone 1 can increase during conditions of decreased pulmonary arterial pressure (e.g., hypovolemia and hemorrhage) and increased alveolar pressure (e.g., positive pressure ventilation).

Zone 2 occurs where arterial pressure increases and surpasses alveolar pressure ($P_{art} > P_{alv} > P_v$). Pulmonary blood flow is re-established and so is gas exchange. This zone of well-matched ventilation and perfusion contains most alveoli.

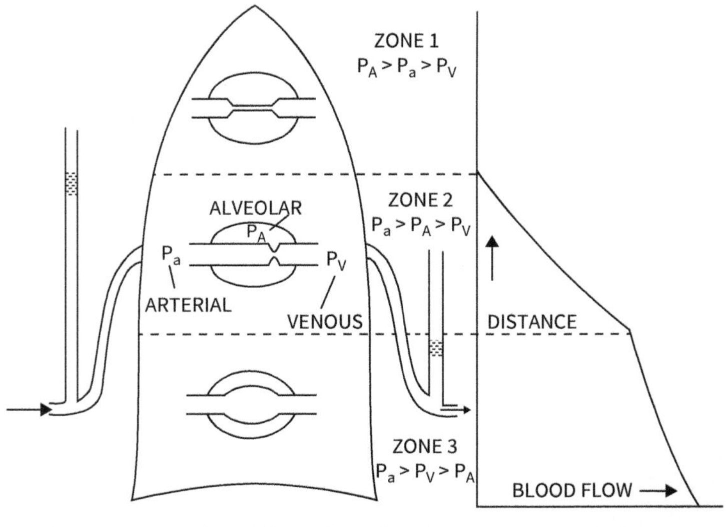

Figure 3.1 West lung zones: regional blood flow distribution zones in the lung.
From West JB, Dollery CT, Naimark A. Distribution of blood flow in isolated lung; relation to vascular and alveolar pressures. *J Appl Physiol.* 1964;19:713–724.

Zone 3, the most dependent lung region, is where pulmonary venous pressure exceeds pulmonary alveolar pressure ($P_{art} > P_v > P_{alv}$). Because vascular pressures are much greater than alveolar pressure, very little alveolar ventilation occurs in Zone 3. The presence of perfusion in the absence of ventilation is termed "shunt." The West zones and relationships between alveolar pressure, pulmonary arterial pressure, and pulmonary venous pressure apply to the static upright lung. Although a simplification, they are a good starting point to understand the distribution of perfusion in the lungs.

To understand the dynamic nature of ventilation, it is necessary to discuss pleural pressure and compliance. The apex of the lung tends to collapse inward creating very negative pleural pressure in the upper chest. The lung base however tends to bulge outward, producing less negative pleural pressure. The transpulmonary pressure, or alveolar distending pressure, can be described as $P_{transpulmonary} = P_{alveolar} - P_{pleural}$. While alveolar pressure is uniform throughout the lung, the pleural pressure increases closer to the lung base, decreasing transpulmonary pressure. This, in turn, leads to increased compliance at basilar alveoli.

Compliance refers to the change in unit volume of lung tissue per unit change in pressure, $C = \Delta V/\Delta P$ Compliant tissues require little pressure to inflate, whereas poorly compliant tissues require very high pressures. Nondependent alveoli tend to be maximally inflated and relatively noncompliant. Dependent alveoli, on the other hand, are compressed and smaller but are more compliant and therefore receive a larger proportion of alveolar ventilation.[2] Lung compliance changes with patient position, restriction of chest wall excursion, and general anesthesia.[3] The alteration of lung compliance plays an important role in ventilation changes during thoracic surgery.

Alveolar ventilation and perfusion mismatch is common during the perioperative period. Perfusion in areas that are not ventilated is termed shunt, and ventilation in areas that do not receive blood flow is termed "dead space." While absolute dead space and shunt exist, areas with reduced ventilation or blood flow are more common, and they are termed "relative shunt" and "relative dead space," respectively. Some degree of shunt is obligatory; "anatomic shunt" or "venous admixture" refers to the deoxygenated blood from the bronchial, pleural, and thebesian circulations that mixes with and dilutes the oxygen concentration of pulmonary arterial blood. In healthy spontaneously breathing patients, this is estimated to be about 1% to 2% of total cardiac output.[4] However, in the lateral position under general anesthesia, venous admixture equals about 10% of cardiac output.[5]

Mismatch between ventilation and perfusion leads to decreased gas exchange and oxygenation. During thoracic surgery the ventilation/perfusion (V/Q) relationship is disrupted by several factors, including induction of general anesthesia, lateral decubitus positioning, OLV, and the opening of the chest wall. The effect of each of these factors will be explored more in-depth.

The Awake State

Ventilation and perfusion are well-matched in awake, spontaneously breathing patients. While upright, alveoli in the dependent lung are better ventilated and perfused than non-dependent alveoli. In the lateral decubitus position, the same occurs. Perfusion to the dependent lung is higher due to gravity, while ventilation to the dependent lung is increased because the alveoli are more compliant, and there is an upward shift of the dependent hemidiaphragm making its contraction more efficient.[6] Thus, in the awake state, V/Q matching is preserved despite changing body position.

General Anesthesia

Induction of general anesthesia with neuromuscular paralysis leads to decreased diaphragmatic and inspiratory muscle tone, in turn decreasing lung expansion and causing atelectasis. Function residual capacity drops by 15-20%.[7]

Most thoracic surgeries are done in the lateral decubitus position for optimal surgical exposure. Once the patient is turned lateral, the now-paralyzed diaphragm is pushed up higher by abdominal contents. In addition, the weight of mediastinal structures and the rigid bean bag used for positioning further impede expansion of the dependent lung, resulting in a 35% drop in dependent lung functional residual capacity.[8] The nondependent lung, on the other hand, is much less restricted and preferentially ventilated. This leads to V/Q mismatch because the dependent lung continues to be more perfused.

Open Pneumothorax and One-Lung Ventilation

When the chest wall is opened, the operative lung would herniate out of the surgical incision if it were not deliberately collapsed. OLV diverts ventilation to the dependent lung, which is already receiving more perfusion, and improves V/Q mismatch in the dependent lung at the expense of a large right to left intrapulmonary shunt in the nondependent lung.

The nondependent lung receives about 40% of the cardiac output in the lateral decubitus position, minus 5% for anatomic shunt. With selective lung collapse and hypoxic pulmonary vasoconstriction (HPV), the blood flow to the nondependent lung is reduced by half, or 35/2 = 17.5% cardiac output. Because anatomic shunt to each lung is 5%, or 10% combined, this makes a total shunt of 27.5% cardiac output during OLV. This leads to a PaO_2 of 150 mmHg at FiO_2 1.0. Since the majority of the cardiac output is directed to the dependent lung, care must be taken to maximize ventilation to improve V/Q match and oxygenation.[9]

V/Q Modifying Factors

Hypoxic Pulmonary Vasoconstriction

HPV reduces perfusion to poorly oxygenated lung tissue. Much has been studied about HPV. Low partial pressure of oxygen triggers a cellular cascade that leads to increased intracellular calcium and smooth muscle contraction, particularly in the smallest pulmonary arteries.[10] The degree of HPV is proportional to the degree of hypoxia and the amount of hypoxic lung tissue. Maximal HPV occurs when between 30% to 70% of lung tissue is hypoxic.[10,11] HPV is biphasic; the early response starts in seconds and peaks 20 to 30 minutes after initiation of OLV and the delayed response peaks after the next 2 hours.[12] The overall shunt flow to the nondependent lung is reduced by about 40% to 50%, allowing the body to tolerate OLV.[11] Factors that inhibit HPV and therefore worsen shunt include very high or low pulmonary artery pressures, hypocapnia, very high or low mixed venous PO_2 vasodilators, pulmonary infection, and inhalational anesthetics at high minimum alveolar concentration.[6] Factors that lead to hypoxia and vasoconstriction in the ventilated lung, such as high airway pressures and low FiO_2 and auto positive end expiratory pressure (PEEP), divert blood flow to the nonventilated lung and also increase shunt[6] (see Table 3.1). Although numerous drugs, including almitrine, inhaled nitric oxide, and prostaglandin E_1, have been studied to alter HPV, none have proven clinically useful yet.[13–15]

Table 3.1 Factors that can affect HPV

Increased HPV	Decreased HPV
Hypoxia	Inhaled anesthetics
Acidosis	Alkalosis
Hypercapnia	Hypocapnia
Vasoconstrictors	Vasodilators: sodium nitroprusside, nitroglycerin, calcium channel blockers, B-agonists
	Pulmonary infection
	High or low pulmonary artery pressure
	High or low mixed venous P_{O2}

Position

Patient position during OLV can have a profound effect on the degree of V/Q mismatch and therefore oxygenation. The lateral decubitus positioning is preferred for most thoracic surgeries, and it maximizes perfusion of the dependent, ventilated lung causing the least V/Q mismatch of all possible positions. Furthermore, if the patient is in a reverse Trendelenburg position while lateral, perfusion of the lower lung is accentuated. A few thoracic surgeries are done in the supine position including sympathectomies and chest wall resections. This results in an increased shunt fraction because of less gravitational redistribution of blood flow causing the collapsed lung to receive much greater blood flow than in the lateral position.[16] Albeit rare, prone thoracic surgery is sometimes required, as in certain minimally invasive esophagectomies. In the prone position, lung compliance is improved. But because gravitational redistribution of blood is absent, shunt and hypoxemia with OLV are worse than when lateral.[16]

Other Modifying Factors

Certain other surgical and patient related factors can also affect oxygenation during OLV. Surgical retraction can increase pulmonary vascular resistance in the nondependent lung, but paradoxically vasoactive substances released during this manipulation may cause vasodilation and counteract HPV.[17] Additionally, surgical ligation of blood vessels in the operative lung decreases blood flow and can thus lead to decreased shunt fraction.[17]

The side of lung collapse affects the degree of V/Q mismatch. The right lung is larger and receives 10% more cardiac output, so shunt fraction is higher when the right lung is collapsed.[18] Restoration of low cardiac output to normal values improves oxygenation. However, supranormal cardiac output results in increased PvO_2 and decreased HPV, causing a rise in shunt fraction and worse oxygenation.[19,20]

Strategies to Address Hypoxia

V/Q mismatch is inevitable during selective lung ventilation, even if every effort is made to minimize the degree of shunt. This V/Q mismatch will decrease oxygenation to varying degrees in different patients. Hypoxemia during thoracic surgery is defined as a decrease in oxygen saturation below 85% to 90%, or PaO_2 <60 mmHg while inspired FiO_2 is 1.0.[21] Such episodes occur in about 5% to 10% of patients, do not last more than a few minutes, and are usually well tolerated by those with normal lung function.[22]

If hypoxemia is severe, prolonged or occurs in patients with compromised lung function, several steps should be undertaken to address the problem. First, the patient should be stabilized. FiO_2 should be increased to 1.0, any nonurgent procedure should be temporarily stopped, and dual-lung ventilation should be restored until oxygenation improves. The most frequent cause of oxygen desaturation is malpositioning of the double-lumen tube or bronchial blocker, so correct position should be confirmed with a fiberoptic bronchoscope once the patient is stabilized. Next, strategies to maximize ventilation of the dependent lung and improve V/Q matching should be undertaken. This includes suctioning of secretions, recruitment maneuvers, and PEEP to the ventilated lung. Maneuvers to improve oxygenation to the nondependent lung can also be initiated. These include apneic oxygen insufflation, with a low flow of oxygen from supplemental tubing to the nonventilated lung, and continuous positive airway pressure or intermittent ventilation to the nonventilated lung, although these are more likely to interfere with the surgical field. Finally, the main pulmonary artery to the nondependent lung can be clamped to halt shunt, but this will cause an acute increase in right heart afterload. As a last resort, extracorporeal membrane oxygenation can be utilized to ventilate a patient during thoracic surgery when no other route for adequate oxygenation is possible.[12]

The V/Q relationship changes during thoracic surgery as a result of induction of anesthesia, lateral positioning, and selective lung ventilation. Knowledge of one lung physiology can help in the management of hypoxia when it occurs.

Acknowledgments

The authors thank Yani Papanikos and John Mekail for their contributions to this chapter.

References

1. West JB, Dollery CT. Distribution of blood flow and the pressure-flow relations of the whole lung. *J Appl Physiol.* 1965;20(2):175–183.
2. Milic-Emili J. Regional distribution of gas in the lung. *Can Respir J.* 2000;7(1):71–76. doi:10.1155/2000/768271.
3. Bartz RR, Moon RE. Physiology of One Lung Ventilation. In: Barbeito A, Shaw AD, Grichnik K, eds. *Thoracic Anesthesia:* New York: McGraw-Hill Professional; 2011: 45–62.
4. Jaeger JM, Titus BJ, Blank RS. Essential anatomy and physiology of the respiratory system and the pulmonary circulation. In: Slinger PD, Blank RS, Campos J, Lohser J, McRae K., eds. *Principles and Practice of Anesthesia for Thoracic Surgery.* Cham, Switzerland: Springer; 2019: 65–92.
5. Neustein SM, Eisenkraft JB, Cohen E. Anesthesia for thoracic surgery. In: Barash PG, ed. *Clinical Anesthesia.* 6th ed. New York: Wolters Kluwer; 2009: 1042.
6. Butterworth JF, IV, Mackey DC, Wasnick JD. Anesthesia for thoracic surgery. In: *Morgan & Mikhail's Clinical Anesthesiology.* 6th ed. New York: McGraw-Hill; 2018: 533–581.
7. Wabha RW. Perioperative functional residual capacity. *Can J Anesth.* 1991;38(3):384–400.
8. Chang H, Lai-Fook SJ, Domino KB, et al. Ventilation and perfusion distribution during altered PEEP in the left lung in the left lateral decubitus posture with unchanged tidal volume in dogs. *Chin J Physiol.* 2006 49(2):74–82.
9. Benumof JL. Isoflurane anesthesia and arterial oxygenation during one-lung ventilation. *Anesthesiology.* 1986;64:419–422.
10. Weir EK, Lopez-Barneo J, Buckler KJ, Archer SL. Acute oxygen sensing mechanisms. *N Engl J Med.* 2005;353(19):2042–2055.
11. Lumb AB, Slinger P. Hypoxic pulmonary vasoconstriction: physiology and anesthetic implications. *Anesthesiology.* 2015; 122(4):932–946.
12. Campos JH, Feider A. Hypoxia during one-lung ventilation—a review and update. *J Cardiothor Vasc Anesth.* 2018;32(5): 2330–2338.
13. Bermejo S, Gallart L, Silva-Costa-Gomes T, Valles J, Aguillo R, Puig MM. Almitrine fails to improve oxygenation during one-lung ventilation with sevoflurane anesthesia. *YJCAN.* 2014;28(4):919–924.

14. Rocca GD, Passariello M, Coccia C, et al. Inhaled nitric oxide administration during one-lung ventilation in patients undergoing thoracic surgery. *J Cardiothor Vasc Anesth.* 2001;15(2):218–223.
15. Della Rocca G, Coccia C, Pompei L, et al. Inhaled aerosolized prostaglandin E1, pulmonary hemodynamics, and oxygenation during lung transplantation, *Minerva Anesthesiol* 2008;74(11):627–633.
16. McLean SR, Lohser J. Physiology of the lateral decubitus position, open chest, and one-lung ventilation. In: Slinger PD, Blank RS, Campos J, Lohser J, McRae K, eds. *Principles and Practice of Anesthesia for Thoracic Surgery.* Cham, Switzerland: Springer; 2019: 93–103.
17. Szegedi LL. Pathophysiology of one-lung ventilation. *Anesthesiol Clin N Am.* 2001;19(3):435–453.
18. Slinger P, Suissa S, Triolet W. Predicting arterial oxygenation during one-lung anesthesia. *Can J Anesth.* 1992;39:1030–1035.
19. Benumof JL, Wahrenbrock EA. Blunted hypoxic pulmonary vasoconstriction by increased lung vascular pressures. *J Appl Physiol.* 1975;38(5):846–850.
20. Malmkvist G, Fletcher R, Nordström L, Werner O. Effects of lung surgery and one-lung ventilation on pulmonary arterial pressure, venous admixture and immediate postoperative lung function. *Brit J Anaesth.* 1989;63(6):696–701.
21. Inoue S, Nishimine N, Kitaguchi K, Furuya H, Taniguchi S. Double lumen tube location predicts tube malposition and hypoxaemia during one lung ventilation. *Brit J Anaesth.* 2004;92(2):195–201.
22. Karzai W, Schwarzkopf K. Hypoxemia during one-lung ventilation. *Anesthesiology.* 2009;110: 1402–1411.

4
Bronchoscopic Anatomy

Geoffrey D. Panjeton, W. Kirk Fowler, Hess Panjeton, Yi Deng, and Jeffrey D. White

Introduction

Navigating the pulmonary system with knowledge, skill, and efficiency is essential to the safe practice of thoracic anesthesiology. With continued advances in thoracic and interventional pulmonary techniques, the ability to identify key landmarks and anatomical structures is necessary to facilitate these procedures, create a customized anesthetic plan, and provide appropriate anesthetic care. This chapter will focus on the normal anatomy of the trachea and bronchi, as well as include important anatomical and pathological variants that may appear in the course of a busy thoracic anesthesia practice. Key features of the tracheobronchial anatomy can be seen in Table 4.1.

Basic Anatomy

The anesthesiologist's window into the lungs starts at the larynx and vocal cords. Figure 4.1 is an image of the vocal cords taken via fiberoptic bronchoscopy.

After the bronchoscope passes through the vocal cords, it enters the trachea. The trachea comprises cartilage and muscles that extend from the inferior aspect of the cricoid cartilage to the carina (Figure 4.2), the origin of the two main bronchi.[1] Figure 4.3 provides an overview of the bronchial system, along with corresponding fiberoptic images. Figure 4.4 provides a clinical correlation of a chest radiograph and the corresponding anatomic structures.

Trachea

The trachea allows for ventilation and the clearance of respiratory secretions.[2] It is a long tube-like structure that begins just past the vocal cords and extends caudally into the superior mediastinum (Figure 4.5). Its position lies anterior to the esophagus and posterior to the aortic arch. In adults, the average distance from the vocal cords to the tracheal carina is 12 cm.[3] The trachea consists of 16 to 22 cartilaginous C-shaped rings made of hyaline. These rings are visible on the anterior and lateral aspects,[1] and they are linked posteriorly by fibrous and connective tissue supported by trachealis muscle, which can be identified by its longitudinal striations.[3,4] The trachea is generally midline, although in some patients it can

Table 4.1 Key Features of Tracheobronchial Anatomy

Structure	Key Features
Trachea	• 16 to 22 C-shaped cartilaginous rings on anterolateral aspects. • Cartilaginous rings linked posteriorly by fibrous and connective tissue supported by trachealis muscle identified by longitudinal striations. • Typically midline, but may be displaced to the right by the aortic arch. The degree of displacement can increase with atherosclerotic aorta, advanced age, or severe chronic obstruction pulmonary disease. • Proximal trachea is superficial but runs further posterior and narrows as it moves inferiorly to the level of the carina. • Diameter is typically between 19.5 and 22 mm in adult males and 17.5 and 19 mm in adult females. Narrowest at the cricoid cartilage—17 mm in men and 13 mm in women. • Average distance from vocal cords to tracheal carina is 12 cm.
Carina	• Lies at the level of the sternal angle anteriorly and the T5 vertebra posteriorly. • Right main bronchus lies in a more vertical orientation (branches approximately 25°) and left main bronchus lies more horizontal orientation (branches at about 45°) relative to the trachea. • Average distance from carina to right upper lung bronchus take-off is 2 cm in men and 1.5 cm women. • Average distance from carina to bifurcation of left upper lung and left lower lung is 5 cm in men and 4.5 cm in women.
Right lung	• The right upper lobe bronchus is the first take-off along the right main bronchus. • The right upper lobe bronchus consists of apical, anterior, and posterior divisions. • The remainder of the right main bronchus continues as the bronchus intermedius. • Bronchus intermedius gives rise to the: • Right middle lobe bronchus with corresponding medial and lateral divisions. • Right lower lobe bronchus, consisting of the superior, anterior basal, medial basal, lateral basal, and posterior basal divisions.
Left lung	• Left upper lobe bronchus divides into the superior division, consisting of the apicoposterior and anterior segments and the inferior division (lingular bronchus), consisting of superior and inferior segments. • Left lower lobe bronchus, consisting of superior, anteriomedial basal, lateral basal, and posterior basal segments.

be slightly displaced laterally to the right as it approaches the level of the aortic arch.[1] Such displacement can be increased due to atherosclerotic changes of the aorta, advanced age, thryomegaly, as well as chronic obstructive pulmonary disease (COPD).[3] The trachea passes through the neck superficially before diving posteriorly into the superior mediastinum. It narrows slightly as it approaches its distal end near the carina.[1] Its average diameter is 19.5 to 22 mm in adult males and 17.5 to 19 mm in adult females.[1,3] The narrowest section of the adult trachea occurs at the level of the cricoid cartilage, typically to 17 mm in men and 13 mm in women.[1,3]

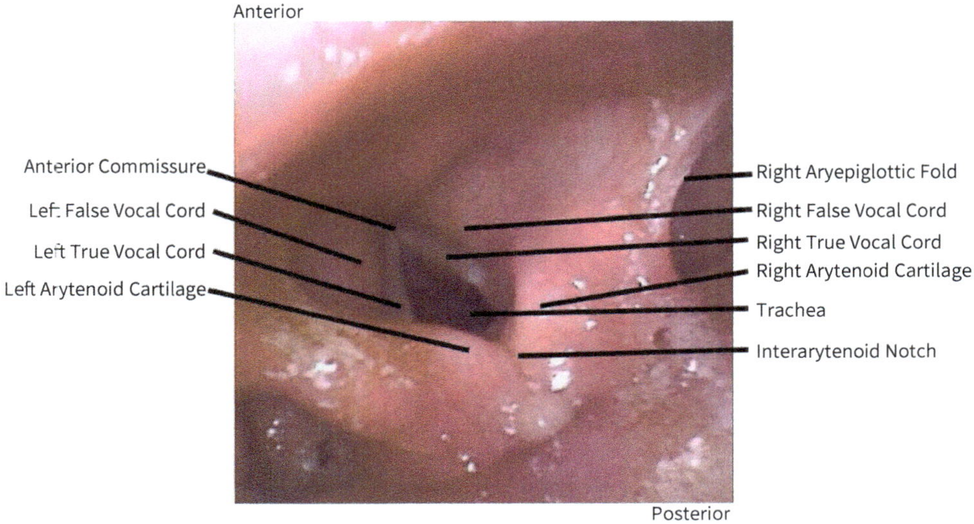

Figure 4.1 Fiberoptic image of the vocal cords and arytenoids.

The Carina

The carina can be found at the distal end of the tracheal border, at the level of the sternal angle anteriorly and the T5 vertebra posteriorly.[3] The carina marks the location of the first branching point of the airway. It is at this level that the airway splits into right and left main bronchi. The right main bronchus lies in a more vertical orientation compared to the left

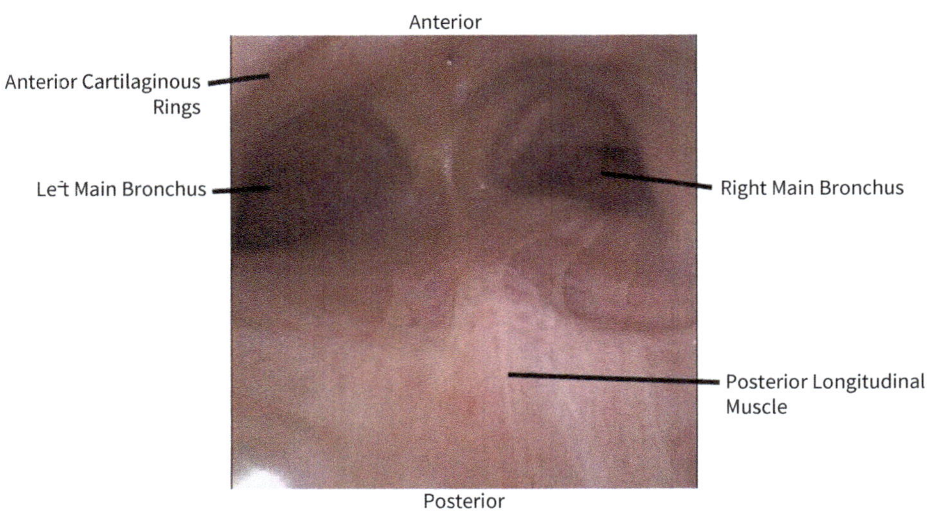

Figure 4.2 Fiberoptic image of the primary carina with right and left main bronchi.

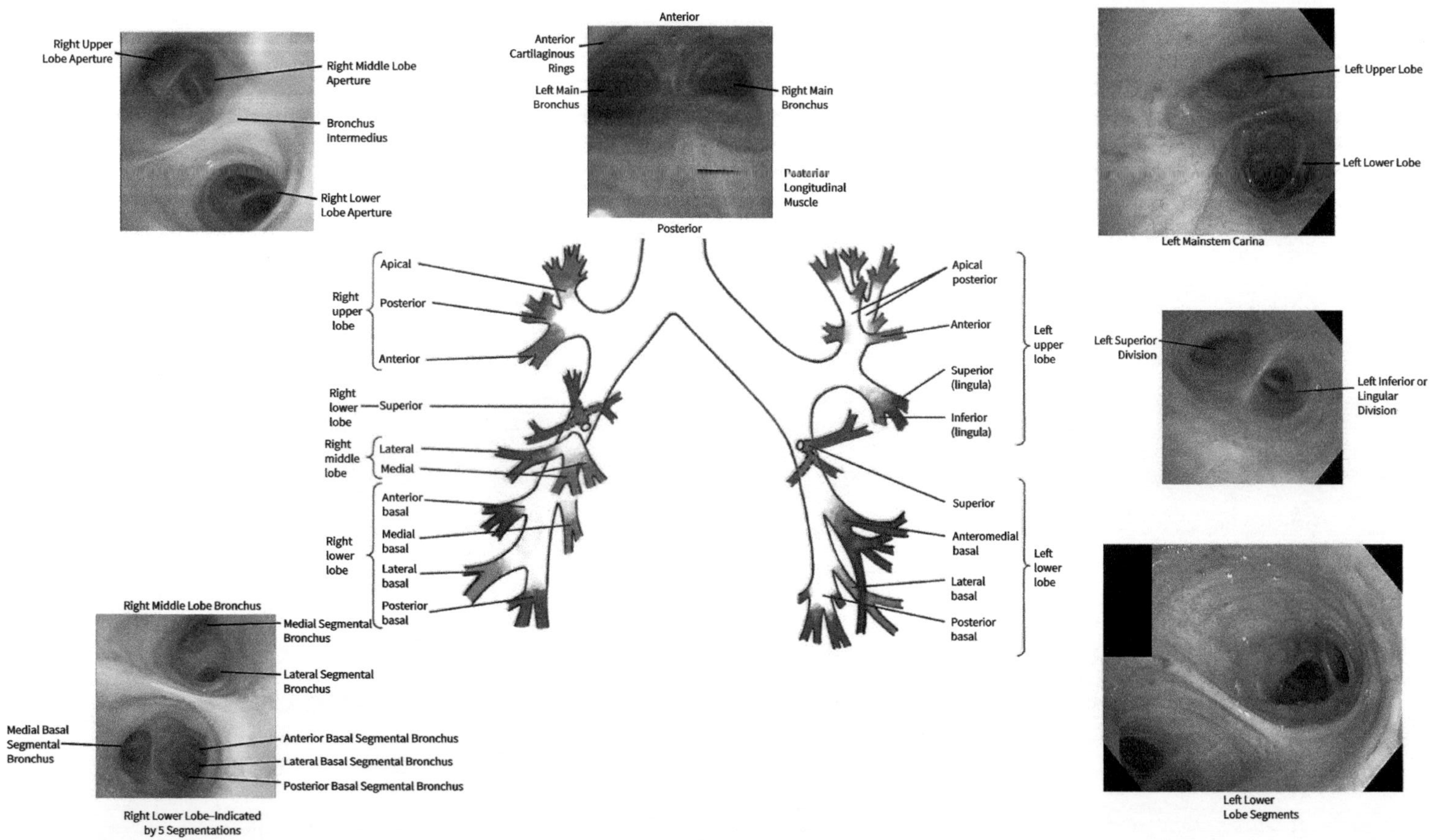

Figure 4.3 Overview of the bronchial system, with corresponding fiberoptic images.

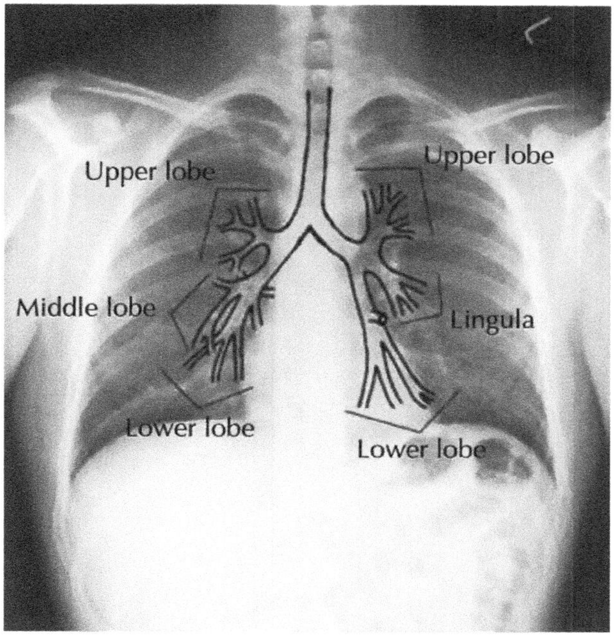

Figure 4.4 Chest X-ray image with outline of bronchi.
Reproduced from *Atlas of Human Anatomy*, 7th edition, Plate 208; chest radiograph from Major NM, *A Practical Approach to Radiology*, Philadelphia: Saunders; 2006.

main bronchus, which tends to have a more horizontal orientation. In addition, the right main bronchus tends to be wider than the left main bronchus, and it branches at approximately a 25° angle compared to the left main bronchus, which generally branches at a 45° angle relative to the trachea.[4] This anatomy explains why aspirated material more readily passes into the right lung via the right main bronchus.

Right Lung and Bronchial Anatomy

The right main bronchus in normal individuals further divides into the deeper airways and serves as an important landmark for distal bronchoscopic identification. In individuals with normal anatomy, the right lung contains three distinct lobes: upper, middle, and lower, with their corresponding secondary or so-called lobar bronchi. The anatomic architecture further subdivides each lung lobe into bronchopulmonary segments; the right lung has 10 (three in the upper lobe, two in the middle, and five in the lower lobe). For purposes of anatomic identification, the bronchi supplying these bronchopulmonary segments are considered the third generation, or tertiary, bronchi. Coursing distally within the lung parenchyma, they continue to divide into ever smaller-diameter airways called bronchioles that ultimately, after approximately 25 divisions (also called generations), are considered to be terminal bronchioles terminating in alveolar sacs that participate in respiratory gas exchange.

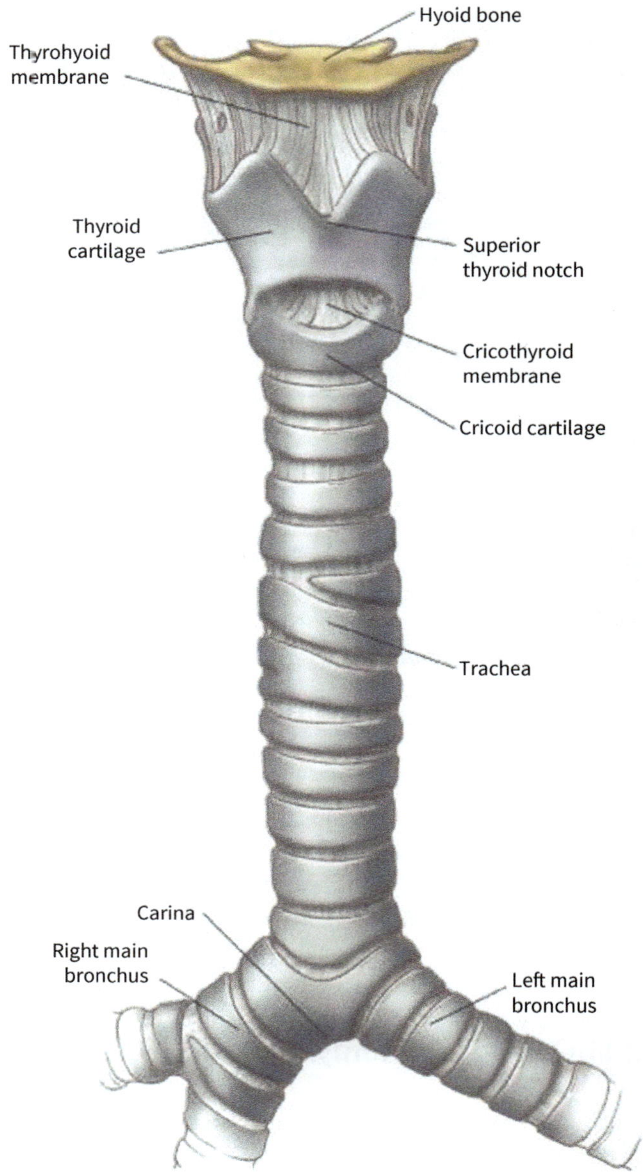

Figure 4.5 Overview of anatomy of trachea and related structures.
Reproduced with permission from Minnich DJ, Mathisen DJ. Anatomy of the trachea, carina, and bronchi. *Thorac Surg Clin*. 2007;17:571–585.

The right upper lobe bronchus normally has a take-off from the right main bronchus at approximately 2 cm from the carina in men and 1.5 cm from the carina in women. The right upper lobe bronchus splits into three lobar bronchi that supply the apical, anterior, and posterior divisions of the right lung. Immediately distal to the right upper lobe bronchus is a feature that is unique to the right side of the bronchial tree. This portion of the right-sided airway is a continuation of the right main bronchus that is often referred to as the bronchus

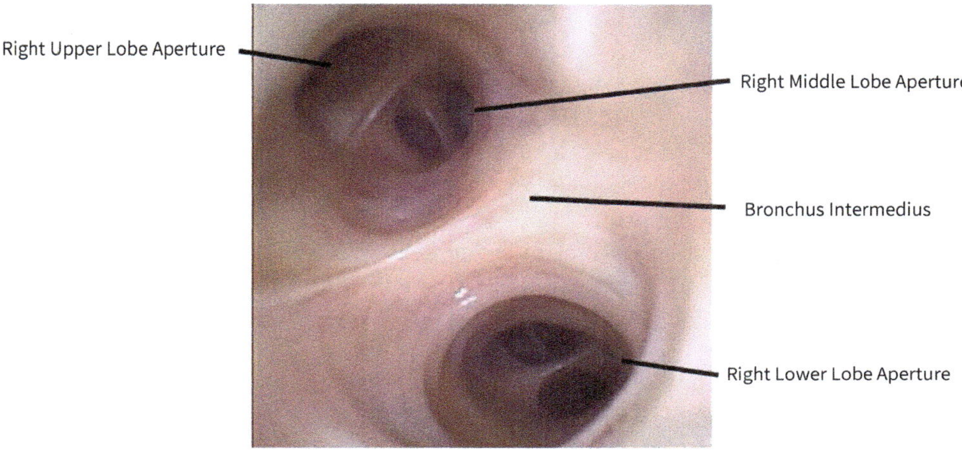

Figure 4.6 Fiberoptic image of the proximal right lung.

intermedius (Figure 4.6).[2] At the distal end of the bronchus intermedius, the airway bifurcates into right middle and right lower bronchi. The right middle bronchus supplies the medial and lateral divisions (Figure 4.7). The right lower bronchus supplies the superior, anterior basal, medial basal, lateral basal, and posterior basal divisions (Figure 4.7).

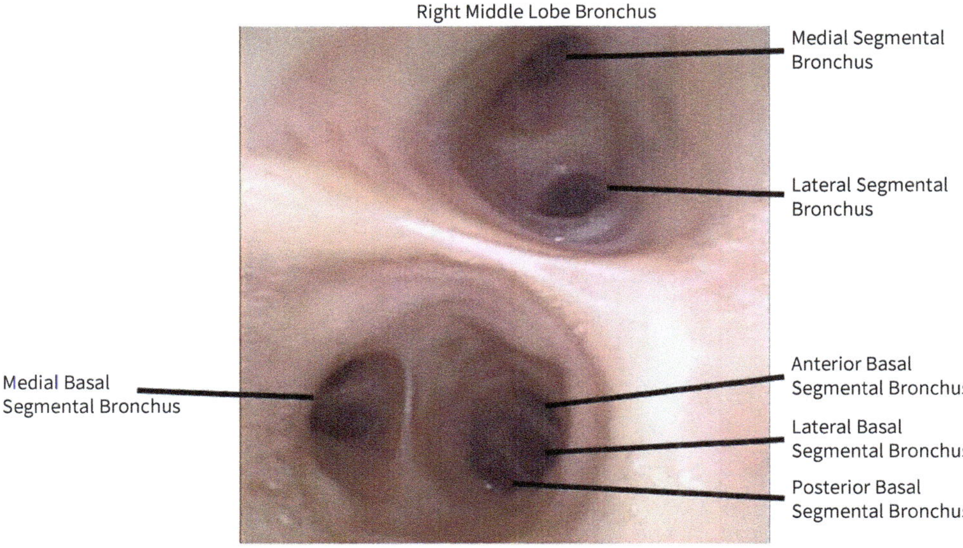

Figure 4.7 Fiberoptic image of the distal right lung.

Left Lung Bronchial Anatomy

The left main bronchus is longer than the right, measuring approximately 5 cm in men and 4.5 cm in women. At the end of the left main bronchus, the airway bifurcates into the left upper lobe bronchus and the left lower lobe bronchus (Figure 4.8). The left lung is considered to have between 8 and 10 bronchopulmonary segments, with the disparity due to the fact that fusion of some of the segments is variable yet quite common. According to the widely accepted Boyden classification scheme, the left upper lobe has four bronchopulmonary segments and the left lower lobe also has four bronchopulmonary segments. Accordingly, the left upper lobe bronchus divides into a superior division supplying the apicoposterior (from fusion of the superior anterior and superior posterior segments) and the anterior segments, and an inferior division (the lingular bronchus) supplying the superior and inferior segments (Figure 4.9). Meanwhile, the left lower lobe bronchus supplies the superior, anteriomedial basal (from fusion of the anterior basal and the medial basal segments), lateral basal, and posterior basal segments (Figure 4.10).

Vascular Supply to the Trachea and Bronchial Tree

The cervical trachea receives its blood supply from the inferior thyroid artery[2] (Figure 4.11), and the carina and lower trachea receive their vascular supply from the bronchial arteries[2] (Figure 4.11). These bronchial arteries are responsible for blood flow from the carina to the terminal bronchioles as well as blood that supplies the nerves and lymphatic structures.[3] Beyond this level, there is often great variation in blood supply, however, the right and left main bronchi are generally supplied by arterial branches from the aorta or intercostal

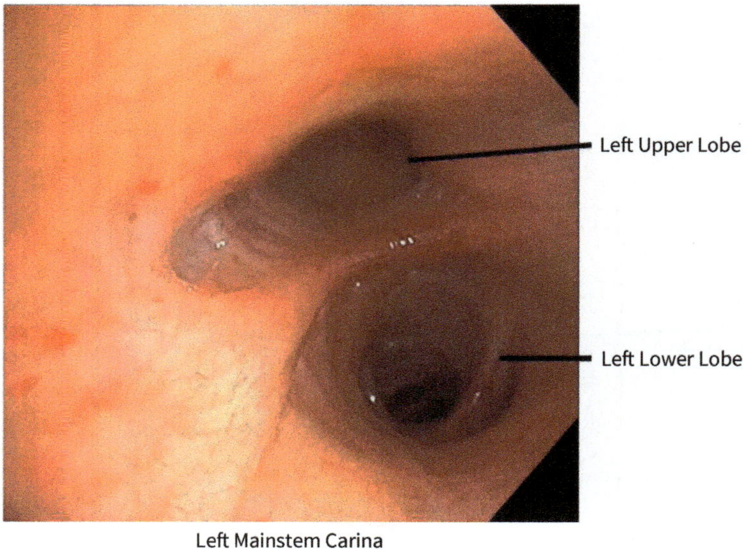

Figure 4.8 Fiberoptic image of the left mainstem carina with left upper and lower lobe apertures.

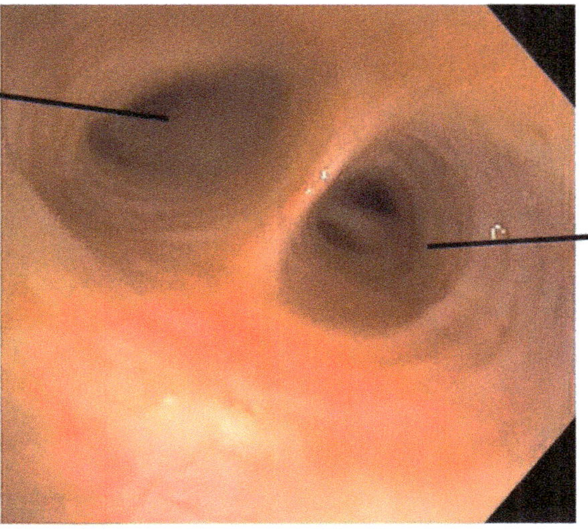

Figure 4.9 Fiberoptic image of the left superior and inferior (lingular) division apertures.

arteries.[2,4] Overall, the bronchial circulation receives between 0.5% and 1.5% of the cardiac output, with one-half directed toward the lung parenchyma and the other one-half toward the trachea and bronchi.[3] The venous blood supply from the trachea and large airways collects via bronchial venules, which subsequently form bronchial veins. Ultimately, this bronchial venous flow reaches the azygos, hemiazygos, or accessory hemiazygos veins, which empty into the superior vena cava or the left brachiocephalic vein, and finally into the right atrium.[3] In contradistinction to the path just described for the blood flow within the bronchial veins, the venous supply originating from the more distal bronchial capillaries passes through anastomotic bronchopulmonary veins that ultimately join pulmonary venules and finally the pulmonary veins that drain into the left atrium (Figure 4.12).[3] Therefore, deoxygenated

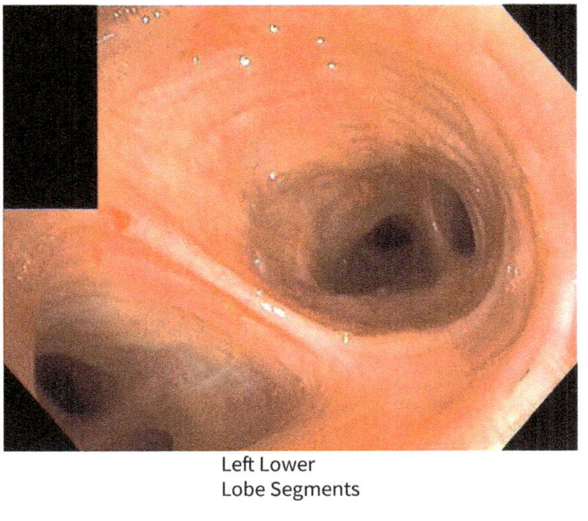

Figure 4.10 Fiberoptic image of the left lower lobe segment apertures.

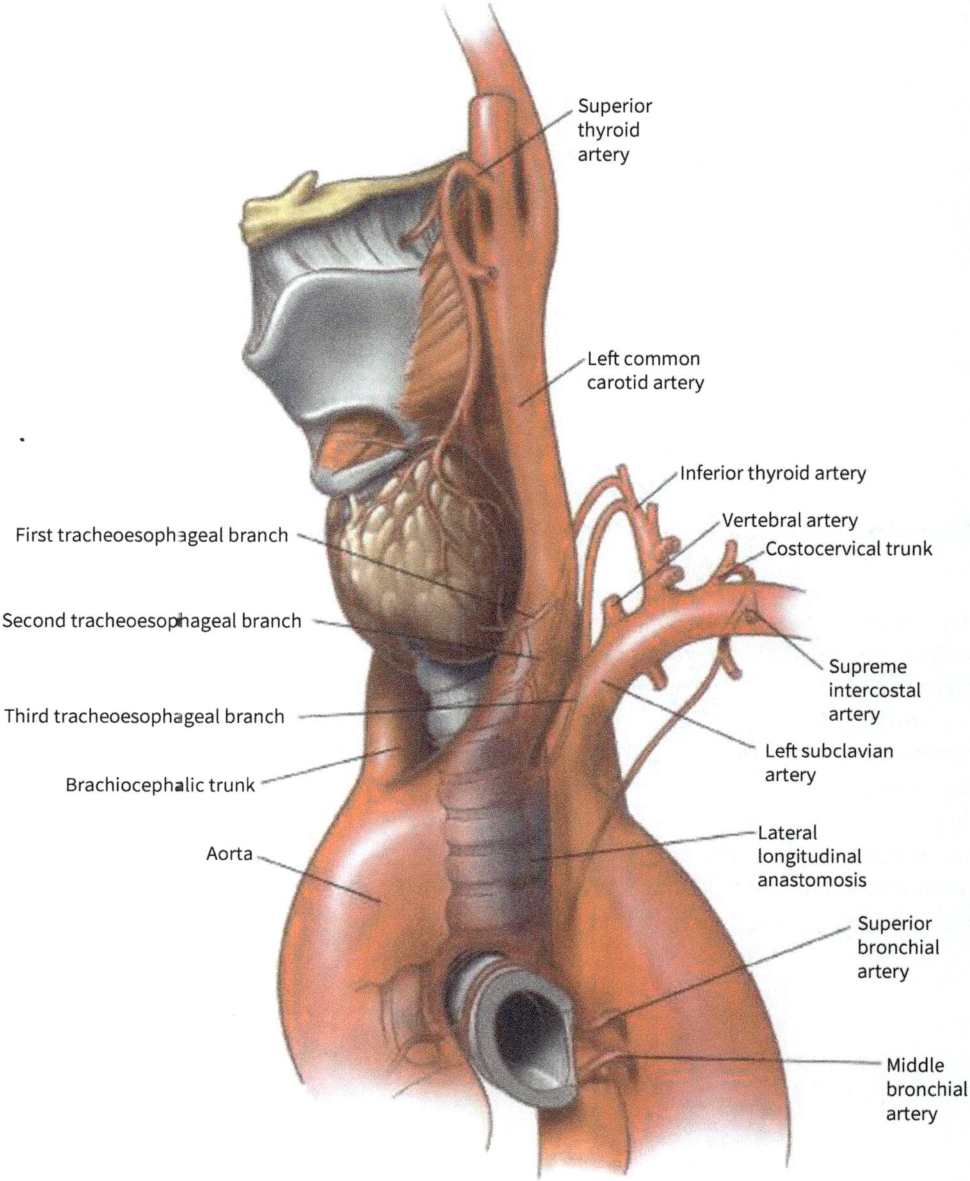

Figure 4.11 Trachea and bronchial arterial vascular supply.

Reproduced with permission from Minnich DJ, Mathisen DJ. Anatomy of the trachea, carina, and bronchi. *Thorac Surg Clin*. 2007;17:571–585.

bronchial capillary venous return mixes with freshly oxygenated blood and accounts in part for physiologic shunt. Although not well studied in humans, animal studies indicate that the right atrium receives 25% to 33% of bronchial venous supply via the bronchial veins and the left atrium receives the remainder 67% to 75% via the pulmonary veins.[3]

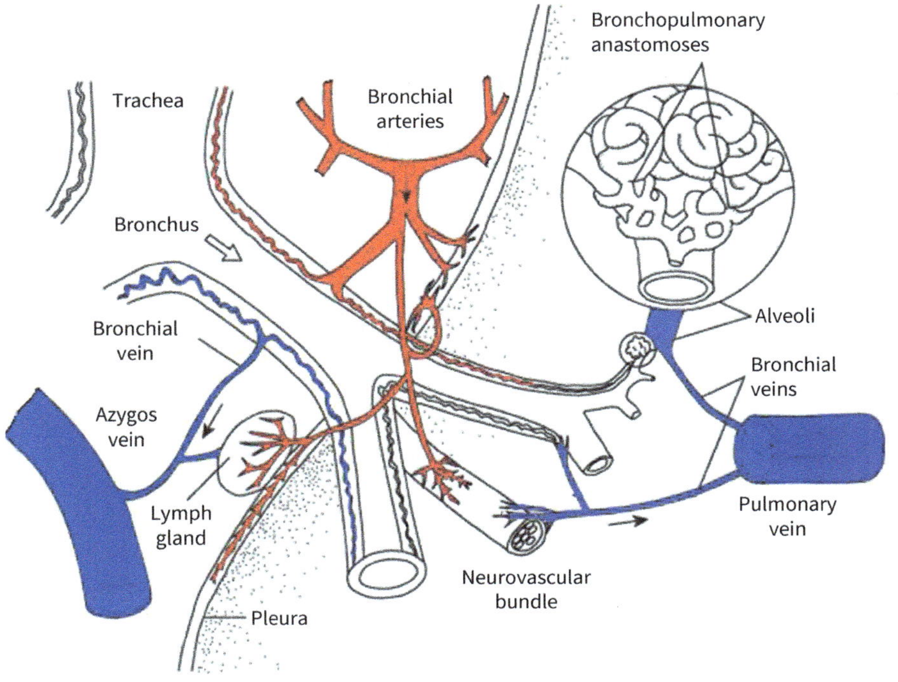

Figure 4.12 Overview of arterial and venous supply to the bronchial tree.
Modified and reproduced with permission from Deffebach ME, Charan NB, Lakshminarayan S, Butler J. The bronchial circulation. Small, but a vital attribute of the lung. *Am Rev Respir Dis*. 1987;135:463–481.

Anatomical and Pathological Variations

Variations along the tracheobronchial tree are often noted during bronchoscopic examinations and are relevant when planning airway procedures, notably intubation, selective lung isolation, pulmonary resections, and interventional pulmonary procedures. These variations arise from anomalies that occur during development of the lungs specifically related to a congenital change in the number of lung buds or their atypical origins. The prevalence of these variations differs widely, with studies quoting anywhere between 1% and 27% of the population.[5] Variations are more often discovered on the right side, with the most common variant being a bifurcated right upper lobe bronchus followed by the presence of four segmental bronchi in the right upper lobe bronchus.[5,6] The most common variant in the left-sided airway is the presence of a further bronchial division in addition to the lingular division.[7] The second most common left lung variant is the presence of three orifices in the lingular division.[7]

A less common yet clinically relevant variant is a tracheal bronchus, which occurs with an incidence of 0.1% to 3% and is often associated with other congenital anomalies, many of them involving the heart. The name "tracheal bronchus" refers to an aberrant bronchial origin typically arising directly off the right lateral wall of the trachea. When this occurs, such an anomalous airway will usually supply the entire right upper lobe lung parenchyma as its sole bronchus (in which case, it is also referred to as a "pig bronchus" due to its similarity to porcine bronchial anatomy)[8]; in other instances, it occurs as an additional, supernumerary bronchus supplying a limited segmental amount of right upper lobe lung. In yet other rare instances, the tracheal bronchus is found to end as a blind airway within the lung parenchyma. When present, the tracheal bronchus usually arises within 2 cm of the carina, but its origin has been reported as high as 6 cm above the carina.[6,8] Tracheal bronchi are clinically relevant because, in some instances, their presentation on fiberoptic bronchoscopy can be confusing.[7] Obstruction of an unidentified tracheal bronchus by an endotracheal tube can cause segmental atelectasis or obstructive pneumonia.[6]

Interventional pulmonary procedures and pulmonary resections are often called for in patients with a comorbid diagnosis of COPD. In these patients, the intrathoracic tracheal rings can soften, which results in a decreased anteroposterior diameter and a widening of the posterior wall, often referred to as a saber sheath trachea.[1] This condition is an example of tracheobronchomalacia, also called tracheomalacia, and its diagnosis can be made via fiberoptic bronchoscopy (considered the diagnostic gold standard) as well as computed tomography. It is clinically very relevant as these anatomic changes can cause obstruction of the lumen of the trachea with coughing or expiration. Tracheomalacia is a common consequence of COPD[7] and is considered to be one of COPD's pathognomonic features. Other common causes of tracheomalacia include long-term intubation, tracheal trauma, congenital abnormalities, chronic extrinsic compression, chronic inflammation, infection, and other etiologies ascribed to being idiopathic.[7] Tracheomalacia commonly manifests with greater than 50% collapse of the trachea's cross-sectional diameter during forced expiration.[7]

As mentioned earlier, congenital abnormalities of the vascular tree can result in symptomatic or asymptomatic extrinsic tracheomalacia in children and adults. Such vascular compression of the tracheobronchial tree caused by aortic arch anomalies accounts for 1.2% of congenital heart disease in children.[8] Certain vascular abnormalities can cause varying degrees of airway compression in specific locations. For example, innominate artery abnormalities can present with anterior mid-tracheal compression. A double aortic arch can compress the right anterior and posterior distal trachea. A pulmonary artery sling can compress the right anterior distal trachea and right mainstem bronchus.[9]

Most congenital cases are identified while patients are children. Approximately 50% to 80% of congenital cases present as double aortic arch or right aortic arch.[8] Pulmonary artery sling and aberrant right subclavian artery account, respectively, for another 4% and 5%.[8] Acquired tracheobronchial compression that manifests in adult patients can be detected on fiberoptic bronchoscopy in patients with advanced atherosclerosis.[8]

Conclusion

A functional understanding of normal tracheobronchial anatomy as well as its clinically relevant variations is essential to effective, safe perioperative anesthetic evaluation and management for thoracic procedures. This chapter provides the information necessary to achieve that in preparation for the thoracic patient who presents with expected, normal tracheobronchial anatomy or, instead, an anomalous variation based on congenital versus disease-related etiology.

References

1. Boiselle PM. Imaging of the large airways. *Clin Chest Med.* 2008;29:181–193.
2. Minnich DJ, Mathisen DJ. Anatomy of the trachea, carina, and bronchi. *Thorac Surg Clin.* 2007;17:571–585.
3. Garcia JGN. Pulmonary circulation and regulation of fluid balance. In: Broaddus VC, Ernst JD, Lzarus SC, et al (eds), *Murray and Nadel's Textbook of Respiratory Medicine.* 6th ed. New York: Elsevier; 2016:92–110.e8.
4. Levitzky MG. Chapter 4. Blood flow to the lung. In: Levitzky MG, ed. *Pulmonary Physiology.* 8th ed. New York: The McGraw-Hill Companies; 2013.
5. Kumar A. Retrospective study of the variations in tracheobronchial tree through bronchoscopy. *Chest.* 2018;154:575A.
6. Gonlugur U, Efeoglu T, Kaptanoglu M, Akkurt I. Major anatomical variations of the tracheobronchial tree: bronchoscopic observation. *Anat Sci Int.* 2005;80:111–115.
7. Lawrence DA, Branson B, Oliva I, Rubinowitz A. The wonderful world of the windpipe: a review of central airway anatomy and pathology. *Can Assoc Radiol J.* 2015;66:30–43.
8. Kanabuchi K, Noguchi N, Kondo T. Vascular tracheobronchial compression syndrome in adults: a review. *Tokai J Exp Clin Med.* 2011;36:106–111.
9. Rogers DJ, Cunnane MB, Hartnick CJ. Vascular compression of the airway: establishing a functional diagnostic algorithm. *JAMA Otolaryngol Head Neck Surg.* 2013;139:586–591.

5
Preoperative Evaluation and Optimization

Alexandra L. Belfar, Kevin Duong, Yi Deng, and Melissa Nikolaidis

Introduction

According to the American Cancer Society, lung cancer is currently the second most common cancer and the leading cause of cancer deaths in both men and women, exceeding mortality rates for colon, breast, and prostate cancers combined.[1] In 2016 alone, 218,229 cases of newly diagnosed lung and bronchus cancer were reported, with incidence remaining roughly stable for the preceding decade.[2] With the updated recommendations of the US Preventive Service Task Force in 2014 for more aggressive lung cancer screening, it is likely that a substantial number of patients will continue to require complex thoracic surgical procedures for the foreseeable future.

Intrathoracic surgery falls within the "elevated-risk" procedural category in the Revised Cardiac Risk Index (a tool commonly used for perioperative risk stratification), and outcomes may be heavily dependent on the patient's baseline status and pulmonary function. In a population whose health is often compromised due to a malignant process, it is imperative to appropriately evaluate and optimize these patients. This chapter will address the preoperative evaluation, risk stratification, and anesthetic planning for thoracic surgical procedures.

Preoperative Evaluation

History and Physical Examination

A comprehensive preoperative assessment should begin with a focused but thorough history and physical examination. A detailed account of patients' pulmonary symptoms, including degree of dyspnea, cough, and exercise tolerance should be elicited. Ongoing tobacco use should be addressed if applicable. In addition to obtaining a broader view of the patient's overall health, this information allows the perioperative care team to gauge the patient's level of pulmonary reserve and ability to tolerate the planned procedure. Severe dyspnea on exertion, for instance, may be correlated with a reduced forced expiratory volume in 1 second (FEV_1), which has unfavorable prognostic implications for postoperative outcomes.[3] A history of a significant productive cough may result in a diagnosis of an acute infection requiring medical treatment prior to surgery. An elderly patient's ability to exercise may cause them to be classified as having reduced or increased risk of perioperative morbidity and mortality.[4,5]

Additional comorbidities that may affect the patient's perioperative course or anesthetic planning should also be addressed appropriately.

On physical exam, signs of chronic hypoxemia or compromised ventilation should be sought. These include cyanosis, clubbing, and abnormal breath sounds on auscultation. Wheezing may be a sign of a poorly controlled long-standing disease process such as chronic obstructive pulmonary disease (COPD), versus an acute exacerbation or infectious process. Decreased breath sounds could indicate the presence of a pleural effusion. Tracheal alignment and symmetry of diaphragmatic excursion should also be noted, as asymmetry or distortion could signal conditions warranting serious concern.

Additional Testing

As with any procedure, additional testing that is clinically appropriate and/or consistent with current guidelines should be completed prior to surgery. This includes electrocardiograms, echocardiograms, and laboratory studies such as a complete blood count, and basic metabolic panel. Data from room-air arterial blood gases (ABGs) were frequently used in the past to risk stratify, or, in some cases, exclude patients from pulmonary resection procedures (specifically, those with PaO_2 <60 or $PaCO_2$ >45 mmHg). While this information may be valuable to assess baseline respiratory status or estimate increased risk, arterial blood gases values are no longer used as sole exclusionary criteria, as they have not been shown to adequately predict how patients will fare postoperatively.[4]

In patients with large endobronchial tumors or mediastinal masses, further imaging, including a computed tomography scan or chest X-ray, may be appropriate to determine the extent of anatomic distortion present and to predict any potential difficulties with intubation, ventilation, or double-lumen tube placement.

Cardiac Risk Stratification

The first and most important step in the comprehensive preoperative assessment is the cardiovascular evaluation. This should occur before more advanced pulmonary testing takes place, as increased cardiovascular risk and/or active cardiac conditions are independent predictors of poor perioperative outcomes. Many of these patients are at elevated risk for cardiovascular disease due to an extensive smoking history. In addition, there is significant overall risk (2%–3%[6,7]) of major cardiac morbidity after resectional surgery, including arrhythmias, cardiac arrest, myocardial ischemia, and cardiac death.

The American College of Cardiology/American Heart Association guidelines on perioperative cardiovascular evaluation for noncardiac surgery are traditionally used to risk stratify and determine the need for additional cardiovascular testing preoperatively. For patients in whom an acute coronary syndrome is not of immediate concern, the Revised Cardiac Risk Index (RCRI) is often utilized to quantify the degree of cardiac risk, as it is fairly simple to use and has been well validated. It was recalibrated in 2010 for the thoracic surgical population as the thoracic RCRI (ThRCRI), with data derived from a group of patients that exclusively underwent major lung resections.[6] The American College of Chest Physicians (ACCP) currently advises that this refined score, ThRCRI, be used in place of the RCRI for

Table 5.1 Thoracic Revised Cardiac Risk Index

Thoracic Revised Cardiac Risk Index	
Risk factors	**Points**
History of coronary artery disease	1.5
History of cerebrovascular disease	1.5
Pneumonectomy	1.5
Serum creatinine > 177 μmol/L or 2 mg/dL	1
Risk of major cardiac event	
Points	**Risk (%)**
0	0.9
1–1.5	4.2
2–2.5	8
>2.5	18

The Thoracic Revised Cardiac Risk Index has four components, each of which is weighted. Patients with a score ≥2 be should referred to a cardiologist for risk stratification and additional testing if needed.

risk stratification in the thoracic surgery population. Once the details of the patient's history are obtained, the points are added together, and a determination of risk class is made (Table 5.1). It is recommended that any patient with a ThRCRI score of 2 or greater be referred to a cardiologist for further evaluation,[8] while those with lower scores may proceed with necessary pulmonary testing (Figure 5.1).

Assessment for Lung Resectability

The primary goal of the remaining preoperative evaluation is to identify those at increased risk of perioperative morbidity and mortality, as well as those who may require ventilator support in the acute postoperative period. Postoperative pulmonary complications (PPCs) account for the majority of these events and are associated with increased 30-day readmission rates, prolonged length of stay, and decreased overall survival.[9] PPCs include atelectasis, pneumonia, bronchospasm, pulmonary edema, acute respiratory distress syndrome, and acute respiratory failure. Risk stratification for PPCs may be completed preoperatively via a thorough assessment of respiratory function. This is typically accomplished by a three-pronged approach, classically known as the "three-legged stool" (Figure 5.2) and encompasses evaluation of lung mechanical function, pulmonary parenchymal function, and cardiopulmonary reserve.

While this model is useful in constructing a framework for evaluation, it can be difficult to synthesize the information obtained in a way that makes sense for preoperative testing and surgical risk stratification. In 2013, the ACCP published an algorithm for the cardiopulmonary preoperative assessment of patients planned to undergo thoracotomy or major resection surgery (Figure 5.3).[10] This incorporated components of the three-legged stool into a

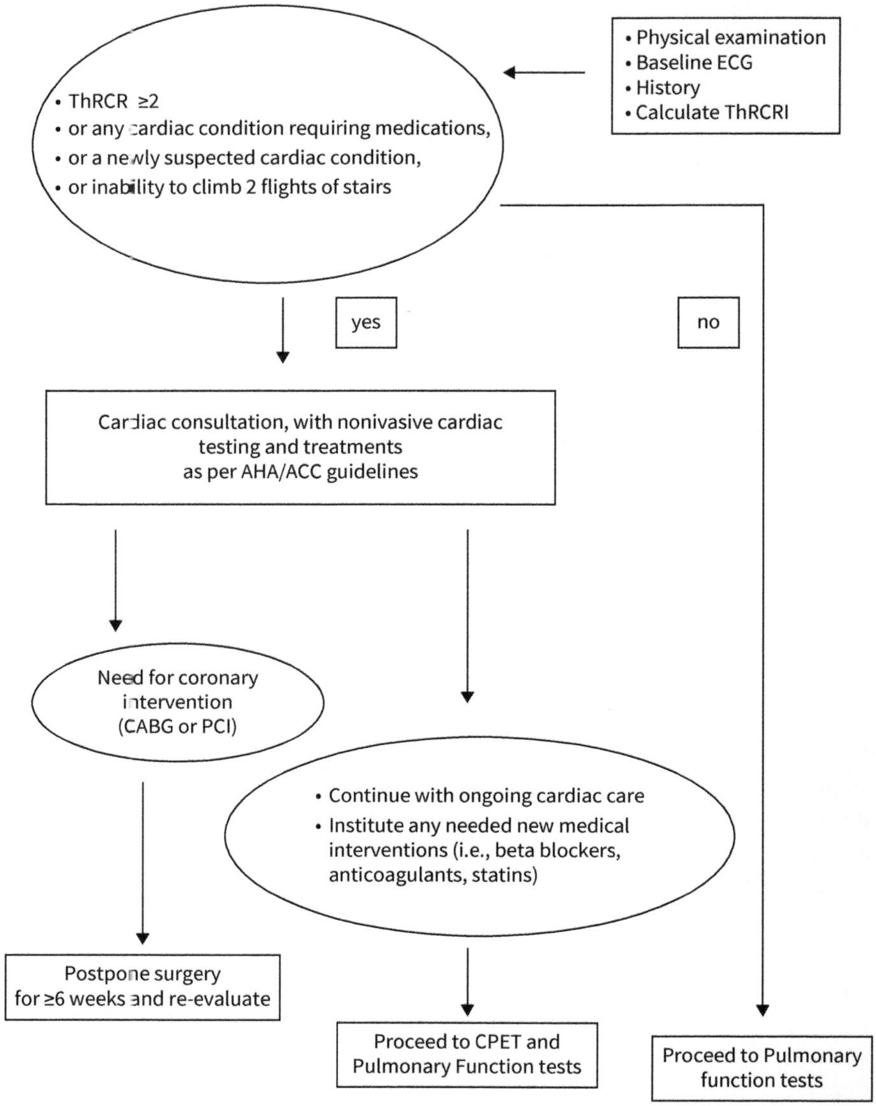

Figure 5.1 Physiologic evaluation and cardiac algorithm for thoracic surgical patients based on the Thoracic Revised Cardiac Risk Index.
ThRCRI = Revised Cardiac Risk Index (RCRI); CPET = cardiopulmonary exercise test; ECG = electrocardiogram; AHA = American Heart Association; ACC = American College of Cardiology; CABG = coronary artery bypass grafting; PCI = percutaneous coronary intervention
Reprinted with permission from Brunelli A, Kim A, Burger KI, Addrizzo-Harris, DJ. Physiologic evaluation of the patient with lung cancer being considered for resectional surgery: Diagnosis and Management of lung CANCER, 3rd ed: American College of Chest Physicians evidence-based clinical practice guidelines." *Chest.* 2013;143(5 Suppl):e166S–e190S.

cohesive format that can be used to determine the need for further cardiopulmonary testing preoperatively and for surgical risk stratification, which can aid in the planning of intra- and postoperative management.

The initial step, as mentioned previously, is cardiac risk stratification with appropriate treatment as needed using the ThRCRI. Assuming that patients are deemed low-risk from

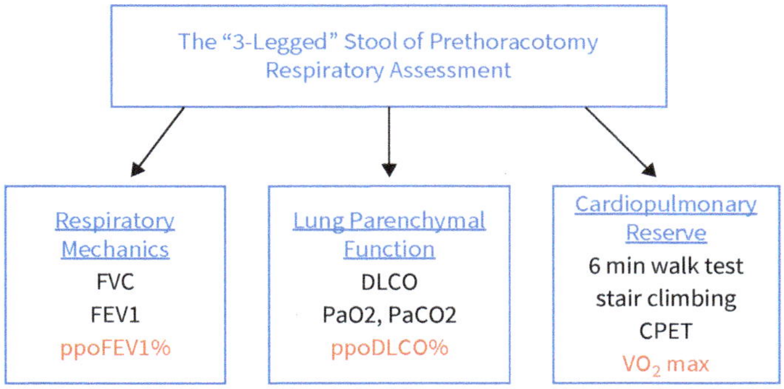

Figure 5.2 The "3-legged" stool involves evaluation of respiratory mechanics, lung parenchymal function, and cardiopulmonary reserve. Several of these measurements, including functional vital capacity, FEV_1, and DLCO can be obtained from pulmonary function testing, while formal or informal exercise testing can be used to assess cardiopulmonary reserve. This pre-thoracotomy respiratory assessment can be used to guide intra- and post-operative management, and to predict those patients more likely to have postoperative complications, including difficulty with ventilator weaning.

Abbreviations: CPET, cardiopulmonary exercise test; DLCO, diffusing capacity of the lungs for carbon monoxide; FEV1, forced expiratory volume in first second; FVC, functional vital capacity; ppo, predicted postoperative; VO_2 max, maximal oxygen consumption.

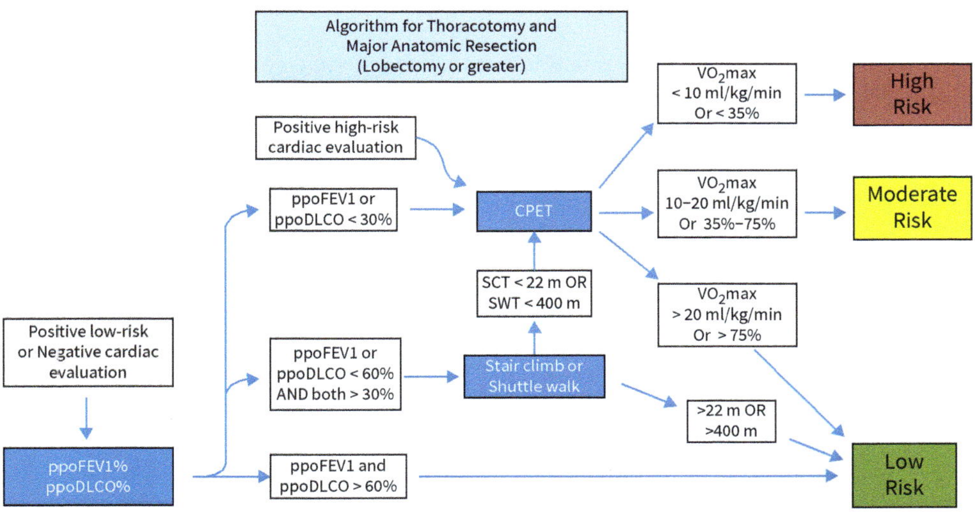

Figure 5.3 ACCP algorithm for cardiopulmonary pre-operative assessment of patients requiring lung resection. According to the ACCP, low risk indicates a mortality rate below 1%. In patients deemed moderate risk, morbidity and mortality rates vary based on pulmonary function, exercise tolerance, and extent of resection. High-risk patients may have perioperative mortality rates in excess of 10%.

Reprinted with permission from Brunelli A, Kim A, Burger KI, Addrizzo-Harris, DJ. Physiologic evaluation of the patient with lung cancer being considered for resectional surgery: Diagnosis and Management of lung CANCER, 3rd ed: American College of Chest Physicians evidence-based clinical practice guidelines." *Chest.* 2013;143(5 Suppl):e166S–e190S.

Abbreviations: ACCP, American College of Chest Physicians; CPET, cardiopulmonary exercise test; DLCO, diffusing capacity of the lungs for carbon monoxide; FEV1, forced expiratory volume in first second; FVC, functional vital capacity; ppo, predicted postoperative; SCT, stair climbing test; SWT, shuttle walk test; VO_2 max, maximal oxygen consumption.

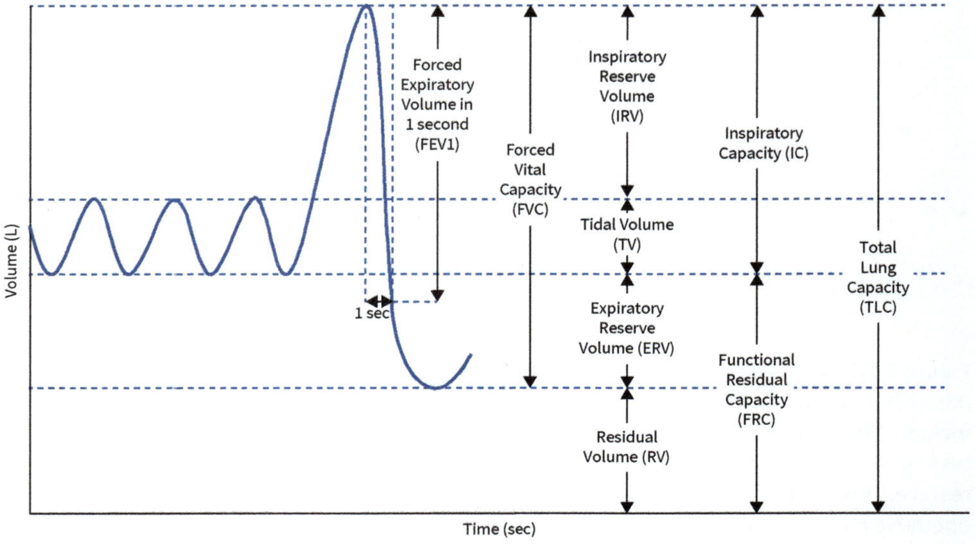

Figure 5.4 Lung volumes and capacities graph showing various volumes at different stages of the respiratory cycle. Measurements of pulmonary mechanics can help to differentiate obstructive from restrictive disease. Data such as FEV_1, FVC, and FRC can be used to predict postoperative pulmonary complications.

a cardiac standpoint, pulmonary function tests are then used to obtain data regarding the status of the patient's pulmonary mechanical function and parenchymal function. This is typically accomplished by spirometry or body plethysmography and can provide the perioperative team additional valuable information (Figures 5.4 and 5.5). Key measurements utilized in the ACCP algorithm include FEV_1 (mechanical function) and diffusing capacity for CO_2 (DLCO; parenchymal function). Predicted postoperative values (ppoFEV_1 and ppoDLCO)

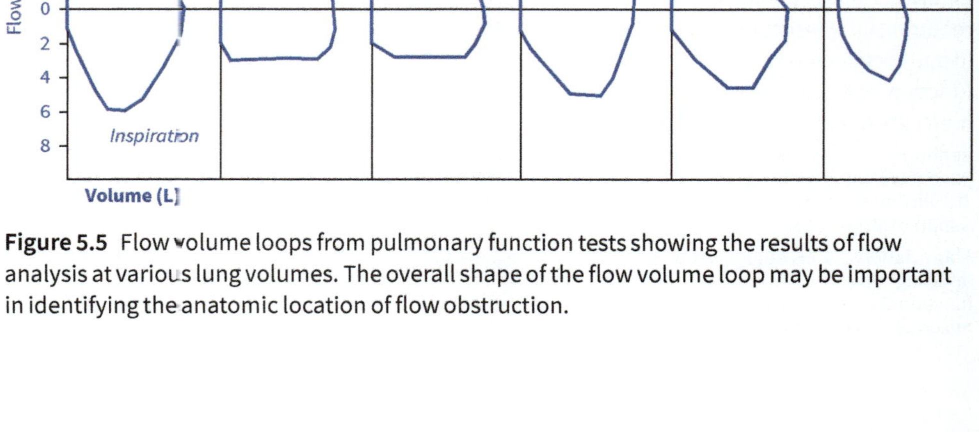

Figure 5.5 Flow volume loops from pulmonary function tests showing the results of flow analysis at various lung volumes. The overall shape of the flow volume loop may be important in identifying the anatomic location of flow obstruction.

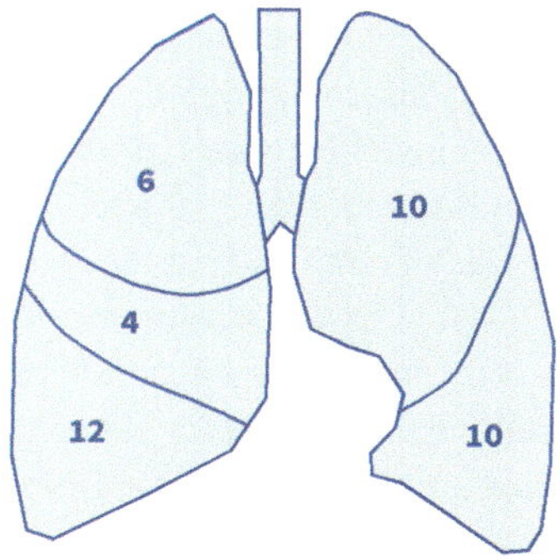

Figure 5.6 The number of subsegments planned for resection is used in the calculation of ppoFEV$_1$ and ppoDLCO. Note that there are 20 subsegments within the left lung and 22 subsegments in the right (for a total of 42), with the right therefore 10% larger. If, for example, a patient with a preoperative FEV$_1$ of 70% were planned to have the entire left lower lobe removed, the patient would be expected to lose 10/42 (24%) of presumably functional pulmonary tissue. Therefore, the ppoFEV$_1$ = 70% × (1 – 24/100) = 53%. The same method may be used for the calculation of ppoDLCO.

Abbreviations: DLCO, diffusing capacity of the lungs for carbon monoxide; FEV1, forced expiratory volume in first second; FVC, functional vital capacity; ppo, predicted postoperative.

are then calculated based on the maximum proposed number of subsegments to be removed as follows Figure 5.6):

$$ppoFEV_1\% = \text{preoperative } FEV_1\% \text{ x } (1 - \%\text{functional lung tissue removed}/100)$$
$$ppoDLCO\% = \text{preoperative } DLCO\% \times (1 - \% \text{ functional lung tissue removed}/100)$$

Reductions in either ppoFEV$_1$ or ppoDLCO are associated with increased risk of PPCs, though ppoDLCO is perhaps more reliable, as it can independently predict PPCs and mortality, regardless of the ppoFEV1.[11–17]

According to the ACCP, patients with ppoFEV$_1$ and ppoDLCO >60% are considered low risk for PPCs and do not require additional cardiopulmonary testing. Those with ppoFEV$_1$ or ppoDLCO <60% and >30% are recommended to undergo informal evaluation of their cardiopulmonary reserve. This could include the stair climbing test, shuttle walk test, 6-minute walk test, or exercise oxygen desaturation test. Conversely, those with a high-risk cardiac evaluation, poor results on informal exercise testing, or a ppoFEV$_1$ or ppoDLCO <30% are recommended to undergo formal laboratory exercise testing, or cardiopulmonary exercise testing. This is considered the gold standard of exercise testing, as it allows the maximum rate of oxygen consumption (VO_2 max), and thus overall patient conditioning, to be quantified. Those with a VO_2 max <10 mL/kg/min or <35% predicted are considered to be at high risk from a cardiopulmonary standpoint, and per the ACCP should be counseled on sublobar resections, less invasive surgical options (video-assisted thoracoscopic surgery, robotic surgery), or nonoperative treatments. Patients with a VO_2 max between 10 and 20 mL/kg/min or 35% to 75% predicted are considered moderate risk, while those with VO_2 max >20mL/kg/min or >75% predicted are at low risk of PPCs. The official recommendations of the ACCP for preoperative evaluation and risk assessment are fully summarized in Figure 5.3.

Of note, the previous equations reflect the typical relationship between the extent of resection and postoperative complications: the ppoFEV_1 and ppoDLCO both decrease as the amount of functional lung tissue removed increases, thus increasing the likelihood of postoperative morbidity and mortality. A notable exception to this may be in patients with severe COPD, in whom resecting segments of emphysematous lung may actually improve the degree of ventilation/perfusion (V/Q) mismatch postoperatively.[8] In these cases, regional lung function studies may be useful, providing a more accurate prediction of postoperative pulmonary function. This is especially true in patients planned to undergo pneumonectomy who are known to be at higher risk for PPCs based on spirometric data. Studies may include radionuclide V/Q scanning, quantitative computed tomography lung scans, or 3D dynamic perfusion magnetic resonance imaging. V/Q scanning is currently the gold standard in regional lung function studies. Other modalities mentioned are relatively new and, at present, not as widely utilized.[4]

Apart from the components of the "three-legged stool," there may be additional risk factors for PPCs that warrant consideration. These include American Society of Anesthesiologists physical status of 3 or higher, age ≥75, history of smoking, body mass index (BMI) ≥30, and history of COPD.[18] While none of these factors should exclude a patient from having surgery, they are helpful in further risk stratification, especially for those planned to undergo significant resections.

Special Considerations

As many thoracic surgical procedures are related to existing cancer diagnoses, it is important to have some familiarity with the anesthetic implications of various malignancies. Broad categories of common pulmonary malignancies include small cell and nonsmall cell lung cancers. Other malignancies may include carcinoid tumors, metastatic lesions from other primary cancers, adenoid cystic carcinoma, and primary pleural tumors, such as mesotheliomas.

Generally, nonsmall cell tumors are more amenable to surgical treatment than small cell cancers. The type of tumor may also have implications for airway and intraoperative management due to size, location, and/or potential to cause metabolic or hormonal disturbances. It is therefore important to perform a focused evaluation of what is often referred to as the "4 *M*'s" in all patients with pulmonary masses: mass effects, metabolic abnormalities, metastases, and medications (Table 5.2). Mass effects may be due to large endobronchial or apical tumors

Table 5.2 The 4 M's in Pre-Operative Assessment of Patient With Lung Cancer

M's	Anesthetic Considerations in Lung Cancer Patients
Mass effects	Obstructive pneumonia, lung abscess, superior vena cava syndrome, tracheobronchial distortion, Pancoast syndrome, recurrent laryngeal nerve or phrenic nerve palsy, chest wall or mediastinal extension
Metabolic effects	Lambert–Eaton syndrome, hypercalcemia, hyponatremia, Cushing's syndrome
Metastases	Particularly to brain, bone, liver, and adrenal glands
Medications	Chemotherapy agents: pulmonary toxicity (bleomycin), cardiac toxicity (doxorubicin), renal toxicity (cisplatin)

and can include anatomic distortion of the tracheobronchial tree, obstructive pneumonias, or effects due to superior vena cava syndrome or Pancoast syndrome. Metabolic effects are often seen with squamous cell or small cell cancers, including electrolyte imbalances (e.g., hyponatremia, hypercalcemia), and/ or paraneoplastic syndromes (Lambert–Eaton, etc.). Metastases may be seen and most commonly result in spread to the liver, brain, bones, and adrenal glands. Finally, it is necessary to determine previous exposure to potentially toxic chemotherapeutic agents, including bleomycin, doxorubicin, or cisplatin, which can cause pulmonary (especially if paired with exposure to a high FiO_2), cardiac, and renal toxicity, respectively.

Preoperative Optimization

Lifestyle Modification

Nutrition

While there is a paucity of recommendations specific to thoracic surgery for preoperative nutritional optimization, it is known that optimizing general nutritional status improves postoperative outcomes in elective surgery.[19] Although cancer surgery is not truly "elective," it is likely that this observation can still be applied to most thoracic surgery patients.

Patients at high risk for nutritional compromise include those who are underweight (BMI of 18.5 or less),[20] those with weight loss of >10% or >5% of total body weight prior to surgery in three months,[21] and those who are obese (BMI ≥30).[21] Potential interventions recommended for these patients include preoperative nutritional therapy for 7 to 14 days, limitation of preoperative fasting to the minimum allowed by nil per os guidelines, immunonutritional supplementation, and nutritional counseling.[19]

Smoking Cessation

Smoking is the most common cause of the majority of lung cancers and is associated with an increased postoperative 30-day mortality rate as well as increased risk of PPCs (with both figures being directly proportional to the number of pack-years smoked).[22] It is therefore prudent for patients undergoing thoracic surgery to attempt smoking cessation preoperatively. Unfortunately, the duration required to mitigate the increased risk is unclear. While it is known that carboxyhemoglobin concentration and the cardiovascular effects of nicotine decrease within hours, return of normal ciliary function and subsequent improvement in mucous clearance takes several weeks.[23] Most recent studies, however, suggest that smoking cessation is beneficial even in those abstaining for less than eight weeks, with no increased complication rates within this timeframe (Table 5.3).[24] Thus, it is recommended that patients be counseled to stop smoking preoperatively for as long as possible and for clinicians to be aggressive in smoking cessation methodologies, as patients may be more motivated to stop permanently in this context.[25] Strategies may include counseling and behavioral therapy, nicotine-replacement therapy, and pharmacological options like varenicline or bupropion.

Exercise and Pulmonary Rehabilitation

Preoperative rehabilitation programs are typically divided into three categories: aerobic exercise training, resistance training, and respiratory/inspiratory muscle training.[26]

Table 5.3 Benefits of Smoking Cessation and Time Course

Time After Smoking	Physiologic Effects
12–24 hours	Fall in carbon monoxide and nicotine levels
48–72 hours	Carboxyhemoglobin levels normalize Right shift in oxyhemoglobin dissociation curve
2–4 weeks	Decreased sputum production Decreased airway reactivity
4–8 weeks	Improvement in pulmonary function tests Reduced wound healing complications Reduced post-op respiratory complications
8–12 weeks	Decreased overall post-operative morbidity and mortality

Smoking cessation in the 2 to 4 weeks prior to surgery is associated with decreased secretions, decreased airway reactivity, and improved wound healing. The greatest benefit for thoracic surgical patients is achieved with a cessation period of 8 weeks or more, which is associated with an overall decrease in post-operative morbidity and mortality.

Unfortunately, the optimal length and content of these programs to achieve postoperative benefit is not known. While overall study quality at this time is low, available evidence suggests postoperative benefit from rehabilitation programs with very low risk of adverse events. The ACCP therefore recommends preoperative or postoperative rehabilitation for those patients at increased risk of postoperative complications (i.e., those with decreased ppoFEV_1 or DLCO or VO_2max <10 or 35% predicted; grade IC level of evidence).[10]

Management of Chronic Conditions

Many patients presenting for thoracic surgery have pre-existing COPD. While the chronic pathophysiologic changes associated with the disease may be difficult to reverse, it is advisable to postpone surgery in the setting of an acute exacerbation or infection, both of which should be treated before proceeding. Optimization of a bronchodilator regimen may be considered in patients who frequently need to use a rescue inhaler. This may include long-acting beta agonists, steroids, or parasympatholytic drugs. This is especially true in the setting of a low preoperative oxygen saturation, as this is an independent predictor for increased risk of PPCs.[27]

Conclusion

In patients undergoing lung resection surgery, a thorough preoperative assessment is imperative for adequate risk stratification and optimization of chronic and acute medical conditions. A comprehensive evaluation begins with a focused history and physical examination, during which concerns or comorbidities that could affect the anesthetic or intraoperative management are addressed. Subsequently, it is crucial to assess cardiovascular risk. The remainder of the ACCP algorithm, using the components of the "three-legged stool," is then used to determine the risk of perioperative morbidity and mortality attributable to PPCs. Those with active respiratory infections or acute COPD exacerbations may benefit from delaying the planned procedure and defining an optimal bronchodilator regimen. Finally, for all patients, but especially those with elevated risk, there is some evidence to suggest benefit from optimizing nutritional status, smoking cessation, and preoperative rehabilitation programs.

References

1. American Cancer Society. Facts and figures 2019. https://www.cancer.org/research/cancer-facts-statistics/all-cancer-facts-figures/cancer-facts-figures-2019.html. Published 2019.
2. US Cancer Statistics Working Group. US cancer statistics data visualizations tool, based on November 2018 submission data (1999–2016). *Centers for Disease Control and Prevention*. www.cdc.gov/cancer/dataviz. Published June 2019.
3. Barash P, Cullen B, Stoelting R, et al. *Clinical Anesthesia*. 7th ed. Philadelphia: Wolters Kluwer Health, 2013.
4. Slinger PD, Johnston MR. Preoperative assessment for pulmonary resection. J *Cardiothorac Vasc Anesth*. 2000;14(2):202–211.
5. Brunelli A, Monteverde M, Al Refai M. Stair climbing as a predictor of cardiopulmonary complications after pulmonary lobectomy in the elderly. *Ann Thorac Surg*. 2004;77:266–270.
6. Brunelli A, Vaela G, Salati M, et al. Recalibration of the revised cardiac risk index in lung resection candidates. *Ann Thorac Surg*. 2010;90(1):199–203.
7. Brunelli A, Cassivi SD, Fibla J, et al. External validation of the recalibrated thoracic revised cardiac risk index for predicting the risk of major cardiac complications after lung resection. *Ann Thorac Surg*. 2011;92(2):445–448.
8. Salati M, Brunelli A. Risk stratification in lung resection. *Curr Surg Rep*. 2016;4(11):37.
9. Lugg ST, Agostini PJ, Tikka T, et al. Long-term impact of developing a postoperative pulmonary complications after lung surgery. *Thorax*. 2016;71:171–176.
10. Brunelli A, Kim A, Berger KI, Addrizzo-Harris DJ. Physiologic evaluation of the patient with lung cancer being considered for resectional surgery: diagnosis and management of lung cancer, 3rd ed: American College of Chest Physicians evidence-based clinical practice guidelines *Chest*. 2013;143 (5 Suppl): e166S–e190S.
11. Nakahara K, Ohno K, Hashimoto J, et al. Prediction of posteoperative respiratory failure in patients undergoing lung resection for cancer. *Ann Thorac Surg*. 1988;46:549–554.
12. Licker MJ, Widikker I, Robert J, et al. Operative mortality and respiratory complications after lung resection for cancer: impact of chronic obstructive pulmonary disease and time trends. *Ann Thorac Surg*. 2006;81:1830–1837.
13. Ferguson MK, Siddique J, Karrison T. Modeling major lung resection outcomes using classification trees and multiple imputation techniques. *Eur J Cardiothorac Surg*. 2008;34:1085–1089.
14. Ferguson MK, Little L, Rizzo L, et al. Diffusing capacity predicts morbidity and mortality after pulmonary resection. *J Thorac Cardiovasc Surg*. 1988;96(6):894–900.
15. Ferguson MK, Reeder LB, Mick R. Optimizing selection of patients for major lung resection. *J Thorac Cardiovasc Surg*. 1995;109(2):275–281.
16. Santini M, Fiorello A, Vicidomini G, Di Crescenzo VG, Laperuta P. Role of diffusing capacity in predicting complications after lung resection for cancer. *Thorac Cardiovasc Surg*. 2007;55(6):391–394.
17. Brunelli A, Refai MA, Salati M, Sabbatini A, Morgan-Hughes NJ, Rocco G. Carbon monoxide lung diffusion capacity improves risk stratification in patients without airflow limitation: evidence for systematic measurement before lung resection. *Eur J Cardiothorac Surg*. 2006;29(4)567–570.
18. Agostini P, Cieslik H, Rathinam S, et al. Postoperative pulmonary complications following thoracic surgery: are there any modifiable risk factors? *Thorax*. 2010;65:815–818.

19. Stokes S, Wakeam E, Antonoff MB, et al. Optimizing health before elective thoracic surgery: systematic review of modifiable risk factors and opportunities for health services research. *J Thorac Dis.* 2019;11(Suppl 4):S537–S554.
20. Weimann A, Braga M, Carli F, et al. ESPEN guideline: clinical nutrition in surgery. *Clin Nutr.* 2017;36:623–650.
21. McClave SA, Taylor BE, Martindale RG, et al. Guidelines for the provision and assessment of nutrition support therapy in the adult critically ill patient. *JPEN J Parenter Enteral Nutr* 2016;40:159–211.
22. Miskovic A, Lumb AB. Postoperative pulmonary complications. *Brit J Anesth.* 2017; 118:317–334.
23. Lumb AB. Preoperative respiratory optimisation: an expert review. *Anaesthesia.* 2019;74 (Suppl 1):43–48.
24. Warner DO. Perioperative abstinence from cigarettes: physiologic and clinical consequences. *Anesthesiology.* 2006;104:356–357.
25. Shi Y, Warner DO. Surgery as a teachable moment for smoking cessation. *Anesthesiology.* 2010; 112:102–107.
26. Cavalheri V, Granger C. Preoperative exercise training for patients with non-small cell lung cancer. *Cochrane Database Syst Rev.* 2017;6:CD012020.
27. Mazo V, Sabate S, Canet J, et al. Prospective external validation of a predictive score for postoperative pulmonary complications. *Anesthesiology.* 2014;121:219–231.

6
Lung Isolation Techniques

William Johnson, Melissa Nikolaidis, and Nahel Saied

Lung Isolation Overview

Lung isolation is a technique used in the operating room or critical care setting to selectively ventilate a single lung for a discrete purpose. There is a spectrum of indications for lung isolation that vary from absolute indications to strongly indicated to preferable but not necessary (Table 6.1). A knowledge of the different indications for one-lung ventilation can help providers to determine whether lung isolation is indicated and what type of technique would be best suited to achieving it. In addition to the different indications for lung isolation, other factors can play a part in decision-making and clinical management such as provider knowledge and skill level, quality and duration of lung isolation needed, setting in which lung isolation will be required, age of patient, and availability of materials and equipment. Three main techniques exist for achieving lung isolation: a bronchial blocker, an intentional mainstem, and a double-lumen tube. Each of these three techniques will be covered in this chapter.

Although there are multiple methods to achieve lung isolation, each method requires a strong understanding of airway anatomy, as well as familiarity with fiberoptic views and techniques to help guide and verify accurate placement.

When performing fiberoptic bronchoscopy for placement and verification of lung isolation, the first and most important view to obtain is an image of the carina which is found at the terminus of the trachea (see Figure 6.1). As it is easy to become disoriented during fiberoptic bronchoscopy, the operator should take care to visualize the anterior cartilaginous rings of the trachea at the top of the screen and the longitudinal smooth muscle at the bottom of the screen. Doing so will aid in orientation and allow for easier identification of the left and right mainstem bronchus. If the operator gets disoriented, the scope can always be withdrawn to the carinal view for reorientation.

Once the carinal view has been successfully identified, the fiberoptic scope can be advanced into the right or left mainstem bronchus. The right mainstem bronchus is usually wider than the left mainstem bronchus, and it branches off from the trachea at a less acute angle (i.e., is more in line with the trachea) than the left side. Because of this, airway tools used for lung isolation will typically pass into the right mainstem over the left mainstem if advanced blindly. Additional verification of the right mainstem bronchus can be made by noting the takeoff for the right upper lobe that occurs just past the carina which is commonly identified by its "Mercedes sign" appearance (see Figure 6.2). If placing airway equipment in the right mainstem bronchus, care should be taken to note the position of the right upper lobe take-off as it can be easily occluded. A view of the left mainstem bronchus should also be obtained during bronchoscopy to verify position (see Figure 6.3).

Table 6.1 Lung Isolation Indications

Absolute Indication	Strongly Consider	May Consider
Lung protection (infection, hemorrhage)	Upper lobectomy	Esophageal surgery
Unilateral lung lavage	Pneumonectomy	Thoracoscopy
Video-assisted thoracoscopic surgery	Thoracic artery aneurysm	Middle lobe lobectomy
Ventilation control (cyst, fistula, bullae trauma)		Lower lobe lobectomy

Source: Purohit, Atul et al. Lung isolation, one-lung ventilation and hypoxaemia during lung isolation. *Ind J Anaesth*. 2015;59(9):606–617.

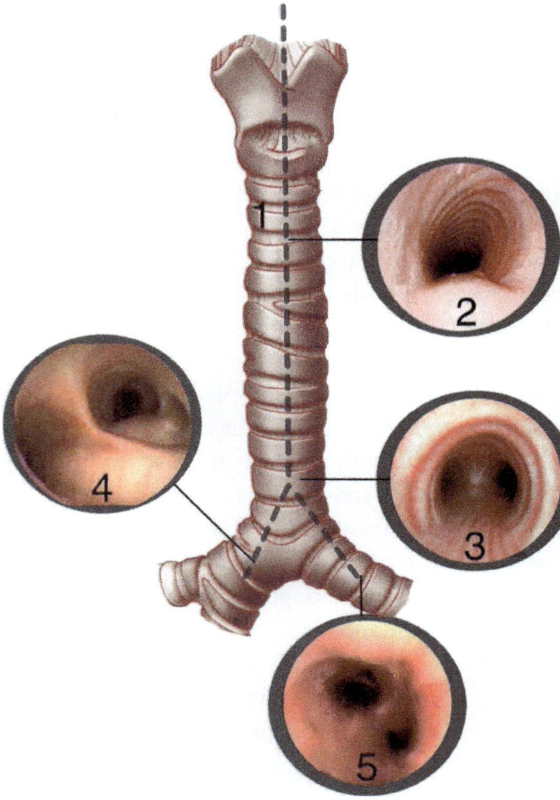

Figure 6.1 Carinal view. Identify: (1) tracheal rings, (2) posterior trachea smooth muscle, (3) left and right main stem bronchi, (4) right upper lobe take-off and continuing right bronchus, (Mercedes sign of right upper lobe), and (5) left bronchus view.

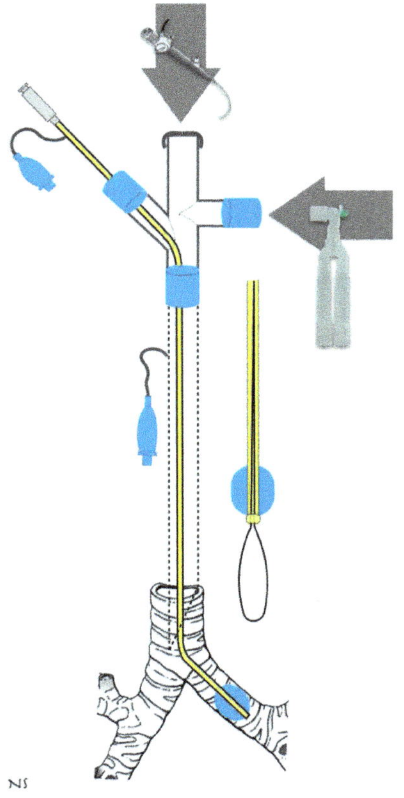

Figure 6.2 A-Arndt™.

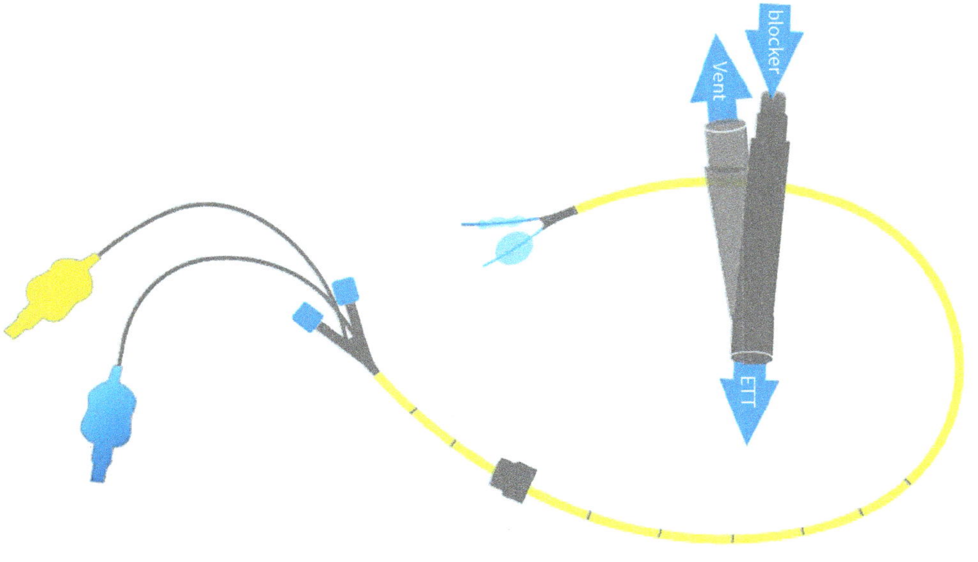

Figure 6.3 Rush E-Z bronchial blocker.

Bronchial Blocker

The first method for obtaining lung isolation is by using a bronchial blocker. In essence, a bronchial blocker is an inflatable balloon on the end of a catheter that is placed into the proximal bronchus to occlude it to achieve lung isolation. Bronchial blockers can be intraluminal (inside the endotracheal tube), extraluminal, or intramural (incorporated into the wall of the endotracheal tube). The most commonly used types of bronchial blockers are the Arndt, the Cohen, and the Univent.

Insertion of Bronchial Blocker

After induction of general anesthesia, the trachea is intubated with a single-lumen endotracheal tube. Once the presence of bilateral breath sounds is confirmed, the blocker can be placed. The distal tip of the bronchial blocker has a wire loop that can be coupled with the distal tip of the fiberoptic scope. Once they are linked, advance the pair down the endotracheal tube until the carina is visualized. Further, direct the fiberoptic scope into the bronchus of choice to block. After the blocker has been directed into the proximal bronchus, the fiberoptic scope can be withdrawn and the bronchial blocker balloon is inflated. Appropriate placement of the bronchial blocker is achieved when the proximal edge of the balloon is resting on the most proximal portion of the bronchus. The Y-shaped terminal end of the E-Z blocker provides two distal balloons, one for each main bronchus. The blocker will stride over carina and each balloon is inflated as needed to isolate the desired lung. Fiberoptic could be used through the provided adapter to confirm precise placement.

Advantages of Using Bronchial Blockers

The use of a bronchial blocker allows for reliable lung isolation using a single-lumen endotracheal tube.[1,2] This is advantageous for patients with difficult airways in which there may be considerable difficulty placing a larger and more rigid double-lumen tube.

Patients that have a bronchial blocker and require postoperative mechanical ventilation can simply have their bronchial blockers removed and continue ventilation through their single-lumen tube. Patients with a double-lumen tube may require an endotracheal tube exchange to a single-lumen tube at the end of the procedure to continue with mechanical ventilation postoperatively.

Bronchial blockers can also be placed in pediatric patients since they come in sizes as small as 5 Fr whereas double-lumen tubes are often too large for this patient population.

They can be used in patients with known difficult airway who are already intubated and patients with tracheostomy in place where double-lumen tubes cannot be used.

Cautions Regarding Bronchial Blocker Placement

The positioning of the blocker should be frequently checked during the procedure, especially after positional changes of the patient. It is not uncommon for the blocker to be inadvertently advanced, which may result in undesired ventilation of the isolated lung, or withdrawn to the point where it is blocking the trachea occluding ventilation to both lungs.

The bronchial blocker has a high volume, low pressure cuff similar to those found in endotracheal tubes. Theoretically, this should reduce the chance of bronchial injury; however, this can still occur, especially with an inappropriately sized or overinflated blocker.

Placement of a bronchial blocker can be very challenging in some patients with distorted airways or airway compression. A back-up plan should be made in the event of the inability to place the bronchial blocker.

Intentional Mainstem

Intentional mainstem is a method of using a single-lumen endotracheal tube to achieve lung isolation without using a bronchial blocker. Instead of inserting a bronchial blocker through a single-lumen endotracheal tube, the cuff establishes a seal in the ventilated lung's bronchus, preventing gas flow (ventilation) of the contralateral lung. Intentional mainstem, also called endobronchial intubation, has limited utility in the adult population and is often an inferior form of lung isolation for several reasons as outlined in the following discussion.

Procedure for Intentional Mainstem

To perform an intentional mainstem, general anesthesia is induced; then, the trachea is intubated with a single-lumen tube. Once initial position has been verified, the fiberoptic scope is inserted and directed into the mainstem bronchus of the ventilated lung. After the fiberoptic scope has been positioned, the endotracheal tube can be advanced further over it, the cuff inflated, and breath sounds auscultated to ensure there is no ventilation of the contralateral lung. Alternatively, the endotracheal tube could be advanced without fiberoptic guidance until unilateral breath sounds occur, but this may not result in isolation of the desired lung.

Advantages of Performing Intentional Mainstem

Performing intentional mainstem provides lung protection in emergency situations (e.g., hemoptysis while patient is already tracheally intubated). Intentional mainstem can be performed for pediatric patients for whom a bronchial blocker or double-lumen tube is too large.

Disadvantages of Intentional Mainstem Technique

It is much more difficult to switch between lung isolation and two-lung ventilation with an intentional mainstem as it involves deflating the endotracheal tube cuff, repositioning the entire tube, and then reinflating the cuff. If there will be multiple changes to type of lung ventilation (one-lung vs. two-lung), this can be cumbersome.

There is no ability to suction or provide continuous positive airway pressure (CPAP) to the nonventilated lung, as there is no access to it. The endotracheal tube cuff is not designed to sit in the bronchus and can either occlude the right upper lobe or not appropriately seal the bronchus, resulting in a lower quality lung isolation when compared with other lung isolation techniques.

Double-Lumen Tubes

The third and most definitive technique for lung isolation is the insertion of a double-lumen tube (Figure 6.4). A double-lumen has two distinct lumens that allow for ventilation of either lung individually or normal two-lung ventilation. Compared to single-lumen endotracheal

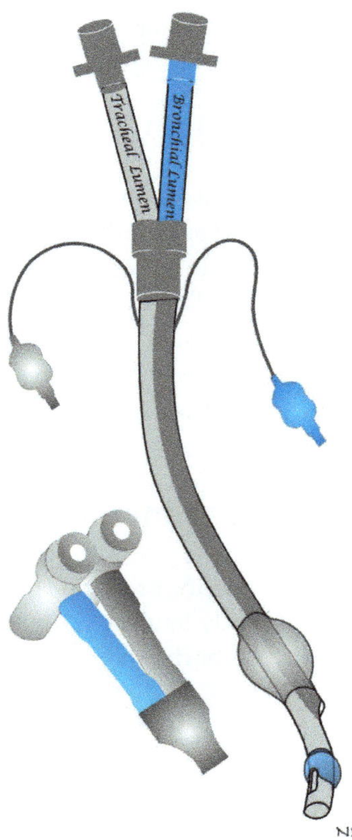

Figure 6.4 Double lumen tube: left endobronchial double lumen tube.

tubes, double-lumen tubes are larger in diameter, longer in length, and less flexible. The two lumens of the double-lumen tube are the bronchial lumen and the tracheal lumen. Double-lumen tubes come in varying lengths for different sized patients and both left and right orientations depending on which bronchus allow intubation by the bronchial lumen. Double-lumen tubes come in the following sizes: 28F, 35F, 37F, 39F, and 41F. Various methods exist for choosing double-lumen tube size but definitive sizing often depends on clinical judgment and fiberoptic confirmation.[3,4]

Placement of Double Lumen Tube

After induction of general anesthesia, direct laryngoscopy with a curved blade (preferred) is performed to obtain a view of the glottis. The double-lumen tube should then be held with the bronchial tip pointed anteriorly. Once the tip of the bronchial lumen has been advanced past the vocal cords, the entire double-lumen tube can be rotated 90° to the desired bronchial side. The fiberoptic scope is inserted into the tracheal lumen until a view of the carina is obtained (Figure 6.5). After verifying pulmonary landmarks, the blue bronchial cuff should be visualized and guided into the appropriate bronchus for lung isolation. Similar to placement of a bronchial blocker, the proximal edge of the cuff should be slightly extending out of the mainstem bronchus. To achieve lung isolation with a double-lumen tube, a clamp is placed across either lumen to occlude flow to the nonventilated/operative lung. Release of the clamp will allow return of two-lung ventilation and placement of the clamp on the other lumen will allow for lung isolation of the contralateral lung.

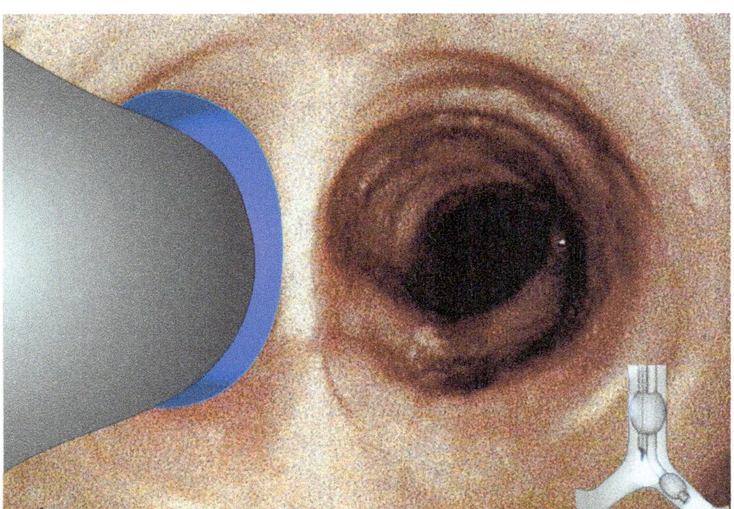

Figure 6.5 Bronchoscopic view of left double lumen tube.

Advantages of Using Double-Lumen Tubes

Double-lumen tubes provide superior lung isolation as compared to bronchial blockers or an intentional mainstem and also allow for easy transition between one- and two-lung ventilation.[1,2]

Placement of a double-lumen tube allows the provider to visualize both lungs with the fiberoptic scope during the procedure whereas the use of a bronchial blocker or intentionally main stemmed tube only allows fiberoptic visualization of the ventilated lung.

Use of CPAP improves oxygenation and/or allows quick deflation of nonventilated lung.

Cautions Regarding Double-Lumen Tubes

If difficulty is encountered during advancing a double-lumen tube through the vocal cords, an intubating or airway exchange catheter could be used to facilitate placement.

If there is difficulty placing a double-lumen endotracheal tube into the correct bronchus, the fiberoptic scope is used to guide placement the bronchial lumen into position.

If postoperative mechanical ventilation is required, the provider may have to exchange the double-lumen tube for a single-lumen tube as there is limited familiarity with double-lumen tube management in certain critical care settings.

Once lung isolation has been achieved with clamp placement, it is necessary to open a distal port of the nonventilated lung to allow it to deflate.

Management of Hypoxia During One-Lung Ventilation

During one-lung ventilation, hypoxia is not an uncommon occurrence. To correct hypoxia, the following steps should be taken.[1,2]

- Increase FiO_2 to 100%.
- Verify placement of the endotracheal device with a fiberoptic scope. When providing lung isolation, a fiberoptic scope should always be immediately available as frequent position checks are often required.
- Suction the endotracheal device to ensure there are no mucous plugs, secretions, edema, or blood obstructing the lumen.
- Provide CPAP to the nonventilated lung.
- Add positive end expiratory pressure to the ventilated lung.
- Return to two-lung ventilation if hypoxia continues or worsens quickly.
- Consider alternative causes for hypoxia that are not immediately related to one-lung ventilation.

Summary

There are multiple indications for one lung ventilation that require one of the three previously discussed techniques. Double-lumen endotracheal tubes are commonly used for lung isolation and are relatively easier to place and allow easy ventilation to one or both lungs compared to other lung isolation techniques. Bronchial blocker may be a better option for patients with difficult airways, patients who require postoperative mechanical ventilation, and patients for whom a double-lumen placement is not possible. Finally, endobronchial placement of a standard endotracheal tube may also be used for lung isolation in the pediatric population or in patients who are not a candidate for double-lumen tubes or bronchial blockers.

References

1. Campos J. Lung isolation. In: Slinger P., ed. *Principles and Practice of Anesthesia for Thoracic Surgery*. New York, NY: Springer New York, 2011; 227–246.
2. "Anesthesia for thoracic surgery." Butterworth JF, Wasnick JD Mackey DC, eds. *Morgan & Mikhail's Clinical Anesthesiology*. 5th ed. New York: McGraw-Hill Education, 2013; 545–571.
3. Zani G, Stefano M, Tommaso BF. How clinical experience leads anesthetists in the choice of double-lumen tube size. *J Clin Anesth* 2016;32:1–3.
4. Amar D, Desiderio DP, Heerdt PM, Kolker AC, Zhang H, Thaler H. Practice patterns in choice of left double-lumen tube size for thoracic surgery. *Anesth Analges* 2008;106(2):379–383.

7
Airway Devices for Thoracic Anesthesia and Ventilatory Techniques

Neeraj Kumar, Priya Gupta, and Indranil Chakraborty

Introduction

Lung isolation techniques are used extensively in modern operating rooms and intensive care units (ICUs). They can be employed in the operating room for several surgical procedures involving the lungs or the mediastinum, out of the operating room for procedures performed by interventional pulmonologists, and in critical care units where a patient's medical or surgical conditions require selective lung isolation or ventilation. A thorough understanding of the anatomy and physiology of human airway and pulmonary function is essential for safe and successful execution of these procedures and techniques. A meticulous preparation of the patient and equipment is a must. Appropriate invasive and noninvasive monitoring of the patient during these isolation techniques and procedures are mandatory. In this chapter, we discuss the basic anatomy we need to know before undertaking these procedures followed by describing the individual equipment and technique being used under current practice. We will then discuss the basic principles and practice of ventilation strategies and techniques

Adult Lung Isolation and Devices

Basic Airway Anatomy

Adult trachea is a tube-like structure composed of multiple C-shaped incomplete cartilaginous rings with the incomplete segment of the C placed posteriorly (Figures 7.1 and 7.2). The trachea bifurcates distally into the right and left main bronchi at the level of the carina, which connect to the right and left lung. It is important to note that in adults the right and the left main bronchi are not identical. The right bronchus is wider in diameter, shorter in length, and more vertical. It also ends in three lobar bronchi for the three lobes of the right lung, with the right upper lobar bronchus branching off within 2 to 3 cm of the carina. The left main bronchus is narrower, longer, and more horizontally oriented. It also ends into two lobar bronchi for the two lobes of the left lung. Most modern lung isolation techniques utilize this difference in anatomy to place a double-lumen tube (DLT) in the left bronchus to avoid inadvertent occlusion of the right upper lobe bronchus.

Anatomy of the tracheobronchial tree

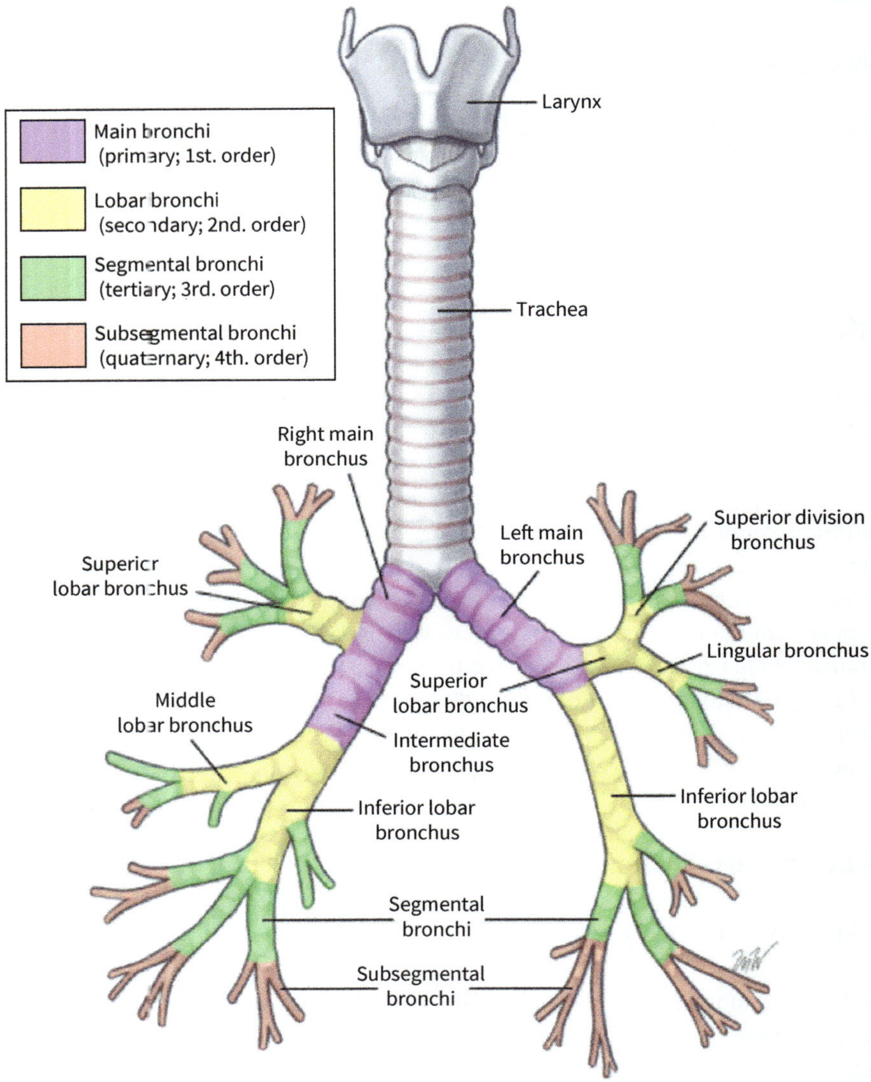

Figure 7.1 Basic adult airway anatomy.

Reproduced with permission from: Herth F. Clinical presentation, diagnostic evaluation, and management of central airway obstruction in adults. In: UpToDate, Post TW (Ed), UpToDate, Waltham, MA. (Accessed on 12/07/2020) Copyright © 2020 UpToDate, Inc. For more information visit www.uptodate.com.

General Preparation

Equipment

Choosing the correct equipment for the correct patient and procedure and ensuring its satisfactory working condition is essential for safe performance of these techniques. It is recommended to keep basic airway management equipment readily available at all times including

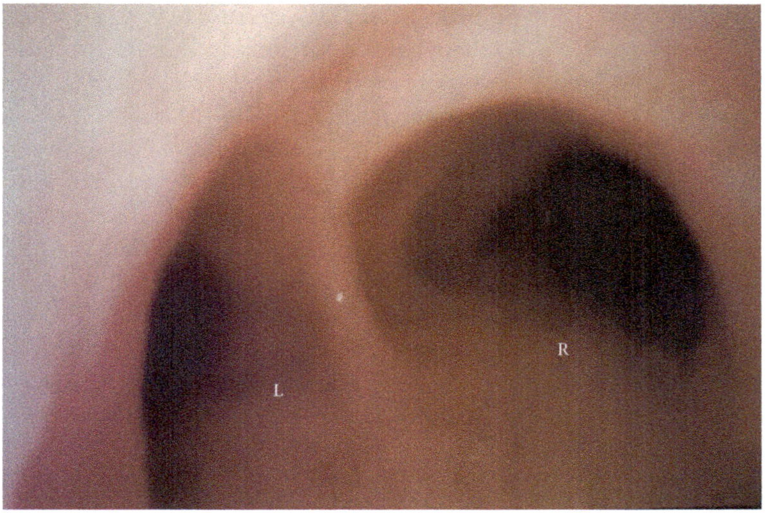

Figure 7.2 Fiberoptic view of the carina and the right and left mainstem bronchi.

an AMBU bag with mask, laryngoscope, appropriate endotracheal tubes, fiberoptic bronchoscope, mechanical ventilation capability with ability to give 100% oxygen, etc. An alternative plan for lung isolation if the first isolation technique fails is always encouraged.

Monitoring

Standard American Society of Anesthesiologists (ASA) monitoring with special emphasis on pulse oximetry and end tidal carbon dioxide tracing is essential for these procedures. Invasive arterial blood pressure monitoring is also highly encouraged, since most of the procedures are at increased risk for hemodynamic instability and may need frequent arterial blood gas analysis.

Adult Lung Isolation Devices

Double-Lumen Tube

These are specially designed endotracheal tubes with two parallel and noncommunicating airway channels (Figure 7.3). Proximally, each channel has its own separate connector for the ventilator. Distally, each airway channel has its own cuff with one channel shorter than the other.

Regular DLT. The various sizes available for adults are 35 Fr, 37 Fr, 39 Fr, and 41 Fr. For successful placement the following equipment is needed apart from standard preparation as previously mentioned:

- Direct Laryngoscope
- Fiberoptic bronchoscope
- Tube clamp

Left-sided DLT is almost exclusively used, irrespective of side of surgery or lung isolation. This is because of the close proximity of the right upper lobe bronchus to carina. Therefore, a right-sided DLT can cause its occlusion and can result in right upper lobe hypoventilation.

Under direct laryngoscopy, the bronchial tip of the DLT is passed beyond the vocal cords. The tube is then rotated 90° to the left of the patient and advanced aiming to direct the bronchial tip toward the left main bronchus. After reaching the recommended depth, the fiberoptic bronchoscope is passed through the tracheal lumen of the DLT to visualize the bronchial part of the DLT going into the left main bronchus. This is aided by visualizing the unobstructed view of the right main bronchus (identified by the right upper lobe bronchus with 2–3 cm of the carina) and the colored cuff of the left bronchial tube going into the left main bronchus. The fiberoptic scope is then passed through the bronchial lumen to verify the correct placement into the left main bronchus. The bifurcation of the left upper and lower lobe bronchi should be clearly visible and tube tip a few centimeters away from it.

Advantages of double lumen tube include one-tube design (left-sided DLT) that can be used for surgeries or isolation on either lung, ease of placement, and very few moving parts.

Disadvantages are tube rigidity, size, and length limitations. It is only suitable for older children and adults and is not suitable for younger pediatric patients.

(A)

(B)

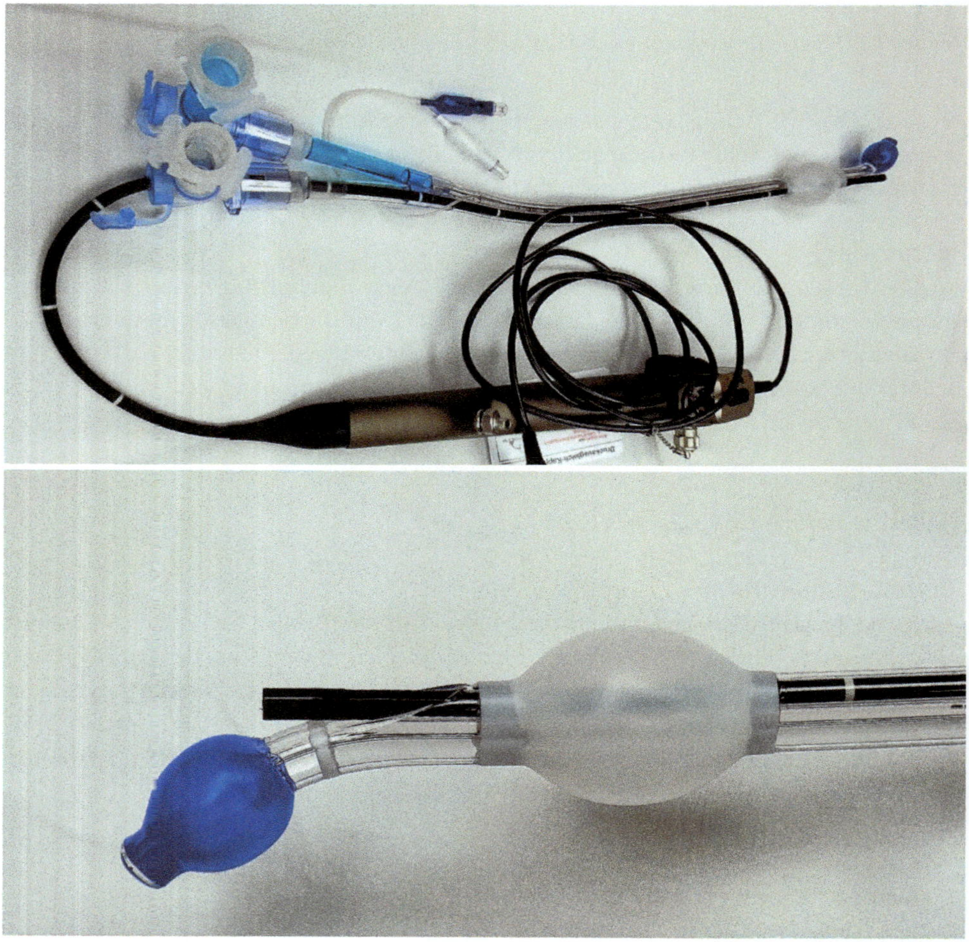

Figure 7.3 Left sided double lumen tube (DLT). (A) shows fiberoptic scope placed via the tracheal lumen of DLT. (B) shows close-up of DLT tip with inflated proximal cuff (white) and distal bronchial cuff (blue). The tip of fiberoptic scope is seen just beyond the tracheal opening of DLT.

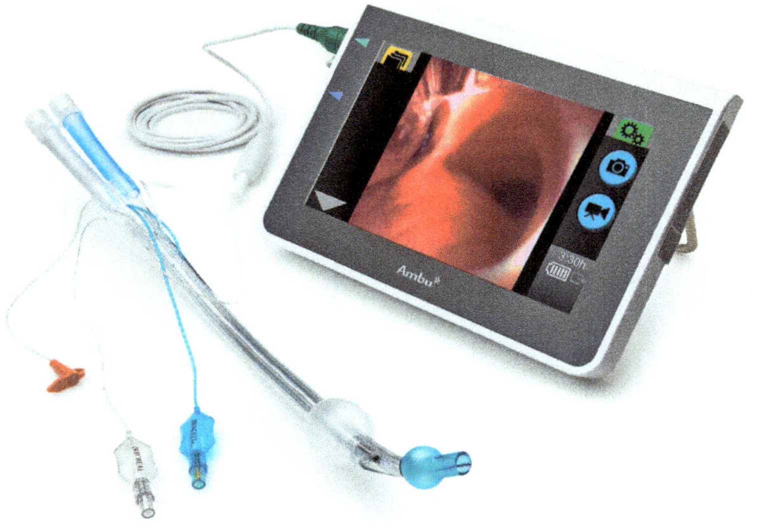

Figure 7.4 Video double lumen tube VivaSightDL.
Image reproduced with permission from Ambu inc.

Complications that can occur include damage to teeth and other airway structures due to rigidity.

Video double-lumen tube: VivaSight-DL® (Figure 7.4). These are variations of standard left-sided DLTs with in-built video camera at the tip of the tracheal tube lumen. Also present is an extra channel to flush saline to clean the camera lens of secretions. The sizes are 35 Fr, 37 Fr, 39 Fr, and 41 Fr.

There is no need for a separate fiberoptic bronchoscope but direct laryngoscopy equipment and a long tube clamp are necessary.

Placement of VivaSight DL involves the following steps:

- The video DLT is checked and its video cable attached with the video monitor.
- The glottis is visualized in usual fashion with a direct laryngoscope.
- The video DLT is then passed beyond the glottis under vision.
- The video DLT is then advanced under live video monitoring and the bronchial tube passed into the left main bronchus.
- The cuffs are inflated, the correct placement of the left bronchial cuff confirmed under video monitoring.

Advantages are that the tube placement can be confirmed live during the intubation process under video monitoring and there is no need for a separate fiberoptic bronchoscope.

Disadvantages are similar to the standard DLT: they are only available in sizes suitable for older children and adults.

Possible complications are higher chances of airway trauma due to stiffness and bigger size compared to a standard single lumen endotracheal tube.

Bronchial Blockers

Uniblocker

The Uniblocker (Figure 7.5) is a device that is capable of blocking either right or the left bronchus when placed through an already present standard single-lumen endotracheal tube under fiberoptic bronchoscopic visualization. The device has a flexible bronchial shaft and comes with a multiport connector that connects to the endotracheal tube and anesthesia circuit; the connector has two ports, one for fiberoptic bronchoscope and the other for the

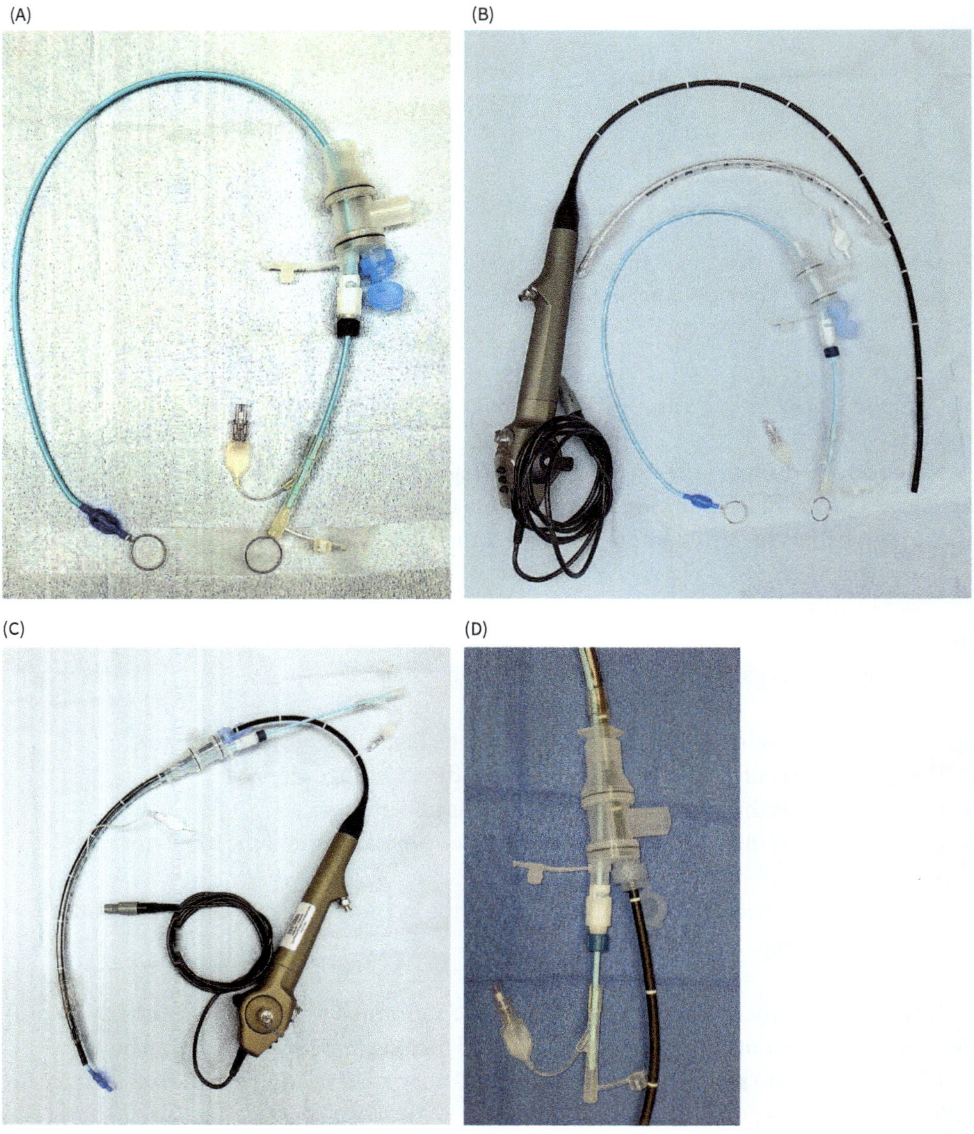

Figure 7.5 Uniblocker; Multiport connector of Uniblocker with the bronchial blocker in place (A); Uniblocker Assembly (B); Uniblocker with fiberoptic scope and bronchial blocker in place via the endotracheal tube (C); and Multiport connector of Uniblocker with the bronchial blocker and fiberoptic bronchoscope (black) in place (D).

bronchial blocker. A single-port swivel connector for the endobronchial tube can also be used for this device. Two sizes are available: 5 F and 7 F.

Uniblocker comes with two stylets. The distal stylet is meant to maintain a slight bend to the tip of the blocker and should be removed prior to use. The Swivel assemble should be checked for integrity. Bronchial cuff should be inflated with 3 mL air for 5 Fr blocker (8 mL air for 9 Fr) and then deflated to ensure proper functioning of the cuff. Lubricant should be applied to the bronchial cuff to ensure smooth insertion.

Technique of Placement

Connect the endotracheal tube port of the multiport connector to the endotracheal tube and anesthesia circuit to the ventilation port. Insert the bronchial blocker into the endotracheal tube via the side port of the multiport connector without applying excessive force. Insert the fiberoptic bronchoscope after the bronchial blocker through the bronchoscope port of the multiport connector and advance both under direct vision. Once the tip of the blocker is seen exiting the endotracheal tube, twist the blocker, and advance the tip into the desired bronchus inserting just past the carina. Inflate the bronchial cuff and visualize the cuff in the desired bronchus. Once the position is confirmed, remove the proximal stylet from the bronchial blocker and lock the blocker in place by twisting the locking cap clockwise. Once the lung collapse is visualized, close the proximal end of the blocker by placing the locking cap into the luer lock. If any adjustments to the position of the blocker is required and during removal, the bronchial cuff must be deflated first and the locking cap released by turning it anti-clockwise. Bronchoscope port can be used to insert a suction catheter if required.

Advantages of using a uniblocker is that it is inserted through a standard endotracheal tube, which is easier to insert due to smaller external diameters compared to a DLT. There is no need to exchange tubes if postoperative ventilation is required. Uniblocker is only available in two sizes, and successful lung isolation may not be possible in all patients. There is no ability to do endobronchial suctioning or to apply continuous positive airway pressure (CPAP) to the isolated lung.

It is possible to cause damage to the bronchial wall with this device if excessive volumes are used to inflate the bronchial cuff.

Arndt Endobronchial Blocker

The Arndt endobronchial blocker (Figure 7.6) uses an adjustable guide loop assembly that connects to a fiberoptic bronchoscope and allows it to be inserted through a single lumen endotracheal tube under direct visualization. It can used to isolate either right of left lung. It is available in 9 Fr, 7 Fr, and 5 Fr sizes. The smallest endotracheal tube sizes for use with this blocker are 7.5 mm for 9 Fr, 6.0 mm for 7 Fr, and 4.5 mm for 5 Fr.

Technique of Insertion

Bronchial balloon cuff should be inflated and deflated prior to use to ensure proper functioning. Appropriate blocker size should be selected based on patient size and size of the endotracheal tube.

Attach the Arndt multiport adaptor that is supplied with the blocker to the endotracheal tube and connect the anesthesia circuit to the ventilator port. Lubricate both the bronchial blocker cuff and the fiberoptic bronchoscope to ensure smooth passage through the endotracheal tube. Insert the bronchoscope through the bronchoscopy port and the blocker through the blocker port on the multiport adaptor connector and advance the blocker into

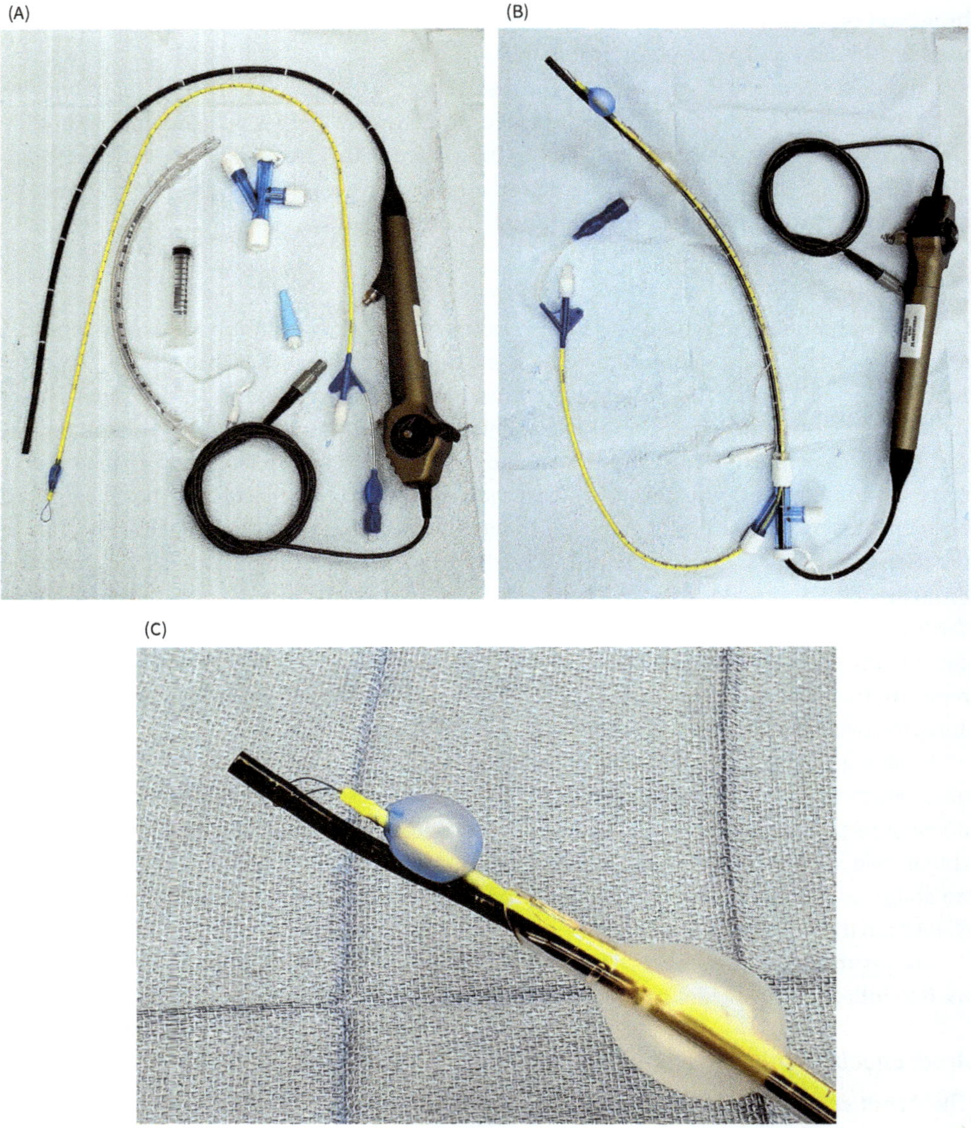

Figure 7.6 Arendt endobronchial blocker assembly with fiberoptic bronchoscope (A); Arendt endobronchial blocker (yellow) and fiberoptic bronchoscope (black) in final position through the multiport connector via the endotracheal tube (B); and magnified distal end of endotracheal tube with Arendt endobronchial blocker (yellow) and fiberoptic bronchoscope (black) in place (C).

the endotracheal tube until the blocker guide loop is seen exiting the adaptor. Advance the bronchoscope through the guide loop and adjust the loop diameter by pulling back on the snare to attach the blocker to the scope. Advance the bronchoscope into either the right or left mainstem bronchus. Once the blocker is seen entering mainstem bronchus, loosen the guide loop to disengage the blocker from the bronchoscope and advance the blocker further while keeping the bronchoscope in place. One the desired placement is achieved, inflate the bronchial cuff; it should be visible in the desired bronchus and not herniate into the mainstem trachea. One the blocker is in place, tighten the blocker port on the multiport adapter and remove the guide loop assembly from the blocker under direct bronchoscopic visualization and ensure that blocker remains in the desired position. When one-lung ventilation (OLV) is no longer required, deflate the bronchial cuff completely prior to the removal of the bronchial blocker.

Similar to the Uniblocker, Arndt blocker is inserted through a standard endotracheal tube; it is not suitable for use in infants as the minimum recommended endotracheal tube size for the 5 Fr blocker is 4.5 mm.

Excessive bronchial cuff pressure or manipulation while cuff is still inflated can cause bronchial or tracheal mucosal injury.

Rusch EZ-Blocker

The Rusch EZ-Blocker (Figure 7.7) is an endobronchial block with two distal extensions, both with a cuff and a lumen. Both the extension and their cuff inflation systems are colored differently to help in identification. The device is inserted through a standard endotracheal tube under fiberoptic guidance and can be used to isolate either right or left lung. It is only available in 7 Fr size.

Technique of Placement

Inflate and deflate both cuffs prior to use with 15 cc max of air to ensure proper functioning of the cuffs and inflation systems. Remove the outer protection tube from the blocker prior to use. Lubricate distal part of the blocker and fiberoptic bronchoscope prior to insertion.

Attach the supplied EZ-Multiport adaptor to the endotracheal tube and attach anesthesia circuit to the ventilator port of adaptor. Introduce the EZ-Blocker through the blocker port and fiberoptic bronchoscope through the bronchoscope port of the multiport adaptor and advance into the endotracheal tube. Advance the EZ-Blocker under direct vision until each extension enters one of the two mainstem bronchi. Inflate the desired bronchial cuff to isolate the lung, do not use more than 15 cc of air to inflate the cuff. Recheck the position of the cuff and the block after repositioning the patient. Once the position of the cuff is confirmed fix the blocker in place by tightening the cap on the shaft of the blocker to the multiport adaptor. Deflate the cuff and loosen the cap from the adaptor prior to removal or if blocker needs to be repositioned.

Similar to other bronchial blockers, EZ-Blocker is designed to be inserted through a standard endobronchial tube. With EZ-Blocker, there is no need to direct the blocker into the desired lung due to the presence of two extensions, either one of which can be used to isolate the desired lung. Minimum recommended endotracheal tube size is 7.0 mm for EZ-Blocker; thus, this device is not suitable for use in the pediatric population.

Minimum possible air volume should be used for cuff inflation; cuff should be deflated prior to removal or repositioning to avoid injury to bronchial or tracheal mucosa.

Endobronchial Intubation with Single-lumen Endotracheal Tubes

This technique can be used for any age but is primarily reserved for young children. Endobronchial intubation with a single-lumen endotracheal tube is the preferred method of lung isolation for the first 6 months of age and is acceptable for ages up to 18 months. It is easier to advance a single-lumen tube into the right bronchus due to less acute angle; fiberoptic bronchoscope can be used to aid and confirm placement.

This technique is simple and does not require use of specialized tubes or blockers but is limited by the potential occlusion of right upper lobe bronchus and inability to apply CPAP or suction to the operative lung.

(A)

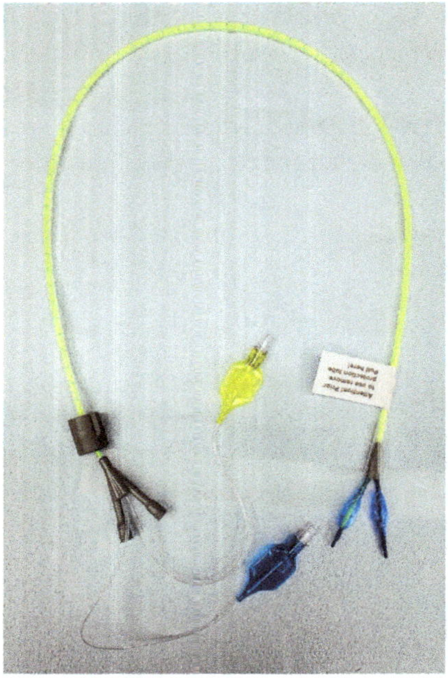

(B)

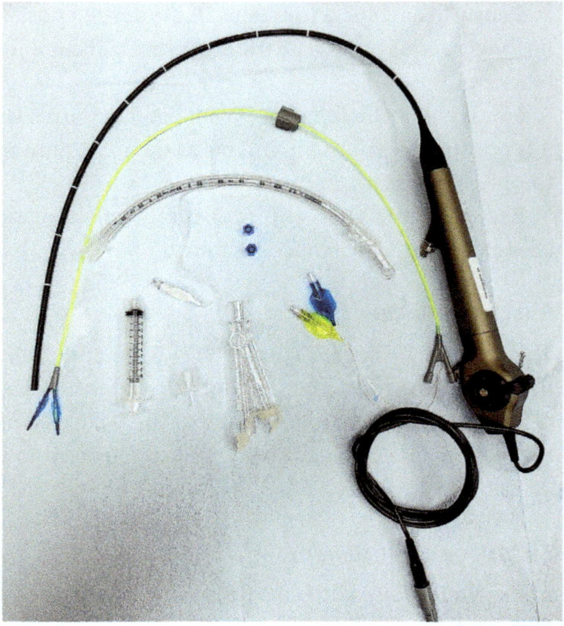

(C)

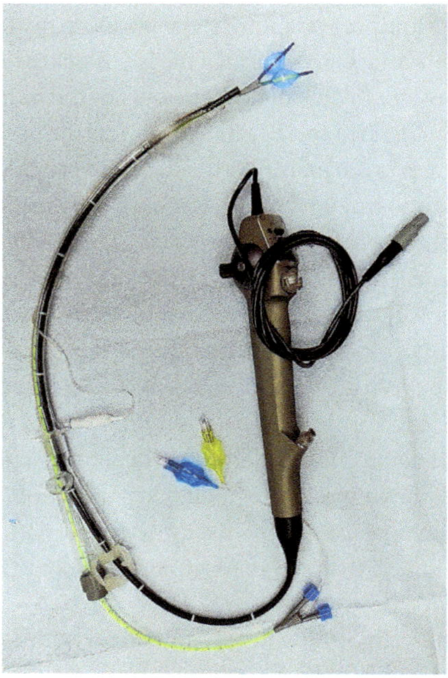

Figure 7.7 Rusch EZ Blocker (A); Rusch EZ Blocker assembly with fiberoptic bronchoscope (B); Rusch EZ Blocker with fiberoptic bronchoscope in final position through the multiport connector via the endotracheal tube; both EZ Blocker cuffs inflated with air (C).

Pediatric Lung Isolation and Devices

Basic Airway Anatomy

Due to the smaller size of the pediatric airway, use of standard lung isolation techniques like DLTs may not be possible in infants and young children. Also, size of the fiberoptic bronchoscope and double- and single-lumen tube must be considered. Average neonatal anterior-posterior diameter of the trachea is 4.3 mm, which increases from 14 to 19 mm in adults.

Preparation

Available imaging such as computed tomography, X-rays, and ultrasound should be reviewed to help guide the appropriate size of fiberoptic bronchoscope and single-lumen tube, DLT, or blockers.

Pediatric Lung Isolation Devices

Endobronchial Intubation With Single-Lumen Endotracheal Tubes

This the preferred method in less than 6 months of age. After placing a standard endotracheal tube, it is advanced under bronchoscopic guidance into the mainstem bronchus. Tube is mostly likely to enter the right mainstem as it comes out at a less acute angle from carina. This technique is limited due to potential of right upper lobe bronchus occlusion and inability to provide operative lung CPAP or suction.

Bronchial Blockers

Uniblocker. Fuji system Uniblocker is available in 5 Fr pediatric size; there is no central lumen for suction or CPAP.

Arndt endobronchial blocker. Available in 5 Fr pediatric size. It has a guiding loop that attaches to fiberoptic bronchoscopy, which can then be used to guide placement. The inner wire can then be removed after placement and channel used for suction or CPAP if required.

Fogarty vascular balloon catheter. Fogarty embolectomy catheter comes in the smallest sizes of 2 and 3 Fr and can be guided under bronchoscope into the desired lung. It has a high pressure balloon and should be inflated with the minimum amount of air required. There is no central channel.

Double-Lumen Tubes

The smallest size DLT available is 26 Fr and can be used in children over 8 years of age, more than 30 kg in weight, and 130 cm in height. As in adults, the left-sided tube is typically used, and fiberoptic bronchoscope used to confirm placement. Advantages of a DLT are ability to provide operative lung CPAP, suction, and ability to quickly switch between one- and two-lung ventilation.

Lung Isolation Ventilatory Techniques

Introduction

The need for lung isolation has increased with more frequent use of video-assisted thoracoscopic surgeries and other complex intrathoracic surgeries and procedures in the operating rooms. This technique is also utilized in the ICUs for ventilatory management. The goal of OLV is to isolate and collapse the operative lung to provide optimal surgical exposure. In the ICU, it may be utilized to separate one lung from the other and thus prevent cross-contamination of infectious material or blood into the pulmonary system. It may also be used to differentially ventilate the two lungs separately to encourage healing of specific lung conditions like bronchopleural fistula. Postoperative acute lung injury is the leading cause of morbidity following lung resection, and current research recommends a protective ventilation strategy during the management of OLV.

Physiology of One-Lung Ventilation

In the lateral decubitus position, used during most thoracic procedures, the dependent lung is better perfused due to gravity whereas ventilation preferentially goes to the nondependent lung, due to decreased compliance of the dependent lung. Commencement of OLV leads to ventilation to only the dependent lung, and any perfusion to the nondependent lung becomes part of the large right-to-left intrapulmonary shunt (20%–30%). This shunt gets progressively worse with induction of general anesthesia, muscle relaxation, positive mechanical ventilation, and thoracotomy with an open nondependent chest wall. Decrease in perfusion to the nonventilated nondependent lung due to hypoxic pulmonary vasoconstriction, surgical manipulation and gravity helps to reduce this shunt. Hypoxic pulmonary vasoconstriction can reduce flow to the nondependent lung by up to 40%. This shunt is primarily responsible for hypoxemia observed during OLV.

Indications

In the operating room, surgeries and procedures that require lung isolation and collapse for surgical access such as lung surgeries including (i) transplantation, (ii) thoracic aorta repair, (iii) esophageal surgeries, (iv) anterior approach to thoracic spine surgeries, and (v) bronchoalveolar lavage procedures. In the ICU, a patient's clinical condition may necessitate the differential ventilation of the two lungs and isolation from each other in conditions like infection, bleeding, bronchopleural fistula and lung trauma.

Ventilatory Techniques

The goal of current recommendations for ventilatory management of OLV is prevention of both hypoxemia and lung injury. Recommended strategies include low tidal volumes in the range of 6 to 8 mL/kg ideal body weight, routine application of positive end expiratory pressure of 5 mmHg or more to the ventilated lung, intermittent recruitment maneuvers, permissive hypercapnia, FiO_2 of less than 1 whenever possible, insufflation of oxygen to the nondependent lung, and application of CPAP to the nonventilated lung in certain situations.

High tidal volume and high peak and plateau pressures can lead to volutrauma and barotrauma to the ventilated lung, contributing to postoperative acute lung injury. Peak pressures should be kept below 30 mmHg. Application of positive end expiratory pressure to the ventilated lung and CPAP to the nonventilated lung helps with oxygenation intraoperatively and has also been shown to provide lung protection. Application of CPAP to the nonventilated lung may interfere with optimal surgical exposure and may not be feasible when complete collapse of the nondependent lung is desired, as in video-assisted thoracoscopic surgeries. Intermittent application of recruitment maneuvers prior to the commencement of OLV and as needed during the maintenance of OLV helps improve oxygenation by opening of atelectatic alveoli. Permissive hypercapnia in the range of PCO_2 of 50 to 70 mmHg can be helpful in preventing postoperative acute lung injury essentially by avoiding hyperventilation. High FiO_2 promotes atelectasis and can cause atelectrauma due to repeated opening and closing of alveoli. Lowest FiO_2 possible to maintain oxygen saturation in the range of 92% to 96% should be used.

8

Patient Positioning and Surgical Considerations

Phi Ho, Yi Deng, and Melissa Nikolaidis

Introduction

Proper positioning requires anesthesiologists, nurses, and surgeons to ensure well-being and safety of the patient while providing appropriate surgical exposure. Patient positioning in thoracic procedures is most commonly in the lateral decubitus position. Other positions include flexed lateral decubitus (kidney), supine, and lateral semiprone. Enhancing surgical access and mitigating risks for neurological injuries make positioning important in thoracic anesthesia.

Initial Positioning

Although the majority of thoracic cases have the patients in the lateral position, most thoracic cases start with the patient in the supine position. Starting in a lateral position would be inconvenient when placing monitors on the patient or inserting new intravenous lines and arterial lines, and it can be technically difficult to intubate in that position. Once the patient is properly monitored and intubated in the supine position, the position change will begin. With the help of the operating room personnel, the patient is carefully rotated 90 degrees with the diseased lung placed in the nondependent position. It is a shared responsibility to ensure that the patient does not get injured during the process.

When in lateral decubitus position, the patient should have a proper alignment of the head, endobronchial tube, and thoracolumbar spine. Additionally, adequate stabilization and support of extremities with padding are tools to minimize circulatory, integumentary, and musculoskeletal injury. When changing the position of the patient, the anesthesiologist should perform a thorough head-to-toe survey of the patient, checking monitors, hemodynamics, lines, oxygenation, and potential nerve injuries (Box 8.1).[1] Hemodynamics are predictably lower in an anesthetized patient due to decreased vascular tone and should be treated appropriately. Ventilation/perfusion mismatch will be more profound, so careful monitoring of oxygenation is prudent. The majority of patients will experience a change in position of their double-lumen tube (DLT) with the transition to lateral positioning. Most will experience an upward shift of the tube on average of 1 cm, but there is little room for a margin of error when it comes to DLT placement.[2] Thus, it is standard practice to assess the location of DLTs through the use of fiberoptic bronchoscope in the tracheal lumen in both the supine and lateral positions.

Box 8.1 Routine Head-to-Toe Survey to Avoid Neurovascular Injury in the Lateral Position

1. Dependent eye
2. Dependent ear pinna
3. Cervical spine in line with thoracic spine
4. Dependent arm (brachial plexus, circulation)
5. Nondependent arm[a] (brachial plexus, circulation)
6. Dependent and nondependent suprascapular nerves
7. Nondependent leg sciatic nerve
8. Dependent leg (circulation)

[a]Neurovascular injuries of the nondependent arm are more likely to occur if the arm is suspended or held in an independently positioned armrest.

Lateral Decubitus Position

Thoracic surgeries most commonly have patients in the lateral position since it provides the most exposure to the diseased lung. Patients are placed on a vacuum mat or a foam mattress with additional support between the knees and arms. The head is placed on a foam pillow or gel ring, paying attention to the alignment of the cervical spine with the thoracic spine (see Figure 8.1). An excessive lateral flexion of the head can cause traction to the brachial plexus, which may result in a brachial plexus injury. Eyes should be covered with tape or a clear plastic eye cover with a self-adhesive foam cushion. It should be visible at all times and avoidant of pressure from lines and pillows. The bottom ear should be free of pressure and placed in a donut head pad made of foam or gel material.

The extremities should be carefully positioned to avoid any nerve injury. The lower leg should be slightly flexed and upper leg straight to avoid stretching of the nerves. Padding is placed under the dependent knee and a pillow or other padding is placed in between the legs to avoid direct pressure on bony prominences. This will mitigate a common peroneal nerve injury, where the nerve is crushed between an external object and the head of the fibula. Excessive tight strapping of the hips can cause sciatic nerve injury of the nondependent leg.

A brachial plexus injury is the most common nerve injury in the lateral position and should be avoided.[3] The dependent arm is placed out in front of the patient on a padded arm board. The nondependent arm is supported over folded pillows or suspended with a padded arm rest. Neither arm should be abducted by greater than 90 degrees to avoid brachial plexus injury.

Another mechanism of brachial plexus injury is direct compression of the nerves. It can occur where the lower arm or shoulder remains directly under the body's weight in the lateral position. To avoid injury, an axillary roll should be placed just caudad to the axilla, *not* in the axilla itself. The purpose of the axillary roll is to lift the weight of the chest wall and avoid compression of the axillary vasculature and nerves. It may be helpful to place an arterial line on the dependent arm to detect positioning compression of the axillary vasculatures.

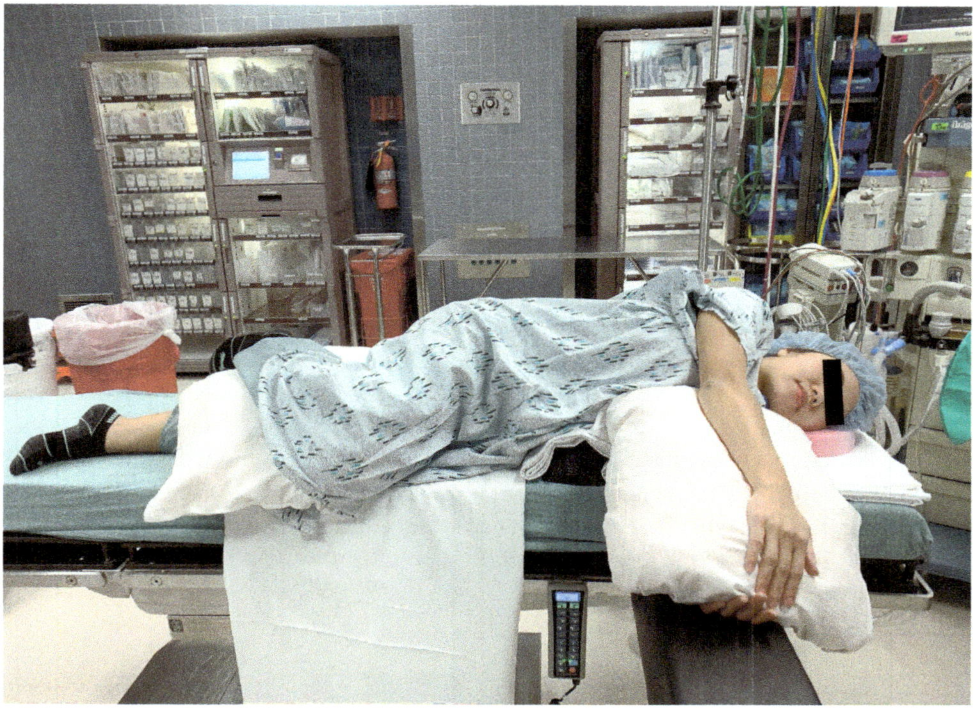

Figure 8.1 Patient in lateral decubitus position. Note that the patient has both arms out and supported with an armrest and pillow. This allows for more surgical exposure. An axillary roll is placed just caudad to the axilla to prevent nerve injuries. The dependent leg is straight and nondependent leg is flexed with a pillow in between.

The brachial plexus is vulnerable to injury due to its lack of mobility, being fixed at the vertebrae, prevertebral fascia, and axillary fascia. It is also in close proximity to bony structures, such as the clavicle, first rib, coracoid process, and the head of the humerus, all of which can cause direct compression of the nerves. The brachial plexus of the nondependent arm is at most risk if it is suspended from an independent arm support. Traction of the brachial plexus and the suprascapular nerve can occur if the patient's trunk slips into a semiprone or prone position while maintaining a fixed nondependent arm. This arm should not be abducted or anteriorly flexed beyond 90 degrees, nor should it be posteriorly flexed beyond the neutral position.

Flexed Lateral Position

Most often, video-assisted thoracoscopic surgery (VATS) procedures require the patient to be in a flexed lateral position, similar to patient positioning for a nephrectomy. After the patient has been placed in a lateral decubitus position, the patient will be aligned at the level of the xiphoid and the flex point of the specialized bed (see Figure 8.2). A little flexion of the bed will bring down the nondependent iliac crest so that it will not interfere with surgical access.

The other benefit of flexion is expanding the thoracic interspaces for the VATS ports.[4] Extra sheets under the patient's head might be necessary to maintain a horizontal plane of the thoracic and cervical spine.

Hemodynamic changes in this position are not vastly different between a lateral decubitus position and supine position. However, with flexion, there is concern for decreased venous return and decreased cardiac index.[5,6] This should be considered in elderly patients or patients with cardiac issues.

Semiprone Position

The semiprone position for VATS procedures has been gaining traction in recent years. This position allows for more operating space, facilitating surgery of the posterior mediastinum. Posteriors lung segments are more easily resected.[7] The hemodynamic effects will be similar to being in a prone position. Hemodynamics are improved, with an increase in abdominal pressure leading to increased systemic vascular resistance and right ventricular preload. This position also decreases hypoxia and pulmonary vascular resistance and thus

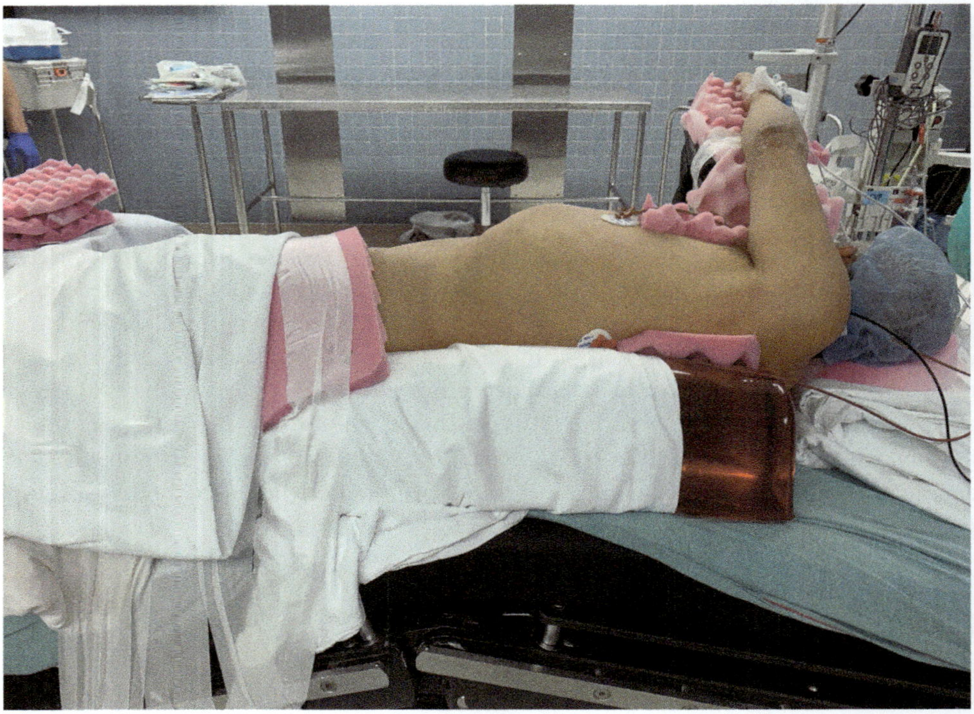

Figure 8.2 Patient in flexed-lateral position. Image is a posterior view and position commonly used for video-assisted thoracoscopic surgical procedures. There is an increase in thoracic interspaces for easier port placements. Forced air warmers are placed on the lower half of the body.

a decrease in right ventricular afterload. Together, these effects will lead to an increase in cardiac output.[8]

The patient will lie on the nondependent side, and the nondependent thigh will be slightly flexed. The dependent thigh will be acutely flexed. The nondependent arm is behind the patient and the dependent arm is flexed at the elbow and arm abduction not exceeding 90 degrees. There are slight variations to the semiprone position where the nondependent arm is placed in front of the patient with an axillary roll slightly caudad to the axilla (see Figure 8.3).

Supine Position

A supine position would be beneficial for several types of thoracic surgeries, such as mediastinal mass resection, lung transplantation, bilateral thoracoscopic procedures, or bilateral wedge resections. A standard supine position would have both arms abducted but not greater than 90 degrees to avoid a brachial plexus injury. Elbows are padded to minimize a risk for an ulnar nerve injury. Hands and forearms are either supinated or kept in a neutral position with palms facing the body to also reduce pressure on the ulnar nerve.

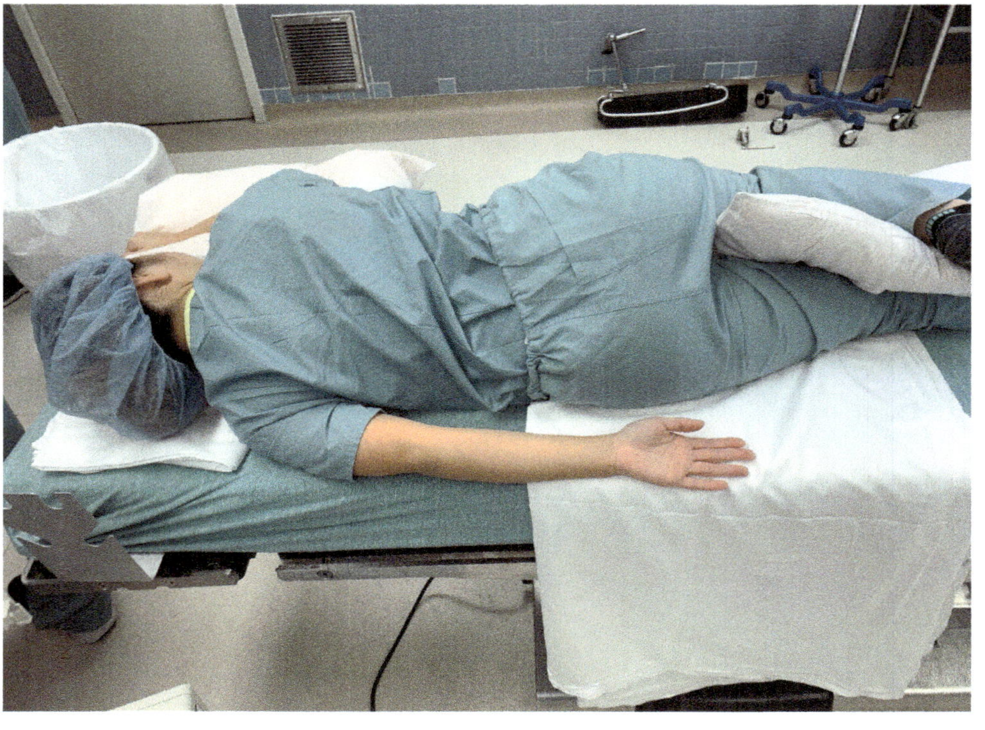

Figure 8.3 Patient in semiprone position. This position is used to access the posterior mediastinum. Patient's head is turned to the side, with ipsilateral arm and leg flexed, supported on pillows. The dependent arm is kept straight and to the side and dependent leg is straight.

Further Reading

Breyer CEW. Patient positioning and associated risks. In: Pardo M, Miller RD, eds. *Basics of Anesthesia.* 7th ed. Philadelphia: Elsevier; 2018: 321–336.

References

1. Hensley J, Frederick A, Martin DE, Gravlee GP. *A Practical Approach to Cardiac Anesthesia.* Philadelphia: Lippincott Williams and Wilkins; 2013.
2. Desiderio DP, Burt M, Kolker AC, Fischer ME, Reinsel R, Wilson RS. The effects of endobronchial cuff inflation on double-lumen endobronchial tube movement after lateral decubitus positioning. *J Cardiothorac Vasc Anesth.* 1997;11(5):595–598.
3. Martin JT. *Positioning in Anesthesia and Surgery.* 2nd ed. Philadelphia: Saunders; 1987.
4. Demmy TL, James TA, Swanson SJ, McKenna RJ Jr, D'Amico TA. Troubleshooting video-assisted thoracic surgery lobectomy. *Ann Thorac Surg.* 2005;79(5):1744–1752; discussion 1753.
5. Jin Y, Ying J, Zhang K, Fang X. Endotracheal intubation under video laryngoscopic guidance during upper gastrointestinal endoscopic surgery in the left lateral position: a randomized controlled trial. *Medicine (Baltimore).* 2017;96(52):e9461.
6. Yokoyama M, Ueda W, Hirakawa M. Haemodynamic effects of the lateral decubitus position and the kidney rest lateral decubitus position during anaesthesia. *Br J Anaesth.* 2000;84(6):753–757.
7. Lin Z, Xi J, Xu S, Wang Q. Uniportal video-assisted thoracic surgery left superior segmentectomy with systematic lymphadenectomy in the semiprone position. *J Thorac Dis.* 2016;8(8):2256–2258.
8. Jozwiak M, Teboul J-L, Anguel N, et al. Beneficial hemodynamic effects of prone positioning in patients with acute respiratory distress syndrome. *Am J Respir Crit Care Med.* 2013;188(12):1428–1433.

9

Anesthetic Management Techniques in Thoracic Surgery

Henry Liu, Xiangdong Chen, Alan D. Kaye, and Richard D. Urman

Introduction: Historical Review

Normal human respiration relies upon an intact chest (intact chest walls and pleural cavities). If the chest is opened by mechanic force, pathological conditions, or surgery, ventilation and oxygenation will be compromised. The exposed lung will collapse, and the mediastinum will shift toward the closed-side lung. The patient will quickly become hypoxemic and tachypneic. This is the pneumothorax challenge that surgeons and anesthesiologists have to overcome for intrathoracic surgical procedures.[1] In the early days of thoracic surgery, surgeons attempted placing the patient's body inside an airtight negative pressure chamber or the patient's head inside a positive pressure chamber, which worked for very limited surgical indications and with short duration.[2] More complicated intrathoracic surgery had not been possible until endotracheal intubation with cuffed tube became a standard airway management technique, and not until the concept of one-lung ventilation (OLV) were developed and adopted.[3] In the mid-20th century, the double-lumen double-cuffed endotracheal tube was developed, which allowed significant progress in managing thoracic surgical patients.[4] Currently anesthesiologists can use lung isolation, selective OLV, more advanced invasive and noninvasive hemodynamic and respiratory monitoring, and multimodal postthoracotomy analgesia, so the thoracic surgeons can perform very complex thoracic procedures on the most debilitated patients. Yet thoracic anesthesiologists may still be challenged by some clinical scenarios, and there are evolving anesthetic techniques such as a nonintubating technique for thoracic surgery while maintaining spontaneous breathing, administration of thoracic spinal anesthesia, and newer peripheral regional analgesic techniques that are being developed and refined.[5–7] Anesthesiologists will need to master the skills needed to deal with perioperative issues, keep themselves abreast with all these new practical techniques and new developments on the horizon.

Anesthetic Management Techniques for Thoracic Procedures in General Anesthesia

Lung Isolation

Absolute Indications

Lung isolation is indicated in patients who suffer from massive hemorrhage or severe lung infection on one side of the lungs. This isolation will offer protective effects to the opposite side of the lungs. Some patients who have a bronchopleural cutaneous or bronchopleural fistula will need lung isolation in order to avoid loss of tidal volume or a pneumothorax. Patient with giant cyst or bullae will need lung isolation to minimize the risk of cyst or bullae rupture. Patients with major bronchial disruption or trauma will obviously need to divert ventilation to the healthy side of the lungs. Lung isolation is also indicated for one-sided pulmonary lavage for severe lung infection or contaminations.[8] Indications for lung isolation are shown in Table 9.1.

Relative Indications

Relative indications for OLV to improve exposure and facilitate surgical procedures include thoracic aortic aneurysm, pneumonectomy, upper lobectomy, esophageal surgery, middle and lower lobectomy, and thoracoscopic procedures.[8] Relative indications are listed in Table 9.1.

Table 9.1 Indications and Relative Contraindications for Lung Isolation

	Purposes of Lung Isolation	Medical Conditions
Absolute Indications	• Protective isolation • Control of ventilation distribution • Unilateral lung lavage	• Massive hemorrhage • Abscess/purulent secretions • Bronchopleural cutaneous fistula • Bronchopleural fistula • Giant cyst or bullae (risk of rupture with PPV) • Major bronchial disruption or trauma • Cystic fibrosis • Lung transplant
Strong relative indications	Improve surgical exposure	• Thoracic aortic aneurysm • Pneumonectomy • Upper lobectomy • Lung volume reduction • Minimally invasive cardiac surgery • Video-assisted thoracoscopy
Weak relative indications		• Esophageal surgery • Middle and lower lobectomy • Mediastinal mass
Relative contraindications		• Unable to tolerate OLV • Intraluminal bronchial mass • Hemodynamic instability • Severe hypoxemia • Severe COPD • Severe pulmonary hypertension.

Sources: Ashok V, Francis J, A practical approach to adult one-lung ventilation, BJA Education, 2018;18(3): 69–74, doi:10.1016/j.bjae.2017.11.007, and Mehrotra M, Jain A, Single lung ventilation, *StatPearls*, https://www.ncbi.nlm.nih.gov/books/NBK538314/, published 2019.

Abbreviations: COPD, chronic obstructive pulmonary disease; OLV, one-lung ventilation; PPV, positive pressure ventilation.

Contraindications

Relative contraindications include patient being unable to tolerate OLV, intraluminal bronchial mass, hemodynamic instability, severe hypoxemia, severe chronic obstructive pulmonary disease, and severe pulmonary hypertension.[9] Relative contraindications are listed in Table 9.1.

The lung isolation techniques, including double-lumen tube, bronchial blocker, mainstem bronchial intubation etc., will be discussed in other chapter(s) of this book.

Intraoperative Monitoring

All American Society of Anesthesiologists standard basic anesthetic monitoring should be used in thoracic surgical procedures.[10] Several routine monitoring parameters are especially important in thoracic anesthesia, especially when OLV is applied (Table 9.2).

Ventilation Monitoring and Management

- SpO_2, $ETCO_2$, and Vmin: These are the three very important parameters that show the patient's ventilatory status. The ventilator setting for the specific patient can be adjusted based on these parameters. If SpO_2 and Vmin are both low, tidal volume, and/or ventilation rate can be increased to increase Vmin, thus improving SpO_2.
- Arterial blood gas analysis: Arterial blood gas will provide very useful information of PaO_2 and $PaCO_2$.
- Airway pressure.

Hemodynamic Monitoring

- Arterial blood pressure
- Cardiac output
- Stroke volume variation
- Heart rate

Table 9.2 Parameters Monitored during Thoracic Procedures

	Parameters
Ventilation monitoring	• SpO_2 • $ETCO_2$ • Vmin • Pairway
Hemodynamic monitoring	• MAP • HR/rhythm • CO/SV
Volume status	• CVP • SV/SVV/PPV • U/O
Anesthetic depth	• BIS

Abbreviations: BIS, bispectral index; CO, cardiac output; HR, heart rate; MAP, mean arterial pressure; PPV, pulse pressure variation; SV, stroke volume; SVV, stroke volume variation; U/O, urine output.

Management of Intraoperative Hypoxemia

FiO_2

If hypoxemia develops during thoracic procedure, increasing FiO_2 is one of the maneuvers to treat hypoxemia Sometimes adding some air will help improve hypoxemia by introducing nitrogen into alveoli to minimize absorption atelectasis (Table 9.3).

Positive End Expiratory Pressure

Increase in positive end expiratory pressure (PEEP) often can improve oxygenation by recruiting more alveoli into participation of oxygenation. However, PEEP can be a "double-sided sword", because PEEP may increase shunt in the down-side lung while recruiting more alveoli for oxygenation in the ventilated lung (Table 9.3).

I:E ratio

Oxygenation takes place during inspiration. Increase in the inspiratory-to-expiratory time (I:E) ratio will simply give more time for oxygenation (Table 9.3).

Goal-Directed Fluid Management

Hypovolemia results in insufficient oxygen delivery and flow-dependent organ dysfunction, whereas hypervolemia leads to pulmonary interstitial edema with impaired oxygen diffusion

Table 9.3 Management of Hypoxemia during One-Lung Ventilation

Increase FiO_2	Increase FiO_2 can often improve oxygenation, but 100%FiO_2 may lead to absorption atelectasis
PEEP	PEEP is a double-sided sword; it can recruit more alveoli to participate oxygenation in non-operative side but it may also increase shunting from non-operative side to operative side
Increase I/E ratio	Oxygenation occurs during inspiration, increase I:E Ratio will potentially help oxygenation
Suction of DLT	If secretions, blood, mucus etc in airway or DLT, suction is very effective
DLT positioning	If DLT shifts position, ventilation and/or lung isolation will be affected
Operative side CPAP	By applying low flow CPAP to operative often improves oxygenation, however it may affect surgical field exposure.
Intermittent two-lung ventilation	If previously described measures not improving oxygenation adequately, intermittent two-lung ventilation is the last resort

CPAP, continuous positive airway pressure; DLT, double-lumen tube; I:E ratio, inspiratory-to-expiratory time; PEEP, positive end-expiratory pressure.

and poor collagen regeneration. The cardiovascular measurements such as stroke volume, stroke volume variations, or pulse pressure variations, along with the application of algorithms and other volume assessment strategies, were used to maximize cardiac output and oxygen delivery and minimize perioperative complications. These parameters can be measured noninvasively as well as invasively (see Table 9.4).[11,12]

Nonintubating Technique for Thoracic Surgical Procedures

Traditionally, all thoracic surgery patients are intubated with an endotracheal tube/double-lumen tube after induction of general anesthesia. However, a nonintubating technique is gaining popularity in recent years. It can be used in general anesthesia with a supraglottic device such as a laryngeal mask airway. Regional anesthesia, such as thoracic epidural anesthesia and intravenous sedation techniques can also avoid endotracheal intubation.

Nonintubating Anesthetic Options for Thoracic Procedure

The main goal is achieving an overall improvement of patients' management and outcomes by avoiding the side-effects related to endotracheal intubation and one-lung ventilation (Figure 9.1). The benefits include reduced postoperative morbidity, faster discharge, decreased hospital costs and a globally reduced perturbation of the patient's well-being. Meta-analysis of collected results suggested that nonintubating general anesthesia for thoracic procedures can reduce operative morbidity and hospital stay when compared to equipollent procedures performed under general anesthesia.[13]

Table 9.4 Hemodynamic Parameters for Volume and Goal-Directed Therapy

Monitoring Parameters	Application in GDT
SV	SV↓ due to hypovolemia, based on Sterling curve. HR↑ as compensatory response.
CO	CO↓ in hypovolemia if no contractility and HR↑
EDLVV/EDLVP	EDLVV likely the best indicator of volume status. EDLVP is often used as parameter of LV volume status instead.
U/O	The oldest indicator of volume status, still useful
SVV	The most commonly used parameter for Goal-directed fluid therapy
PPV	Also used in goal-directed fluid therapy

Abbreviations: CO, cardiac output; EDLVP, end-diastolic left ventricular pressure; EDLVV, end-diastolic left ventricular volume; HR, heart rate; PPV, pulse pressure variation; SV, stroke volume; SVV, stroke volume variation; U/O, urine output.

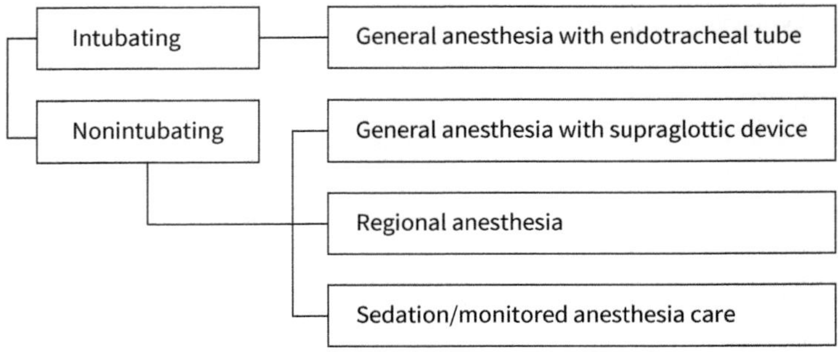

Figure 9.1 Anesthetic options for thoracic surgery.

Indications of Sedation for Thoracic Procedures

See Table 9.5 for indications of sedation for thoracic procedures.

Table 9.5 Indications of Sedation for Thoracic Procedures

Type of surgery	Specific procedures
Surgery on the pleural space	• Drainage of pleural effusion • Pleurodesis under TEA, thoracic paravertebral and local anesthesia • Pleurostomy under TEA • Decortication under TEA or paravertebral block • Treatment of pneumothorax under TEA, including pleurectomy • Empyema drainage under epidural or paravertebral block (9); • Bleb resection
Surgery on the lung	• Pneumonectomy under TEA • Lobectomy via thoracotomy and thoracoscopy under TEA • Bilobectomy under TEA • Wedge resection under TEA or LA • Thoracoscopic lobectomy and segmentectomy under TEA • Lung metastasis resection under TEA • Lung volume reduction surgery and bullectomy under TEA
Biopsies	• Anterior mediastinal mass biopsy • Pleural/ lung biopsy under TEA
Surgery in mediastinum	• Pericardial window • Tracheal resection with cervical epidural C7 to T1 (with local anesthetic to blunt cough response) • Thymectomy under TEA

Source: Kiss G, Castillo M. Nonintubated anesthesia in thoracic surgery: general issues. *Ann Transl Med.* 2015;3(8):110. doi:10.3978/j.issn.2305-5839.2015.04.21

Abbreviations: LA, local anesthesia; TEA, thoracic epidural analgesia.

Table 9.6 Multimodal Analgesia in Thoracic Surgery

Pharmacologic approach	Nonsteroidal anti-inflammatory	Intravenous: diclofenac, ibuprofen Oral: celecoxib, indomethacin, aspirin
	Acetaminophen	Intravenous Oral Rectal
	Opioid	Fentanyl Hydromorphone Morphine, etc
	Other	Gabapentinoids, ketamine etc
Nonpharmacologic approach	Thoracic neuraxial block	Thoracic epidural Intrathecal opioid
	Intercostal block	Transcutaneous approach Thoracoscopic approach
	Truncal block	Paravertebral block Erector spinae plane Serratus anterior plane block Sternal block

Sources: Liu H, Emelife PI, Prabhakar A, et al, Regional anesthesia considerations for cardiac surgery, *Best Pract Res Clin Anaesthesiol*, 2019;33(4):387–406, doi:10.1016/j.bpa.2019.07.008, and Thompson C, French DG, Costache I, Pain management within an enhanced recovery program after thoracic surgery, *J Thorac Dis*. 2018;10(Suppl 32):S3773–S3780, doi:10.21037/jtd.2018.09.112.

Postoperative Analgesia

Multimodal Analgesia

Postoperative analgesia is critical for a successful thoracic procedure, especially when enhanced recovery protocol is implemented. Multimodal analgesia is the analgesic approach most thoracic surgery programs adopt. Multimodal analgesia involves using intravenous analgesics such as nonsteroidal anti-inflammatory agents, acetaminophen, opioids, other pharmacologic agents, as well as thoracic neuraxial approaches such as thoracic epidural analgesia, intercostal blocks, and truncal blocks, as shown in Table 9.6.

Summary

In this chapter we describe the anesthetic management techniques for common thoracic surgical procedures. Ventilation and hemodynamic monitoring and management are critical for thoracic surgery. We listed the most commonly used modalities for ventilation and hemodynamic monitoring and introduced management strategies for intraoperative hypoxemia. Anesthetic options, especially newer nonintubating techniques for thoracic surgical procedures, are also discussed. Goal-directed fluid therapy is increasingly being emphasized in thoracic surgery care, and multimodal analgesia is becoming the norm of postoperative analgesia in the perioperative care of these patients.

References

1. Matas R. Intralaryngeal insufflation. *JAMA*. 1900;34:1468–1473.
2. Brodsky JB, Lemmens HJM. The history of anesthesia for thoracic surgery. *Minerva Anestesiol.* 2007;73(10):513–524.
3. Rovenstine EA. Anaesthesia for intrathoracic surgery: the endotracheal and endobronchial techniques. *Surg Gynecol Obstet.* 1936;63:325–330.
4. White GM. A new double lumen tube. *Br J Anaesth.* 1960;32:232–234.
5. He J, Liu J, Zhu C, et al. Expert consensus on spontaneous ventilation video-assisted thoracoscopic surgery in primary spontaneous pneumothorax (Guangzhou). *Ann Transl Med.* 2019;7(20):518. doi:10.21037/atm.2019.10.08
6. Caruselli M, Michel F. Thoracic spinal anaesthesia: an interesting alternative to general anaesthesia. *Minerva Anestesiol.* 2020;86(3):244–246. doi:10.23736/S0375-9393.19.14117-X
7. Liu H, Emelife PI, Prabhakar A, et al. Regional anesthesia considerations for cardiac surgery. *Best Pract Res Clin Anaesthesiol.* 2019;33(4):387–406. doi:10.1016/j.bpa.2019.07.008
8. Ashok V, Francis J. A practical approach to adult one-lung ventilation. *BJA Education.* 2018;18(3):69e74. doi:10.1016/j.bjae.2017.11.007
9. Mehrotra M, Jain A. Single lung ventilation. *StatPearls.* https://www.ncbi.nlm.nih.gov/books/NBK538314/. Published 2019.
10. American Association for Anesthesiologists. Standards for basic anesthetic monitoring. https://www.asahq.org/standards-and-guidelines/standards-for-basic-anesthetic-monitoring. Published October 21, 1986. Amended October 28, 2015.
11. Licker M, Triponez F, Ellenberger C, Karenovics W. Fluid therapy in thoracic surgery: a zero-balance target is always best! *Turk J Anaesthesiol Reanim.* 2016;44(5):227–229. doi:10.5152/TJAR.2016.006
12. Feng S, Yang S, Xiao W, Wang X, Yang K, Wang T. Effects of perioperative goal-directed fluid therapy combined with the application of alpha-1 adrenergic agonists on postoperative outcomes: a systematic review and meta-analysis. *BMC Anesthesiol.* 2018;18:113. doi:10.1186/s12871-018-0564-y
13. Tacconi F, Pompeo E. Non-intubated video-assisted thoracic surgery: where does evidence stand? *J Thorac Dis.* 2016;8(Suppl 4): S364–S375. doi:10.21037/jtd.2016.04.39
14. Kiss G, Castillo M. Nonintubated anesthesia in thoracic surgery: general issues. *Ann Transl Med.* 2015;3(8):110. doi:10.3978/j.issn.2305-5839.2015.04.21
15. Thompson C, French DG, Costache I. Pain management within an enhanced recovery program after thoracic surgery. *J Thorac Dis.* 2018;10(Suppl 32):S3773–S3780. doi:10.21037/jtd.2018.09.112

10
Bronchoscopy and Mediastinoscopy Procedures

Justin W. Wilson

Introduction

Thoracic and diagnostic procedures such as bronchoscopy and mediastinoscopy are fairly common, especially for patients with thoracic cancer. The typical surgical progression for thoracic cancer patients is performance of bronchoscopy to demonstrate airway anatomy and check tumor burden throughout the airway and then proceed with mediastinoscopy to sample mediastinal lymph nodes and send to pathology; if the nodes are negative for cancer then subsequent tumor resection is warranted. Standard preoperative workup includes the usual preoperative labs (hematology and chemistry), electrocardiogram, chest X-ray, and computed tomography (CT) scan to determine the location of the tumor, especially relative to adjoining structures. In chapter we discuss bronchoscopy and mediastinoscopy in detail and the difficulties and challenges these patients can present from the anesthetic perspective, including preoperative and intraoperative management.

Bronchoscopy

Bronchoscopy is utilized for diagnostic and therapeutic interventions, as well as confirmation of endotracheal tube (ETT) placement. For bronchoscopy, mortality is minimal while morbidity may include barotrauma, airway obstruction, pneumothorax, hemorrhage, perforation and laceration (airways and esophagus), tooth damage, pneumomediastinum, and airway fire if laser or electrocautery is utilized.

Interventional pulmonology has pushed the locations from the operating room to remote anesthetic locations. This has evolved our anesthetic practice and frequently we are called on to treat sicker patients (American Society of Anesthesiologists Physical Status III–V) that we traditionally have cared for in the operating room. Most patients presenting to the interventional pulmonology suite present with some form of central airway obstruction that affects the large bronchi or the trachea, airway obstruction can be intrinsic, extrinsic, or mixed compression.[1] In addition to anesthesia delivery and monitoring equipment, the interventional suite should have advanced airway equipment such as difficult intubation cart and jet ventilation capabilities. Reconsideration of remote locations can include significant comorbidities, predicted need for postop ventilation or prolonged recovery from anesthesia, and multispecialty involvement in the case.[2] Bronchoscopy can be further subdivided into rigid and flexible bronchoscopy.

Rigid Bronchoscopy

Rigid bronchoscopy is utilized to examine hemoptysis, intrabronchial procedures: mechanical dilation of the tracheobronchial tree, tumor debridement, and removal of foreign bodies. Indications for rigid bronchoscopy usually include the preoperative diagnosis of lung carcinoma, hemoptysis, foreign body obstruction, and respiratory papillomatosis. Ventilation strategies for use during rigid bronchoscopy include apneic oxygenation, spontaneous assisted ventilation, controlled ventilation (closed system), manual jet ventilation (Sanders jet ventilator), and high frequency jet ventilation (HFJV).[3]

Flexible Bronchoscopy

Flexible bronchoscopy is used to diagnose and evaluate multiple conditions, most commonly bronchial neoplasm. Flexible bronchoscopy is usually accomplished with sedation and topical anesthesia without utilizing an anesthesiologist. The benefit over rigid bronchoscopy is the ability to examine peripheral lung out to fifth division bronchi; it doesn't require neck extension from the patient and is less stimulating to the patient. In the typical surgical scenario for thoracic tumors, flexible bronchoscopy is performed first, followed by mediastinoscopy, and subsequent resection of lung cancer. Bronchoscopy in the previous situation is used to evaluate the extent of thoracic carcinoma and rule out contralateral lung involvement. For more extensive procedures such as laser ablations, balloon dilation, and stent placement, a general anesthetic will be required as they are more stimulating for a patient. Flexible bronchoscopy is also utilized to facilitate endotracheal intubations for patients with difficult airways. One limitation of the flexible bronchoscope is the small suction channel; this limits the amount of secretions or blood that can be suctioned out of view. When general anesthesia is required, at minimum an 8.0 tube should be utilized to decrease auto positive end-expiratory pressure (PEEP) and allow passage of the flexible bronchoscope. It's important to remember if the auto-PEEP effect can cause hypotension and ultimately barotrauma. If a <8.0 ETT is utilized, use of a pediatric flexible bronchoscope may be indicated to facilitate adequate ventilation (Figure 10.1).

Anesthetic Management for Bronchoscopy

Patients presenting with preoperative hypoxemia (PaO_2 <70 mmHg) and hypercapnia (PCO_2 >45 mmHg) indicate significant pulmonary impairment and likely at increased risk. During these procedures, expect hypoxemia and hypoventilation, as well as the complications that arise from them. Whenever lasers are utilized during the procedure, the FiO_2 should be less than 40% to decrease the risk of airway fire. Premedication with antisialogogues, typically glycopyrrolate, is used to decrease secretions. Premedication with narcotics and benzodiazepines should be used sparingly in patients with limited pulmonary reserve. Bronchoscopy is

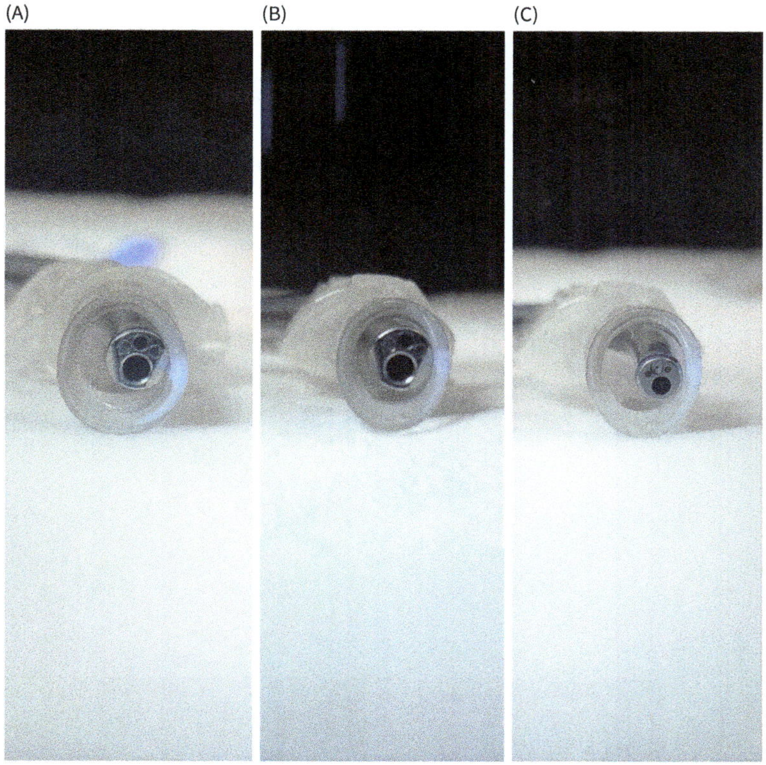

Figure 10.1 Various endotracheal tube sizes with different sizes of bronchoscopes. A: 8.0 ETT with an adult bronchoscope. B: 7.0 ETT with an adult bronchoscope. C: 7.0 ETT with a pediatric bronchoscope.

highly stimulating and usually requires a higher dose of anesthetics; the use of short-acting agents is preferred to make sure the patient can spontaneously ventilate and protect their airway at the end of the procedure. Keep in mind, patients with lung or mediastinal tumors can have extrathoracic manifestations through tumor secretion of hormones or hormone like substances, otherwise known as paraneoplastic syndromes.[4] For instance, a more common manifestation is myasthenic (Eaton–Lambert) syndrome, which is a proximal myopathy associated with small cell lung cancer. There is a reduction in acetylcholine release from the presynaptic motor neurons, and thus patients will be resistant to depolarizing muscle relaxation and sensitive to non-depolarizing muscle relaxants (Table 10.1).[4]

Rigid Bronchoscopy

Rigid bronchoscopy is highly stimulating and a general anesthetic is usually required, and utilizing a total intravenous technique is typical, as is utilizing drugs with rapid on and off effects. Ventilation is through the sidearm of the bronchoscope (when the lens is attached), a cuff is not present on the rigid bronchoscope, so a leak of anesthetic gases will likely be present; high fresh gas flow as well as high volumes may be required (Figure 10.2). Using total

Table 10.1 Extrathoracic Manifestations of Thoracic Tumors

Endocrine	Hyperparathyroidism Cushing's syndrome SIADH Carcinoid syndrome
Neuromuscular	Myasthenia gravis Myasthenic (Eaton-Lambert) syndrome Peripheral neuropathy Autonomic neuropathy
Hematological	Anemia Thrombocytopenia Thrombosis

SIADH = syndrome of inappropriate antidiuretic hormone secretion.

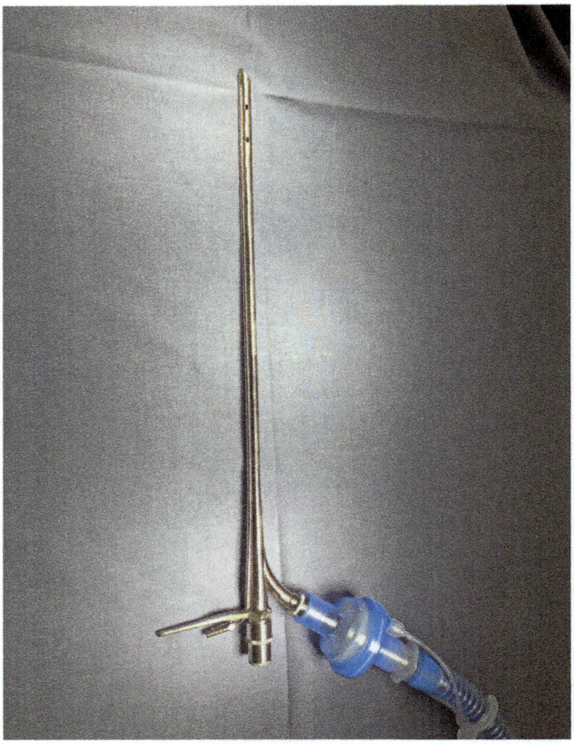

Figure 10.2 Rigid bronchoscope with vent circuit attached.

intravenous techniques helps keep a constant level of anesthesia while minimizing room pollution of anesthetic gases. When the lens is not attached, it results in an open-ended bronchoscope with a large leak of gas necessitating the use of specialized ventilation strategies such as HFJV and low frequency jet ventilation via a Sanders injector (Figure 10.3). The various modes of jet ventilation depend on the Bernoulli principle, which allows the use high flow and low pressure to ventilate and oxygenate with minimal side effects. When jet ventilation is utilized, there is a greater need for muscle relaxation to move the chest wall. When using the Sanders injector, keep in mind the entrainment of room air due to the Venturi effect, which drops the FiO_2 to around 80% at the trachea.[5] The Sanders jet ventilator is connected to the sidearm of bronchoscope; this allows for the generation of 55 cm H_2O with a driving pressure of 30 psi. Start with an initial 30 psi and gradual increase to max of 50 psi, monitoring for chest rise and fall. While using the Sanders jet ventilator, it is important to monitor for chest rise, which helps indicate the adequacy of ventilation, and also chest fall to monitor egress of air. This is important to prevent complications including barotrauma and pneumothorax. Utilizing a specialized ventilator for HFJV (10–15 Hz) decreases barotrauma due to the ventilator halting the inspiratory phase in the presence of high airway pressures; another benefit is it allows for humidification of oxygen, decreasing dryness of airway mucosa. Impediments to HFJV include the requirement of high minute ventilation (around 120 breaths/min) and the risk of hypercapnia.

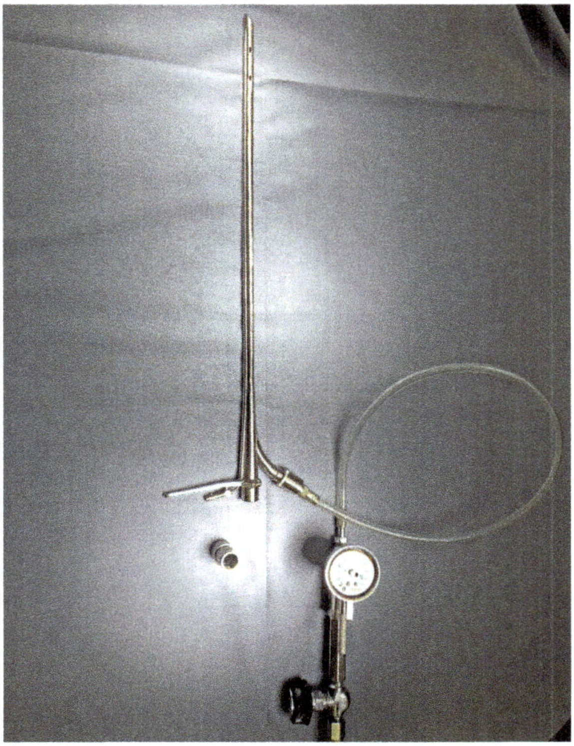

Figure 10.3 Rigid bronchoscope without lens and a Sanders jet injector attached.

Flexible Bronchoscopy

Poiseuille's law states that flow is directly proportional to the fourth power of the radius; thus, small changes in diameter of the ETT will have a large impact on tidal volume delivered. Using an ETT of sufficient size allows the patient to be ventilated adequately without high peak airway pressures and exceeding the pressure limit on the ventilator. The other concern is the limited egress of air from the ETT caused by the flexible bronchoscope; thus, PEEP should be turned off during the procedure. Similar to the rigid bronchoscope, jet ventilation can be achieved through the suction port of the flexible bronchoscope if necessary.

Sedation with various modes of local anesthetic, including topicalization and blocks, is mostly utilized for anesthesia during flexible bronchoscopy. Stimulating procedures (laser ablations, stenting, dilation, etc.) require a general anesthetic with an elbow (right angle) adapter and ETT or laryngeal mask airway (Figure 10.4). The benefit of the laryngeal mask airway is it allows for the examination of the larynx. Before topicalizing the airway, premedicate the patient with an antisialogogue (glycopyrrolate). Inhaled nebulized lidocaine (4–6 mL of 4% in a nebulizer) is a simple way to topicalize the airway; other means of topicalization include lidocaine ointment, local anesthetic droppers, atomizers, and sprays. Keep in mind the maximal does of lidocaine is 5 mg/kg, up to 300 mg without epinephrine, and with epinephrine 7 mg/kg up to 500 mg. Regional anesthesia can also be utilized with glossopharyngeal and superior laryngeal nerve blocks with a transtracheal injection to

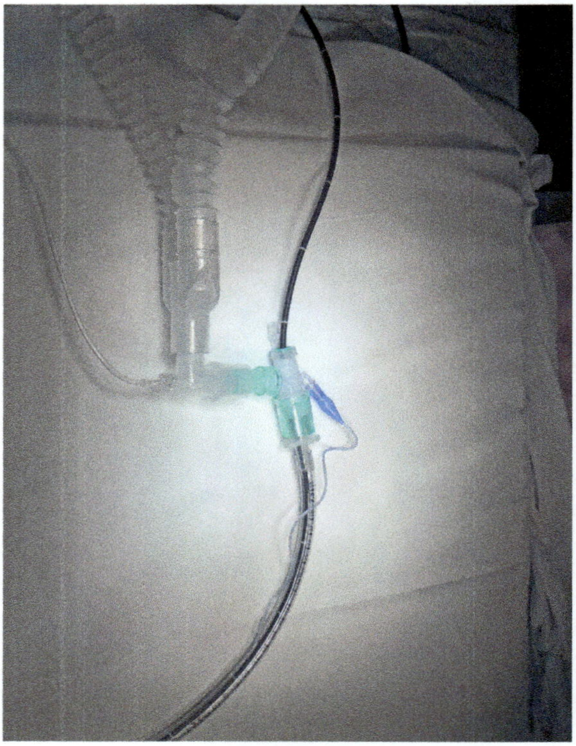

Figure 10.4 Flexible bronchoscope through ETT with right angle adapter.

topicalize below the vocal cords. Anesthesia of the larynx and trachea is relatively contraindicated in patients with a full stomach due to suppression of airway reflexes and aspiration risk. Topicalization and a general anesthetic can be combined, usually decreasing the general anesthetic requirement.

Mediastinoscopy

A mediastinoscope is a Miller-like blade that is used to get under the sternum and into the mediastinum, giving the operator a small field of view into the anatomic subdivisions of the mediastinum (Figure 10.5). Mediastinoscopy is utilized to biopsy mediastinal lymph nodes, and the most common indication is bronchogenic carcinoma; other indications for mediastinoscopy include lymphadenopathy associated with lymphoma and sarcoidosis, and a biopsy of the tissue for diagnosis, such as suspected tumors and infectious disease processes. Mediastinoscopy remains the mainstay for staging due to its high sensitivity (>80%) and specificity (100%).[6] Contraindications include thoracic aneurysm and superior vena cava (SVC) obstruction as they impair anatomy increasing risk of vessel injury and bleeding. While relative contraindications include previous mediastinoscopy, and radiation, this is due to risk of adhesion and increased bleeding. Mortality has been reported as <0.1%, and morbidity includes bleeding, pneumothorax, vocal cord paralysis, esophageal perforation, pleural perforation, and tracheal laceration.

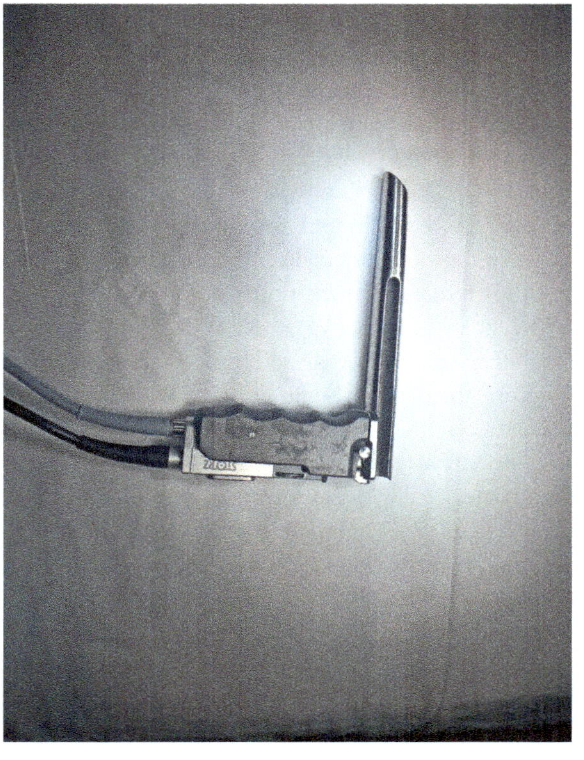

Figure 10.5 Mediastinoscope.

Anesthetic Management for Mediastinoscopy

Most patients that present for mediastinoscopy are smokers with multiple comorbidities such as pulmonary disease, hypertension, coronary artery disease, and peripheral vascular disease. The most challenging aspect of patient care is the potential presence of an anterior mediastinal mass and the possibility of catastrophic airway obstruction or cardiovascular collapse after induction of general anesthesia. Always question the patient on the ability to lay supine and the presence of cough or dyspnea. On physical exam, check for presence of cyanosis, wheezing, cough, stridor, and dyspnea both upright and supine. Preoperative indicators for increased respiratory problems include cardiopulmonary signs (see previous discussion), combined obstructive and restrictive picture, peek expiratory flow rate <40%, and tracheal diameter <50% on CT scan.[7] If the patient presents for mediastinoscopy due to tissue diagnosis of anterior mediastinal mass, the patient should be first referred to interventional radiology for percutaneous needle biopsy. Also check for signs of SVC syndrome (caval obstruction): shortness of breath, cough, edema, venous engorgement of head, neck and upper body, supine dyspnea (orthopnea), headache, and mental status change. If SVC syndrome is present, the airway may be significantly swollen and can bleed even from minor trauma; an awake fiber optic intubation is usually warranted. Preoperative CT scans will demonstrate whether SVC syndrome and anterior mediastinal mass are present. Pulmonary function testing can help delineate variable intrathoracic or extrathoracic obstruction.

If preoperative imaging is suspicious or physical exam warrants (symptomatic in supine position), consider an awake fiberoptic intubation. Loss of muscle tone can precipitate hemodynamic collapse or airway obstruction in asymptomatic patients; use short-acting neuromuscular blockers (succinylcholine) or have sugammadex available to reverse amino-steroid non-depolarizing neuromuscular blockade (rocuronium, vecuronium). A mask induction with inhalation agent (e.g., sevoflurane) or various other intravenous techniques can be utilized to keep the patient spontaneously breathing and prevent hemodynamic collapse or airway obstruction. A surgeon familiar with rigid bronchoscopy should be available to bypass obstruction if warranted, and for high-risk patients where hemodynamic collapse or airway obstruction is highly likely, cardiopulmonary bypass should be utilized. For patients with SVC syndrome, there can be many collaterals and an increase in surgical blood loss; also, with impaired venous return from the upper body, lower body intravenous access is warranted.

Regarding intraoperative monitors, in addition to standard American Society of Anesthesiologists monitors, the patient should have the noninvasive blood pressure cuff on the left arm and a radial arterial line (if used) or pulse oximeter on the right arm. This is due to the possibility of innominate artery compression and impaired cerebral perfusion during surgery, which can easily be detected with the previously described monitor setup (Figure 10.6). A reinforced ETT should be utilized to decrease the chance of kinking. Major bleeding is the most obvious, although relatively rare complication (about 0.4%), with the most likely sources being innominate artery and vein, azygos vein and aorta.[8] Thus, large bore intravenous access should be acquired, and type and cross-matched blood should be available. Other complications that can occur are venous air embolism if the head of bed is elevated to decrease venous congestion, especially in spontaneously breathing patients. In addition, recurrent laryngeal nerve injury can occur during surgery, and if suspected, the vocal cords

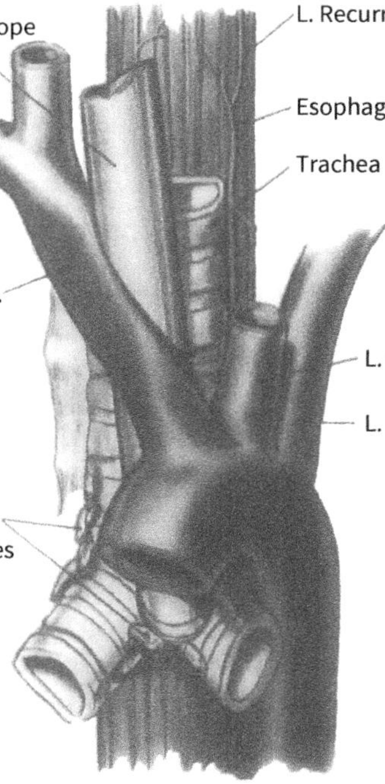

Figure 10.6 Mediastinoscope positioned next to great vessels during mediastinoscopy. (Permission)

should be inspected post intubation. If bilateral vocal cord injury occurs, it may result in airway obstruction, making mask ventilation ineffective and requiring reintubation.

Conclusion

Pulmonic and thoracic procedures continue to be dynamic and ever-changing. As these procedures are being transitioned outside the operating room and into remote anesthesia sites, the anesthetic plan will vary depending on the needs of the proceduralists, the extent of the patient's lung disease including specialized lung ventilation strategies, and, lastly, other patient comorbidities. The one constant through all these changes is that anesthesiologists will continue to be at the forefront, leading the way.

References

1. Pawlowski J. Anesthetic considerations for interventional pulmonary procedures. *Curr Opin Anaesthesiol.* 2013;26:6–12.
2. Jose R, Shaefi S, Navani N. Anesthesia for bronchoscopy. *Curr Opin Anaesthesiol.* 2014;27:453–457.
3. Pathak V, Welsby I, Mahmood K, Wahidi M, MacIntyre N, Schofer S. Ventilation and anesthetic approaches for rigid bronchoscopy. *Ann Am Thorac Soc.* 2014;11(4):628–634.
4. Ahmed-Nusrath A, Swanevelder J. Anesthesia for mediastinoscopy. *Cont Ed Anaesth Crit Care Pain.* 2007;7(1):6–9.

5. Evans E, Biro P, Bedford N. Jet ventilation. *Cont Ed Anaesth Crit Care Pain.* 2007;7(1):2–5.
6. Hammound ZT, Anderson RC, Meyers BF, et al. The current role of mediastinoscopy in the evaluation of thoracic disease. *J Thorac Cardiovasc Surg.* 1999;118(5):894–899.
7. Bechard P, Letourneau L, Lacasse Y, Cote D, Bussieres J. Perioperative cardiorespiratory complications in adults with mediastinal mass. *Anesthesiology.* 2004;100(4):826–834.
8. Park BJ, Flores R, Downey RJ, Bains M, Rusch V. Management of major haemorrhage during mediastinoscopy. *J Thorac Cardiovasc Surg.* 2003;126:726–731.

11
Anterior Mediastinal Masses

Kevin Sidoran, Hanan Tafesse, Tiffany D. Perry, and Tricia Desvarieux

Mr. F is a 54-year-old male with a history of type II diabetes mellitus and hypertension who presents to the emergency department with worsening orthopnea over the past 2 months. Vital signs are significant for mild tachycardia to 95. On exam, he appears plethoric with facial and upper extremity edema. His cardiac exam has regular rate and rhythm, lungs are clear to auscultation bilaterally, and there are dilated superficial veins over his chest. Chest X-ray shows no opacities, and electrocardiogram, basic metabolic panel, complete blood count, and serum troponin are within normal limits.

Anatomy of the Mediastinum

The mediastinum extends from the thoracic inlet superiorly to the diaphragm inferiorly and is bound between the left and right pleural sac and lungs laterally, the sternum anteriorly, and the vertebral column posteriorly. It is divided into the superior and inferior mediastinum by a plane passing through the sternal angle and the fourth thoracic vertebra. The inferior mediastinum is then divided into the anterior mediastinum, which lies between the sternum and the heart; the middle mediastinum, which includes the heart, the major airways, blood vessels, and the esophagus; and the posterior mediastinum, which is between the posterior pericardial sac and the vertebral column. The anterior mediastinum contains the thymus, lymph nodes, vessels, and fat (Figures 11.1 and 11.2). In adults, lymphoma (both non-Hodgkin and Hodgkin types), thymoma, carcinomas (either primary or metastatic) and intrathoracic thyroid masses comprise the vast majority of mediastinal masses (Figures 11.3 and 11.4).[1] Considering the differences between pediatric and adult anatomy, weaker intercostal muscles, and lack of developed cartilage, the pediatric population has a higher mortality rate from anterior mediastinal masses.[2]

Signs and Symptoms

On computed tomography (CT) scan, it is found that Mr. F has an 8 × 9 cm mass in his anterior mediastinum. There is compression of his right ventricle (RV), superior vena cava (SVC), and dilated superficial veins on his chest and neck consistent with exam. Taking into account the patient's presentation and imaging results, the provider decides on a diagnosis of SVC syndrome.

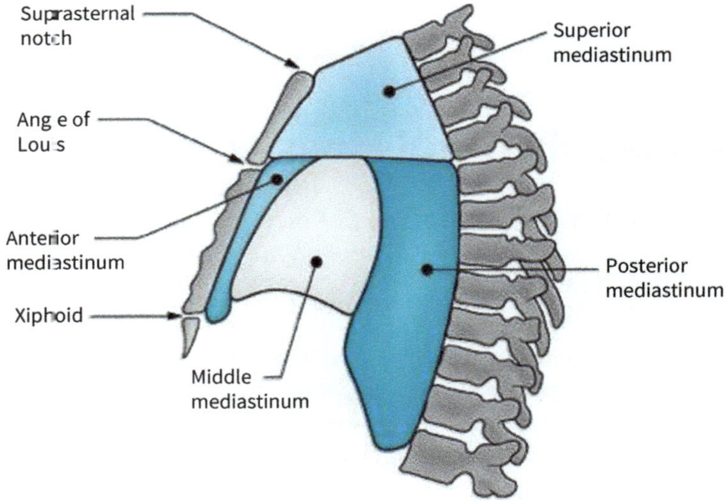

Figure 11.1 Divisions of the mediastinum. The anterior mediastinum is bordered anteriorly by the sternum, posteriorly by the heart, and laterally by the lungs.

Reprinted with permission from Bar-Yosef S. Mediastinal masses: implications for anesthesiologists. In: Barbeito A, Shaw AD, Grichnik K. eds. *Thoracic Anesthesia*. New York, NY: McGraw-Hill; 2012, Chapter 12.

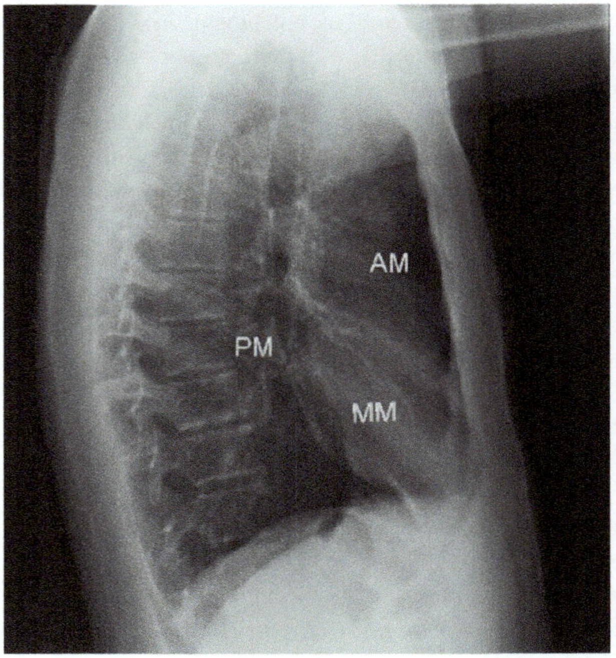

Figure 11.2 Lateral chest radiograph showing different divisions of the mediastinum.

Reprinted with permission from Blank RS, Souza DGD. Anesthetic management of patients with an anterior mediastinal mass: continuing professional development. *Can J Anesth*. 2011;58(9):853–867.

Abbreviations: AM, anterior mediastinum; MM, middle mediastinum; PM, posterior mediastinum.

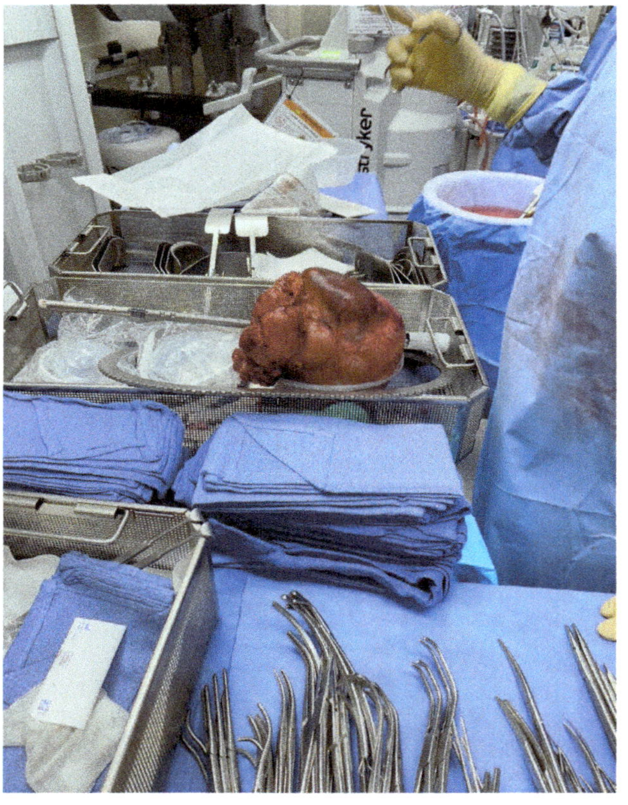

Figure 11.3 Resected thymoma.
Picture taken at the George Washington Hospital operating room.

Among the signs and symptoms which should alert anesthesiologists about increased perioperative risk are increased dyspnea or cough when supine and syncopal episode or pericardial effusion which may indicate an increased risk of cardiovascular complications.[3] Table 11.1 includes common signs and symptoms of an individual with anterior mediastinal mass.

Implications for Anesthesiologist

Preoperative Evaluation

The morning of surgery, Mr. F is hoarse with cough, chest pain and orthopnea when he is placed in the supine position for transportation to the operating room, and suddenly experiences a syncopal episode. The transport team raises the head of his bed, and he regains consciousness.

The anesthetic consideration for patients with anterior mediastinal mass will be different based on the individual anatomy, pathology, and proposed surgical procedure. All patients with anterior mediastinal mass should have a chest X-ray and chest CT scan before any surgical procedures. A chest X ray is used to calculate the ratio between the widest diameter of the mediastinal mass and the width of the thorax at T5–T6, also known as mediastinal

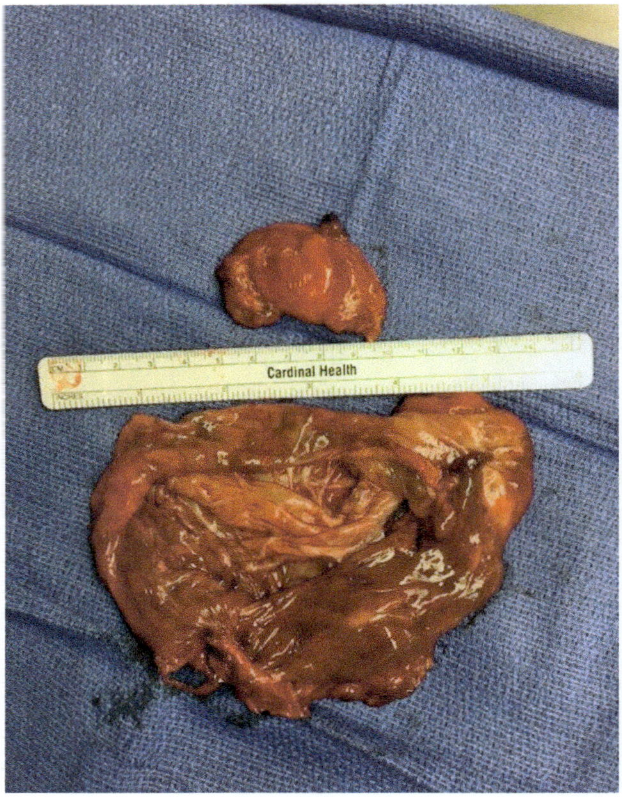

Figure 11.4 Resected thymic cyst.
Picture taken at the George Washington Hospital operating room.

thoracic ratio. A mediastinal thoracic ratio greater than 0.5 is associated with a higher incidence of post respiratory complications. Meanwhile, chest X-rays are not enough to assess involvement of the tracheobronchial tree accurately. Therefore, a CT scan is always necessary. On CT scan, a tracheal narrowing greater than 50% in cross-sectional area is associated with increased airway obstruction during anesthesia (Figures 11.5 and 11.6).

Table 11.1 Presenting Signs and Symptoms of Anterior Mediastinal Masses

Cardiovascular Compression	Airway Compression
Syncope	Orthopnea
Jugular venous distention	Cough
Dilated superficial veins	Chest fullness
Cyanosis	
Tachycardia	

Adapted from Pearson JK, Tan GM: Pediatric anterior mediastinal mass: a review article. *Semin Cardiothorac Vasc Anesth.* 2015;19:248–254.

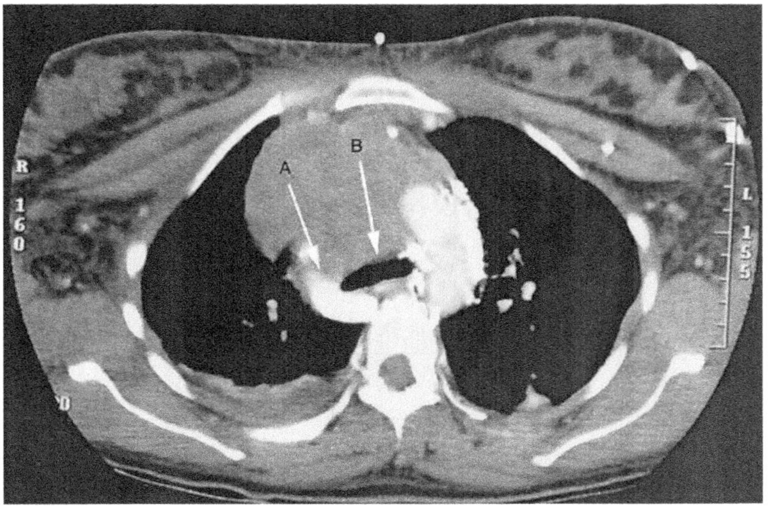

Figure 11.5 (A) Dilated azygos vein due to congestion from superior vena cava obstruction. (B) Tracheal compression (greater than 50%) immediately cephalad to the carina.

Reprinted with permission from Bar-Yosef S. Mediastinal masses: implications for anesthesiologists. In: Barbeito A, Shaw AD, Grichnik K. eds. *Thoracic Anesthesia.* New York, NY: McGraw-Hill; 2012, Chapter 12.

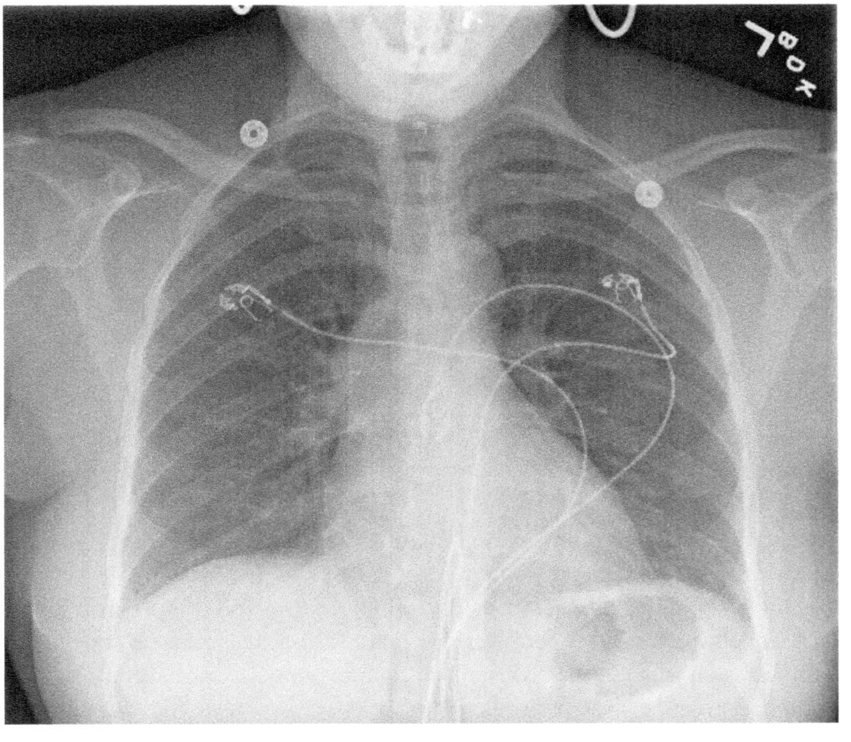

Figure 11.6 Chest X-ray showing right side mass and tracheal narrowing.

Image retrieved from George Washington University Hospital Radiology records.

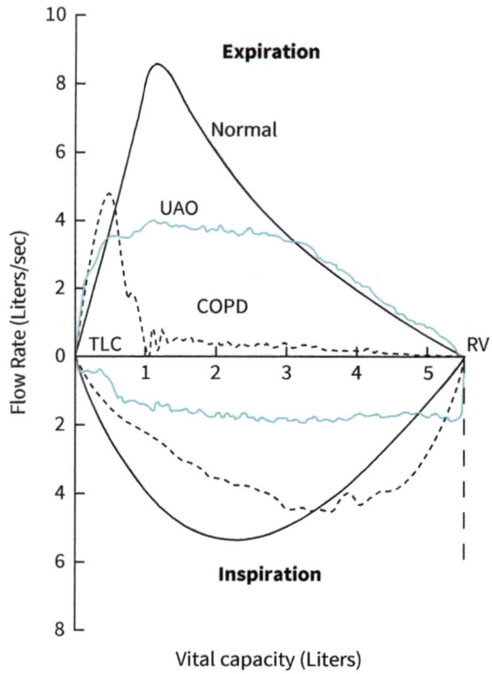

Figure 11.7 Flow-volume loops from a spirometry study of a normal subject, a patient with a fixed upper airway obstruction and a patient with chronic obstructive pulmonary disease. Note the reduction in both inspiratory and expiratory flows and the mid-expiratory flow plateau in the patient with upper airway obstruction.

Reprinted with permission from Bar-Yosef S. Mediastinal masses: implications for anesthesiologists. In: Barbeito A, Shaw AD, Grichnik K. eds. *Thoracic Anesthesia*. New York, NY: McGraw-Hill; 2012, Chapter 12.

Additionally, patients with cardiac symptoms should have a transthoracic echocardiogram to assess for cardiac, systemic, or pulmonary compromise. Although the benefit of preoperative flow-volume loops is not always clear, they are commonly ordered as part of the preoperative assessment. Specifically, an increased mid-expiratory plateau when changing from the upright to the supine position is thought to predict a variable intrathoracic airway obstruction and could be an indicator of people who are at increased risk of airway collapse (Figures 11.7 and 11.8).

A risk stratification of patients with anterior mediastinal mass has been proposed by Blank and de Souza[4]:

- *Low risk*: asymptomatic or mildly symptomatic, without postural symptoms or radiographic evidence of significant compression of structures.
- *Intermediate risk*: mild to moderate postural symptoms tracheal compression <50%.
- *High risk*: Severe postural symptoms, stridor, cyanosis, tracheal compression >50% or tracheal compression with associated bronchial compression, pericardial effusion, or SVC syndrome.

As illustrated in Table 11.2, to avoid anesthetic risk, perioperative plans should be based on the available imaging as well as preoperative assessment including history and physical of each individual patient. It is also important to have a multidisciplinary approach involving

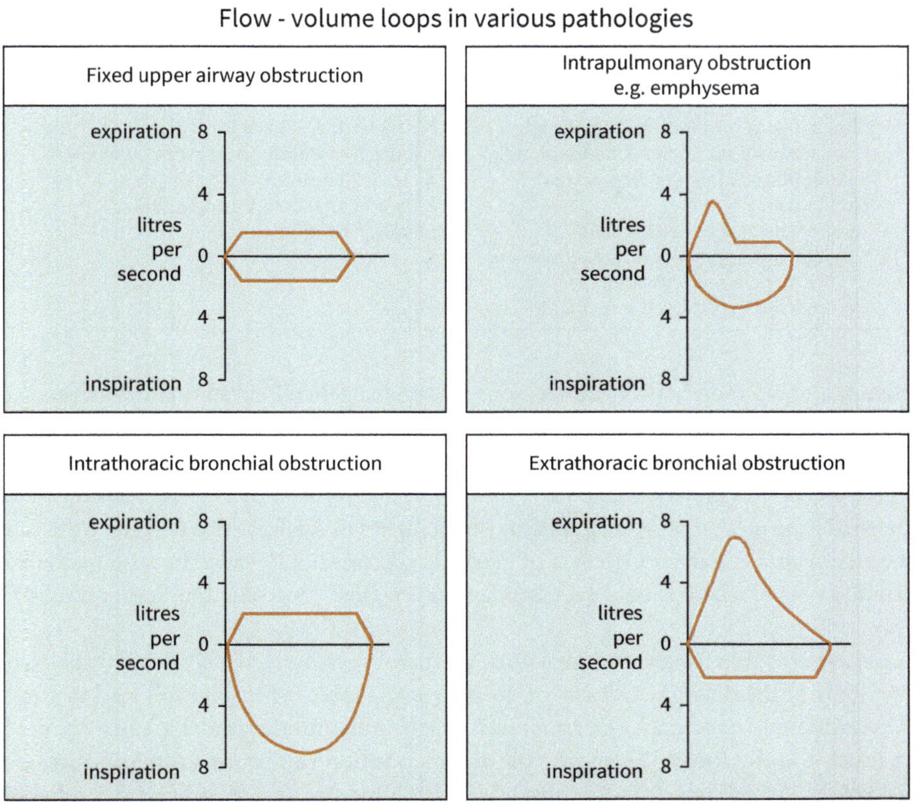

Figure 11.8 Flow volume in various pathologies.

cardiothoracic surgery, anesthesiology, and critical care pulmonology when taking care of a patient with an anterior mediastinal mass.

Induction

Upon induction with propofol, the end tidal CO_2 levels begin to drop, and peak inspiratory pressures rise higher than initial values. Bronchoscopy reveals total occlusion of the right mainstem bronchus, and a stent is placed.

Unexpected and often total airway obstruction can occur on induction of anesthesia in patients with an anterior mediastinal mass, even in patients who are asymptomatic. According

Table 11.2 Pre-Evaluation and Preparation

Risk Assessment	Anesthetics Risk
• Signs and symptoms • Radiographic data Computed tomography X-ray • Spirometry • Echocardiography	• Obstruction of major airway • Cardiac compression (tamponade effect)/Pericardial effusion • Compression of pulmonary artery or right ventricular outflow tract tachycardia • Superior vena cava compression (superior vena cava syndrome)

Table 11.3 Airway Management: Plan a Staged Induction

Mechanism	Options for Induction
• The change of positioning: from upright to supine position (increase tumor blood volume and size by increasing central blood volume • Awake state to anesthetized state • Spontaneous negative pressure ventilation to positive pressure ventilation • Unparalyzed to paralyzed muscular tone	• No induction → local • Awake fiberoptic bronchoscope (intubate distal to stenosis) • Staged IV or inhalation induction • Standard IV induction

to Neuman et al., there are various reasons that make general anesthesia dangerous. Lung volume is reduced as little as 500 to 1,500 mL; second, relaxation of bronchial smooth muscle leads to greater compressibility of the airway from the overlying mass. Moreover, loss of spontaneous diaphragmatic movement with paralysis induced by muscle relaxant reduces the normal transpleural pressure gradient, which dilates the airway. This decreases the caliber of the airway and enhances the effect of extrinsic compression.[5] Thus, the administration of neuromuscular blockers should be considerably weighed for induction and control of the airway.

Additionally, it has been shown that during general anesthesia, the cephalad displacement of the dome of the diagram and loss of the distending forces of inspiration lead to a reduction in pulmonary compliance and airway diameter and limit the available space for the trachea relative to the tumor. Moreover, the supine position can cause an increase in central blood volume, which may increase tumor blood volume size. On the other hand, it has been shown that positive pressure ventilation during induction is dangerous as the increased gas flow across a stenosis decreases intraluminal pressure, leading to further tendency to collapse (Table 11.3).[6] In conclusion, in the case where general anesthesia is required, spontaneous respiration and avoiding paralysis would preserve normal transpulmonary pressure and maintain airway patency.

Intubation

Blank and de Souza discuss that the appropriate strategy for airway management is defined by the anatomy of tracheobronchial obstruction.[4] Tracheal compression with an adequate segment of normal distal trachea usually permits the placement of an appropriately sized reinforced endotracheal tube beyond the site of obstruction. However, if the distal trachea, carina, and/or both mainstem bronchi are compressed, it may not be possible to pass an endotracheal tube beyond obstruction. In this case, rigid bronchoscopy can be used to secure the airway,[4] hence the need of a skilled operator in rigid bronchoscopy and pre-emptive planning with the surgical team. An awake fiberoptic intubation is useful for patients with mediastinal masses to avoid agents compromising respiratory mechanics, maintain airway reflexes, and ensure minimal changes in the forces maintaining tracheal patency. The fiberoptic allows direct visual assessment of the obstruction and of the proximal and distal airway.

Sedation

Intravenous agents that have both analgesic and sedative property with minimal respiratory depression are preferred for sedation and maintenance of spontaneous ventilation via endotracheal tube. Such agents include, among others, dexmedetomidine and ketamine. Additionally, decrease respiratory gas flow may result from an increase in turbulence distal to the site of obstruction. Helium oxygen is used to facilitate the induction of general anesthesia as it helps to promote laminar gas flow in patients with obstruction.[7] In case ventilation becomes difficult, options should include waking up the patient, changing to a rescue position, and using rigid bronchoscopy.

Positioning

The correct rescue position should be determined preoperatively and chosen based on the anatomic relationship between the mass and surrounding compressed structures. Rescue positions include upright, seated position; lateral decubitus; or prone position, depending on the anatomic relation with the mass and airway.[4]

Maintenance

Thirty minutes into the surgery, the patient is responding to surgical stimuli, so the anesthesiologist decides to administer a dose of rocuronium. After the paralytic is given, breath sounds are absent on the right, and peak inspiratory pressures begin to rise to the 40s and 50s.

Spontaneous Ventilation

As with the rest of anesthetic management, the maintenance phase will be approached individually based on patient pathology and the size and mass effect of the anterior mediastinal mass. As mentioned earlier, one of the major concerns during an anterior mediastinal mass procedure is airway collapse (Figure 11.5). Although other common causes of ventilatory failure, like tension pneumothorax and bronchospasm, should be considered, extrinsic obstruction from a mass must be the biggest concern in these cases. Physiologically, airway patency is largely dependent on the negative intrathoracic pressure exhibited by the chest. This takes into account the strength and effort of intercostal muscles. As a patient is paralyzed, the negative force and tension that the intercostals are able to exhibit decreases. This occurs along with a loss of elastic recoil of the chest, leading to an increased chance of cardiac and tracheobronchial compression. This has been shown in a study by Bergman that demonstrates a decreased functional residual capacity and end expiratory position of the diaphragm under paralysis with succinylcholine, indicating a cephalad displacement of the diaphragm with paralysis.[8] Taking the tension that intercostal muscles exhibit on breathing mechanics, positive pressure ventilation under paralysis has been shown to be difficult in several case studies, with spontaneous ventilation proving to be the safer method in pediatric and adult populations.[6,9,10] Although one-lung ventilation has been used on infants during resection of large mediastinal masses, this method has not been described in adults.[11] One unique method of ventilation in the setting of tracheobronchial compression is the use of Heliox in that it reduces the viscosity of air inhaled and would therefore reduce turbulence of air flow that may be caused by airway compression, allowing for improved ventilation.[7]

Access and Extracorporeal Membrane Oxygenation

Given the risk of venous obstruction, and ultimately SVC syndrome, in these cases, access is preferred in the lower extremities. For particularly tenuous cases, extra corporeal membrane oxygenation (ECMO) has been explored as a possible safety net on induction and maintenance.[3,4] There are a couple of reports on having ECMO on standby during cases of large anterior mediastinal mass resections,[12] as well as a couple cases where ECMO was used in these cases successfully.[13–15] Bypass has also been used in similar cases where there is high risk of ventilatory and/or cardiovascular collapse such as severe compression or difficult resection is anticipated (Figure 11.9).

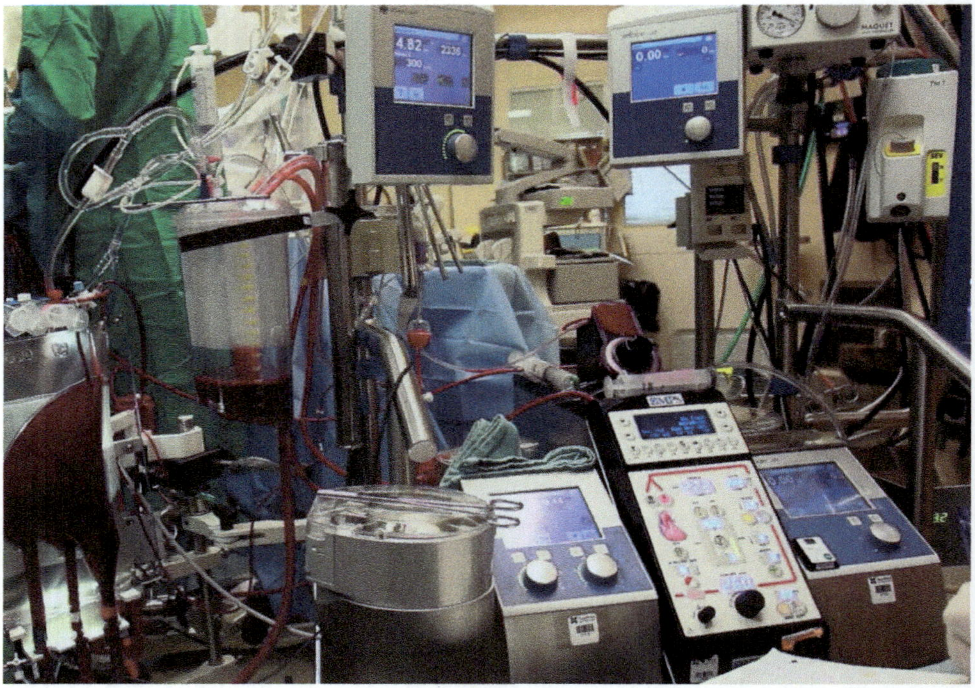

Figure 11.9 Bypass/extra corporeal membrane oxygenation set up in the operating room.
Image retrieved from George Washington University Hospital.

Complications: Cardiovascular Collapse

As discussed previously, the mediastinum contains the most vital components of circulation, including the SVC, heart, pulmonary artery, and aorta. If any of these structures are compressed to a point of severe obstruction of flow, it could prove fatal for a patient. When masses are large enough, compression on the great vessels and the heart can reduce Cardiac Index and Stroke Index, as demonstrated in animal models.[16] Although several case reports with noted cardiovascular compression did not have any complications of mortality or complications,[12,17,18] there have been cases reported that resulted in cardiovascular collapse.[3,13,15,19,20] Similar complications have also been noted in the pediatric population.[21–25] It has also been shown in isolated cases that intraoperative monitoring with transesophageal echocardiography can be useful in anterior mediastinal mass resection where cardiac compromise is present based on symptomology or anticipated based on surgical manipulation (Figures 11.10–11.12).[26] Management must take into account the multiple pathophysiology of the case. Given that ventricular outflow obstruction can lead to RV failure, vasopressors are typically used to preserve coronary flow. Some of the circulatory compromise may be due in part to reduced preload, which can be treated with fluid, although this should be done conservatively given that too much fluid would exacerbate any existing RV dysfunction.

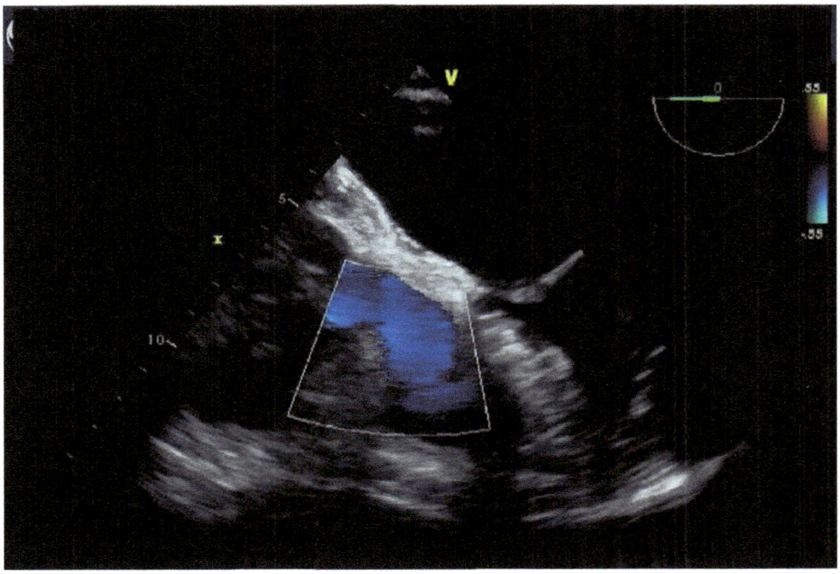

Figure 11.10 Transesophageal echocardiography showing pulmonary artery compression.
Image retrieved from George Washington University Hospital transesophageal echocardiography records.

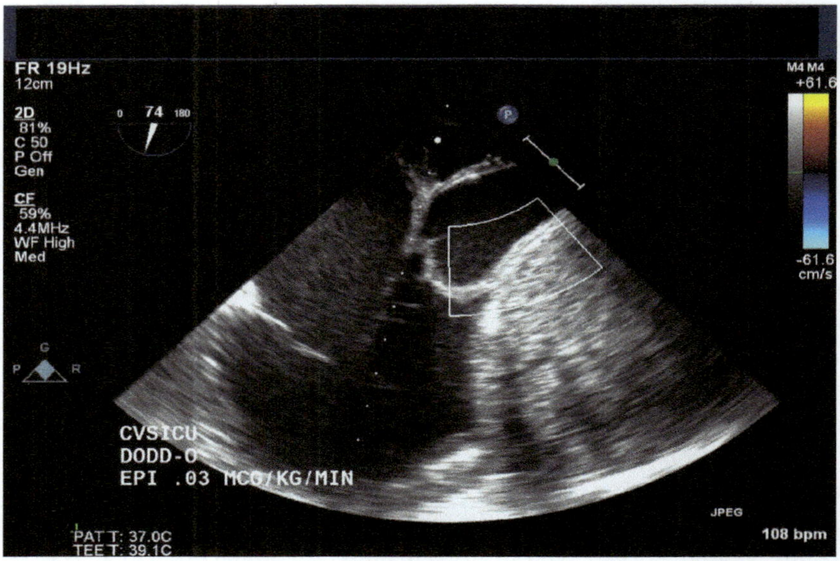

Figure 11.11 Transesophageal echocardiography showing right atrium compression.
Image retrieved from George Washington University Hospital transesophageal echocardiography records.

SVC Syndrome

One clinical manifestation of great vessel compression is SVC syndrome. The pathophysiology of SVC syndrome involves SVC obstruction leading to superficial venous congestion and engorgement. Signs and symptoms of the syndrome are similar to those of right heart failure, including dyspnea, cough, headache, elevated venous pressures, upper body edema, facial plethora, cyanosis, and tachycardia (Figures 11.13 and 11.14).[27] SVC syndrome may be

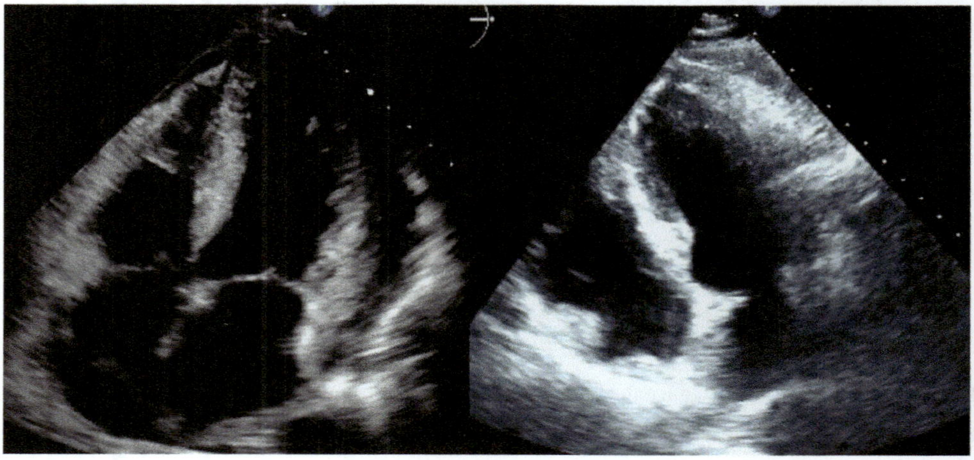

Figure 11.12 Transesophageal echocardiography showing effusion with tamponade.
Image retrieved from George Washington University Hospital transesophageal echocardiography records.

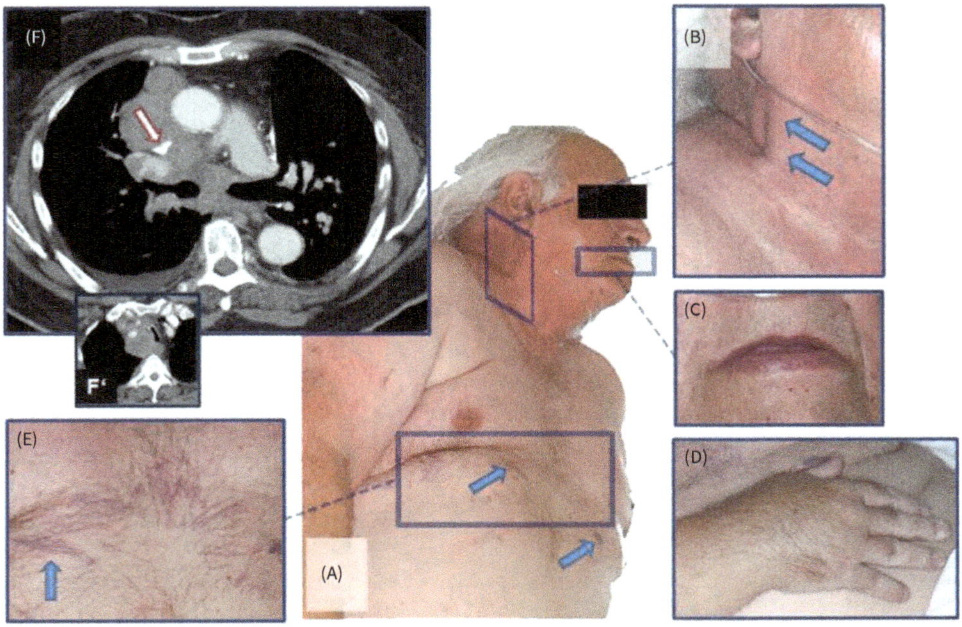

Figure 11.13 Patient with superior vena cava syndrome. (A) Plethora of face and neck. (B) Distended jugular veins. (C) Cyanosis of the lips. (D) Right arm and hand massively swollen. (E) Substantial collateral circulation (arrow). (F) Computed tomogram shows compression of the superior vena cava (arrow) due to a large mediastinal mass, causing tracheal compression and deviation, and stridor.

Reprinted with permission from Lepper PM, Ott SR, Hoppe H, et al. Superior vena cava syndrome in thoracic malignancies. *Respiratory Care.* 2011;56(5):653–666.

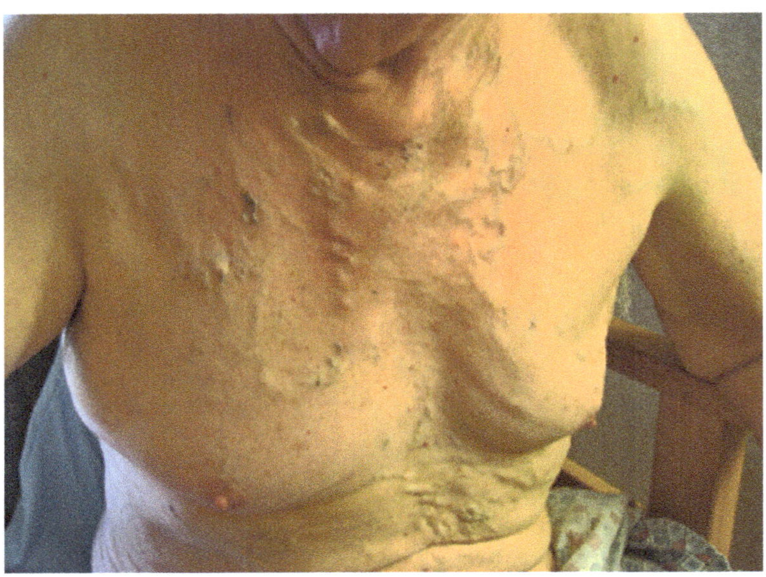

Figure 11.14 Patient with superior vena cava syndrome with substantial co-lateral circulation and venous engorgement.

Picture taken at George Washington Hospital.

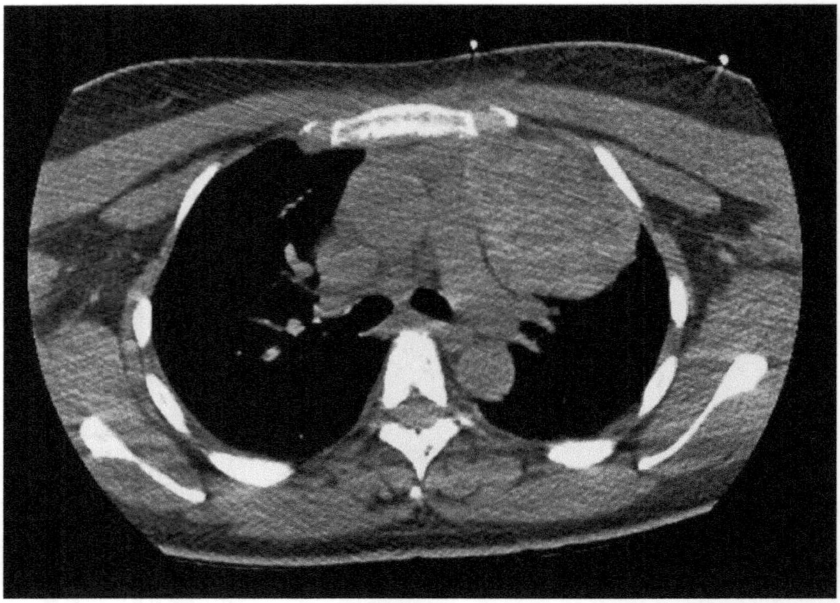

Figure 11.15 Computed tomography showing a large anterior mediastinal mass abutting the main pulmonary artery and compressing the left airway.

Image retrieved from George Washington University Hospital radiology records.

due to intraluminal (i.e., thrombus) or extraluminal (i.e., compressive mass or hematoma) pathologies.[27] Diagnostically, CT can be used to visualize SVC compression (Figures 11.15 and 11.16) and echocardiography has been shown to be useful in diagnosing both the presence and etiology of SVC syndrome in adults[26,28–30] and pediatrics,[31] and management typically involves lower extremity access and blood pressure maintenance to preserve preload. Fluids should be administered judiciously when considering RV failure, and appropriate vasopressors should be given to maintain adequate coronary perfusion.

Emergence

As the patient is awakening from anesthesia, the anesthesiologist extubates in the supine position, oxygen levels begin to drop into the 80s, and the patient is reintubated.

Extubation

As the patient emerges out of anesthesia, the most important consideration for the anesthesiologist is the method of extubation. It is most important to extubate patients with an elevated head of bed and with the patient awake and with full spontaneous respiratory effort to decrease the risk of a compromised negative intrathoracic pressure and elastic chest recoil. This is intuitive since in the upright position, the diaphragm, and whatever mediastinal mass remains after excision is pulled caudad instead of directly compressing the mediastinal

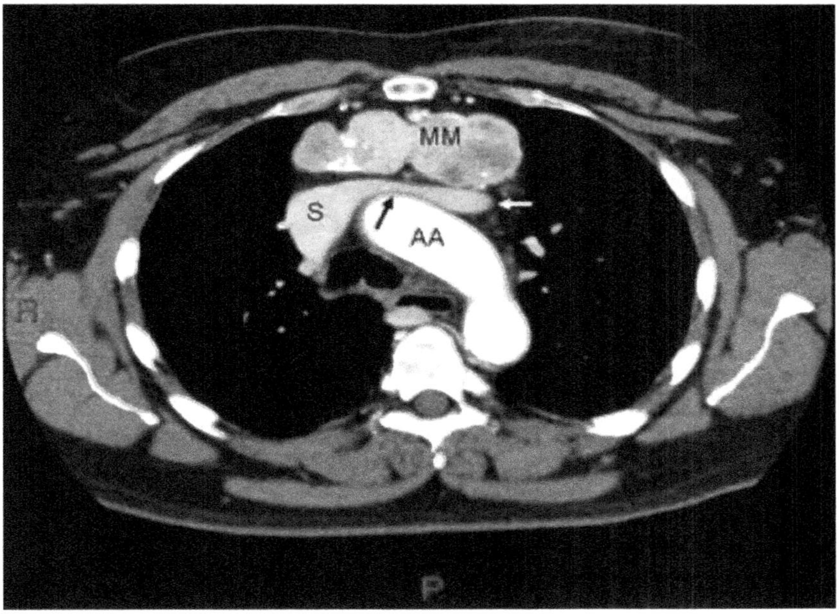

Figure 11.16 Computed tomogram chest of anterior mediastinal mass showing significant superior vena cava compression.

Reprinted with permission from Blank RS, Souza DGD. Anesthetic management of patients with an anterior mediastinal mass: continuing professional development. *Can J Anesth.* 2011;58(9):853–867.

Abbreviations: AA, aortic arch; MM, mediastinal mass; S, superior vena cava.

structures. This principle is shown by signs of obstruction on flow volume loops such as a decreased forced expiratory volume in 1 second and functional residual capacity in the supine position compared to sitting.[32,33] If there is considerable difficulty during extubation, or the patient requires reintubation, it is possible to keep the patient intubated until chemoradiation reduces the mass to a safe size.

Postoperative Considerations

Given the difficulty with extubation in the operating room, the patient is left intubated and undergoes several rounds of chemoradiation to further debulk his mediastinal mass. After the patient is extubated in the ICU, he remains mildly tachypneic to 22 with diminished breath sounds on the right side. Repeat morning chest X ray shows a moderate right-sided pleural effusion. Over the next few days, the effusion resolves spontaneously without chest tube placement. Pain is adequately controlled with ropivacaine paravertebral nerve blocks, and the patient is ambulating normally by postextubation day 2. After a full diet is resumed, and his peripheral nerve blocks are removed, the patient is discharged without further complication.

As with other thoracic procedures, postoperative monitoring should be considered in light of complications such as chylothorax, pneumothorax, hemothorax, and pericardial disease. Typical postoperative care should include chest physiotherapy, adequate pain management, early ambulation, and glycemic control with adequate nutrition.[2]

Conclusion

The surgical management of an anterior mediastinal mass is largely dependent on the size of the tumor and any compression on the structures within the thoracic cavity. With more severe signs and symptoms, such as orthopnea, syncope, and jugular vein distention, there may be a need for more careful measures such as elevated head of bed or alternative intubation techniques. During induction and maintenance, it is important to maintain spontaneous ventilation and the maximum respiratory drive possible for the patient. In all cases, the anesthesiologist needs to be attuned to any rises in peak inspiratory pressures or severe hypotension that may indicate life-threatening cardiorespiratory collapse. The focus should be on minimizing and assessing threats to airway, breathing, and circulation. Therefore, often a multidisciplinary team approach strategized on mitigating risks should be employed. As with many scenarios in medicine, it is vital that all members of the surgical team, including cardiothoracic surgeons, anesthesiologists, and critical care specialists, share a mental model and clinical awareness of the patient to ensure the best care possible.

References

1. Azarow KS, Pearl RH, Zurcher R, Edwards FH, Cohen AJ. Primary mediastinal masses: a comparison of adult and pediatric populations. *J Thorac Cardiovasc Surg.* 1993;106(1):67–72.
2. Bar-Yosef S. Mediastinal masses: implications for anesthesiologists. In: Barbeito A, Shaw AD, Grichnik K, eds. *Thoracic Anesthesia.* New York, NY: McGraw-Hill; 2012: Chapter 12.
3. Slinger P, Karsli C. Management of the patient with a large anterior mediastinal mass: recurring myths. *Curr Opin Anaesth.* 2007;20(1):1–3.
4. Blank RS, de Souza DG. Anesthetic management of patients with an anterior mediastinal mass: continuing professional development. *Can J Anesth.* 2011;58(9):853–867.
5. Neuman GG, Weingarten AE, Abramowitz RM, Kushins LG, Abramson AL, Ladner W. The anesthetic management of the patient with an anterior mediastinal mass. *Anesthesiology.* 1984;60(2):144–147.
6. Rotman HH, Liss HP, Weg JG. Diagnosis of upper airway obstruction by pulmonary function testing. *Chest.* 1975;68(6):796–799.
7. Szokol JW, Alspach D, Mehta MK, Parilla BV, Liptay MJ. Intermittent airway obstruction and superior vena cava syndrome in a patient with an undiagnosed mediastinal mass after cesarean delivery. *Anesth Analg.* 2003;97(3):883–884.
8. Bergman NA. Reduction in resting end-expiratory position of the respiratory system with induction of anesthesia and neuromuscular paralysis. *Anesthesiology.* 1982;57(1):14–17.
9. Hattamer SJ, Dodds TM. Use of the laryngeal mask airway in managing a patient with a large anterior mediastinal mass: a case report. *AANA J.* 1996;64(5):497–500.
10. Stricker P, Gurnaney H, Litman R. Anesthetic management of children with an anterior mediastinal mass. *Anesthesiology.* 2006;105:A970.
11. Vas L, Falguni N, Veena N. Anaesthetic management of an infant with anterior mediastinal mass. *Paediatr Anaesth.* 1999;9(5):439–443.
12. Rath L, Gullahorn G, Connolly N, Pratt T, Boswell G, Cornelissen C. Anterior mediastinal mass biopsy and resection. *Sem Cardiothor Vasc Anesth.* 2012;16(4):235–242.
13. Takeda S-I, Miyoshi S, Omori K-I, Okumura M, Matsuda H. Surgical rescue for life-threatening hypoxemia caused by a mediastinal tumor. *Ann Thorac Surg.* 1999;68(6):2324–2326.
14. Tempe DK, Arya R, Dubey S, et al. Mediastinal mass resection: femorofemoral cardiopulmonary bypass before induction of anesthesia in the management of airway obstruction. *J Cardiothorac Vasc Anesth.* 2001;15(2):233–236.

15. Inoue M, Minami M, Shiono H, et al. Efficient clinical application of percutaneous cardiopulmonary support for perioperative management of a huge anterior mediastinal tumor. *J Thorac Cardiovasc Surg.* 2006;131(3):755–756.
16. Johnson D, Hurst T, Cujec B, Mayers I. Cardiopulmonary effects of an anterior mediastinal mass in dogs anesthetized with halothane. *Anesthesiology.* 1991;74(4):725–736.
17. Shapiro HM, Sanford TJ, Schaldach AL. Fiberoptic stylet laryngoscope and sitting position for tracheal intubation in acute superior vena caval syndrome. *Anesth Analg.* 1984;63(2):161–162.
18. Crosby E. Clinical case discussion: anesthesia for Cesarean section in a parturient with a large intrathoracic tumour. *Can J Anaesth.* 2001;48(6):575–583.
19. Alkhafaji S, Mazhar R, Carr CS, Alkhulaifi AM. Extreme cardiac and pulmonary artery compression causing positional oxygen desaturation. *Emerg Med J.* 2008;25(8):541.
20. Béchard P, Létourneau L, Lacasse Y, Côté D, Bussières JS. Perioperative cardiorespiratory complications in adults with mediastinal mass. *Anesthesiology.* 2004;100(4):826–834.
21. Anghelescu DL, Burgoyne LL, Liu T, et al. Clinical and diagnostic imaging findings predict anesthetic complications in children presenting with malignant mediastinal masses. *Ped Anesth.* 2007;17(11):1090–1098.
22. Ng A, Bennett J, Bromley P, Davies P, Morland B. Anaesthetic outcome and predictive risk factors in children with mediastinal tumours. *Pediatr Blood Cancer.* 2007;48(2):160–164.
23. Hall KD, Friedman M. Extracorporeal oxygenation for induction of anesthesia in a patient with an intrathoracic tumor. *Anesthesiology.* 1975;42(4):493–495.
24. Levin H, Bursztein S, Heifetz M. Cardiac arrest in a child with an anterior mediastinal mass. *Anesth Analg.* 1985;64(11):1129–1130.
25. Lin C-M, Hsu J-C. Anterior mediastinal tumour identified by intraoperative transesophageal echocardiography. *Can J Anesth.* 2001;48(1):78–80.
26. Yang YL, Lu HI, Huang HW, Tseng CC. Mediastinal tumor resection under the guidance of transcesophageal echocardiography. *Anaesth Intensive Care.* 2007;35:312.
27. Narang S, Harte BH, Body SC. Anesthesia for patients with a mediastinal mass. *Anesthesiol Clin North Am.* 2001;19(3):559–579.
28. Ayala K, Chandrasekaran K, Karalis D, Parris T, Ross J. Diagnosis of superior vena caval obstruction by transesophageal echocardiography. *Chest.* 1992;101(3):874–876.
29. Barbeito A, Bar-Yosef S, Lowe JE, Atkins BZ, Mark JB. Unusual cause of superior vena cava syndrome diagnosed with transesophageal echocardiography. *Can J Anaesth.* 2008;55(11):774–778.
30. Dawkins PR, Stoddard MF, Liddell NE, Longaker R, Keedy D, Kupersmith J. Utility of transesophageal echocardiography in the assessment of mediastinal masses and superior vena cava obstruction. *Am Heart J.* 1991;122:1469–1472.
31. Jamshidi R, Weitzel N. Mediastinal mass with superior vena cava syndrome. *Semin Cardiothorac Vasc Anesth.* 2011;15:105–111.
32. Goh MH, Liu XY, Goh YS. Anterior mediastinal masses: an anaesthetic challenge. *Anaesthesia.* 1999;54:670–682.
33. Vilke GM, Chan TC, Neuman T, Clausen JL. Spirometry in normal subjects in sitting, prone, and supine positions. *Respir Care.* 2000;45(4):407–410.

12
Pneumonectomy

Lacey Wood and Antony Tharian

Introduction

History of Pneumonectomy

Pneumonectomy is the surgical removal of one lung in its entirety. See Figure 12.1 for demonstration of a chest X-ray of a patient after pneumonectomy. The first successful staged pneumonectomy was performed by Dr. Rudolph Nissen in Berlin in 1931. On April 5, 1933, the first successful one-stage pneumonectomy for cancer was performed by Dr. Evarts Graham on a 48-year-old gynecologist named Dr. James Gilmore using endotracheal nitrous oxide. Dr. Gilmore's left lung was removed, and pathology revealed epidermoid carcinoma (also known as squamous cell carcinoma) with two peribronchial lymph nodes positive for tumor, T2 N1, or stage IIb by current lung cancer staging.[1]

Indications for Pneumonectomy

The most common indication for pneumonectomy is bronchial carcinoma with tumors involving[2–4]:

- Mainstem bronchus proximal to the bronchus intermedius.
- Hilar structures such as main pulmonary artery or superior or inferior pulmonary veins.
- All lobes or crossing of the major fissures.
- Other locations not appropriate for alternative resections.
- Traumatic injury with uncontrolled hemorrhage.
- Chronic inflammatory or infective disorders such as
  - Bronchiectasis.
  - Multidrug-resistant tuberculosis.
  - Atypical mycobacterial infections.
  - Fungal infections resulting in lung destruction.
  - Other necrotizing or opportunistic infections.

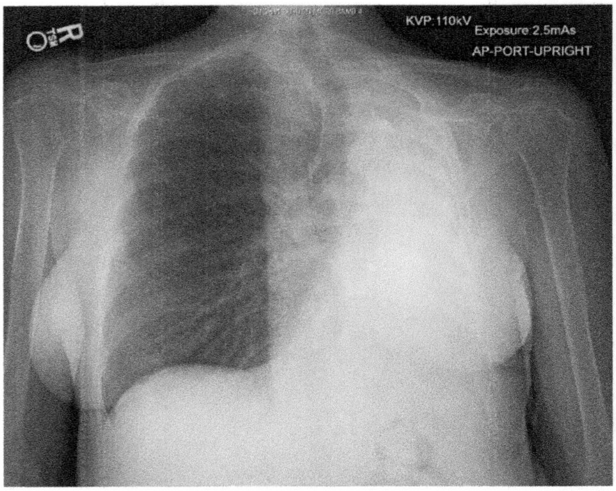

Figure 12.1 Chest X-ray of a patient after pneumonectomy.

Contraindications to Pneumonectomy

The most common contraindications for pneumonectomy are[2,3,5,6]:

- Evidence of distant metastases.
- Tumor invasion into mediastinal structures such as
  - Heart.
  - Great vessels.
  - Aorta.
  - Esophagus.
  - Vertebrae.
  - Proximal to mid trachea.
- Patient factors such as VO_2 max < 10mL/kg/min or < 35% predicted.

Lung Cancer—Staging and Treatment

Lung cancer is one of the leading causes of cancer death worldwide, with an annual incidence of greater than 2 million new cases per year. It has caused over 1.75 million deaths worldwide in 2018.[7] Lung cancer has also been the leading cause of cancer deaths in both men and women in the United States since 1987 and accounts for 25% of all cancer deaths. In 2016, lung and bronchus cancers caused more than 148,879 deaths in the United States alone.[8]

Lung cancer is divided into nonsmall cell lung cancer and small cell cancers. Nonsmall cell lung cancer makes up 75% to 85% of lung cancers and can be divided into adenocarcinoma, squamous cell, and large cell carcinoma. Staging is assessed using the eighth edition of

Table 12.1 T, N, and M descriptors for the eighth edition of TNM Classification for Lung Cancer.

T: Primary tumor	
Tx	Primary tumor cannot be assessed or tumor proven by presence of malignant cells in sputum or bronchial but not visualized by imaging or bronchoscopy
T0	No evidence of primary tumor
Tis	Carcinoma in situ
T1	Tumor ≥3 cm in greatest dimension surrounded by lung or visceral pleura without bronchoscopic evidence of invasion more proximal than the lobar bronchus (i.e., not the main bronchus)*
T1a(mi)	**Minimally invasive adenocarcinoma¶**
T1a	**Tumor ≥1 cm in greatest dimension***
T1b	**Tumor ≥1 cm but ≥2 cm in a greatest dimension***
T1c	**Tumor ≥2 cm but ≥3 cm in greatest dimension***
T2	Tumor ≥3 cm **but ≥5cm** or tumor with any of the following features:$^{\Delta}$ **Involves main bronchus regardless of distance from the carina but without involvement of the carina** Invades visceral pleura **Association with atelectasis or obstructive pneumonitis that extends to the hilar region, involving part or all of the lung**
T2a	**Tumor ≥3 cm but ≥4 cm in greatest dimension**
T2b	**Tumor ≥4 cm but ≥5 cm in greatest dimension**
T3	**Tumor ≥5 cm but ≥7 cm in greatest dimension** or associated with separate tumor nodule(s) in the same lobe as the primary tumor or directly invades any of the following structures: chest wall (including the parietal pleura and superior sulcus tumor), phrenic nerve, parietal pericardium
T4	**Tumor ≥7 cm in greatest dimension** or associated with separate tumor nodule(s) in a different ipsilateral lobe than that of the primary tumor or invades any of the following structure: **diaphragm**, mediastinum, heart, great vessels, trachea, recurrent laryngeal nerve, esophagus, vertebral body, and carina.
N: Regional lymph node involvement	
Nx	Regional lymph nodes cannot be assessed
N0	No regional lymph node metastasis
N1	Metastasis in ipsilateral peribronchail and/ or ipsilateral hilar lymph and intrapulmonary nodes, including involvement by direct extension.
N2	Metastasis in ipsilateral mediastinal and/or subcarinal lymph node(s)
M: Distant metastasis	
M0	No distant metastasis
M1	Distant metastasis present
M1a	Separate tumor nodule(s) in a contralateral lobe; tumor with pleural or pericardial nodule(s) or malignant pleural or pericardial effusion✓

Table 12.1 *Continued*

T: Primary tumor			
M1b	**Single extrathorcic metastasis[§]**		
M1c	**Multiple extrathorcic metastases in one or more organs**		
Stage groupings			
Occult carcinoma	TX	N0	M0
Stage 0	Tis	N0	M0
Stage IA1	**T1a(mi)**	**N0**	**M0**
	T1a	**N0**	**M0**
Stage IA2	**T1b**	**N1**	**M0**
Stage IA3	**T1c**	**N1**	**M0**
State 1B	T2a	N1	M0
Stage IIA	T2b	N1	M0
Stage IIB	**T1a to c**	**N1**	**M0**
	T2a	**N1**	**M0**
	T2b	N1	M0
	T3	N1	M0
Stage IIIA	T1a to c	N2	M0
	T2a to b	N2	M0
	T3	N2	M0
	T4	N2	M0
Stage IIIB	**T1a to c**	**N3**	**M0**
	T2a to b	**N3**	**M0**
	T3	N2	M0
	T4	N2	M0
Stage IIIC	**T3**	**N3**	**M0**
	T4	**N3**	**M0**
Stage IVA	**Any T**	**Any N**	**M1a**
	Any T	**Any N**	**M1b**
Stage IVB	**Any T**	**Any N**	**M1c**

Note: changes to the seventh edition are in bold.

TNM: tumor, node, metastasis; Tis:carcinoma in situ; T1a (mi): minimally invasive adenocarcinoma.

* The uncommon superficial spreading tumor of any size with its invasive component limited to the bronchial wall, which may extend proximal to the main bronchus, is also classified as T1a.

¶ Solitary adenocarcinoma, ≥3 cm with a predominately lepidic pattern and ≥5mm invasion in any one focus.

Δ T2 tumors with these features are classified as T2a if ≥4cm in greatest dimension or if size cannot be determined, and T2b if ≥5cm in greatest dimension.

✓ Most pleural (pericardial) effusions with lung cancer are due to tumor. In a few patients, however multiple microscopic examinations of pleural (pericardial) fluid are negative for tumor and the fluid is nonbloody and not an exudate when these elements and clinical judgment dictate that the effusion is not related to the tumor, the effusion should be excluded as a staging descriptor.

§ This includes involvement of a single distant (nonregional) lymph node.

Source: Goldstraw P, Chansky K, Crowley J, et al. The IASLC lung cancer staging project: proposals for revision of the TNM stage groupings in the forthcoming (eighth) edition of the TNM Classification for Lung Cancer. *J Thorac Oncol*. 2016;11(1):39– 51. doi:10.1016/ j.jtho.2015.09.009. Table 1 and Table 9 used with the permission of Elsevier Inc. © All rights reserved.

Abbreviations: T, tumor; N, node; M, metastasis.

the *Tumor, Node, Metastasis Staging System* as can be seen in Table 12.1.[9] Patients with stage IIb and below are generally considered operable with a chance of cure by surgery alone.[6,10] Patients with stage T4 or N2 can also be considered for resection.[2,6] Computed tomography (CT) scanning and positron emission tomography CT are used to assess for lymph node status and distal metastases. Mediastinal lymph nodes are biopsied using modalities such as mediastinoscopy, bronchoscopy with transbronchial needle aspiration, endobronchial ultrasound-guided transbronchial needle aspiration, or transthoracic percutaneous needle aspiration.[6,11] Patients confirmed to have N2 disease are commonly treated with a combination of surgical resection, chemotherapy, and radiation, whereas presence of distant metastases is usually a contraindication to resection.[3,6,10]

Preoperative Assessment

Preoperative Considerations

Pneumonectomy has the highest morbidity of all pulmonary resections with a mortality rate of 3.7 % to 7.8%.[5,12] Hence, it is chosen as a last resort when other procedures such as sleeve lobectomy, vascular sleeve resection, and nonanatomical resections such as wedge resections are not adequate to remove local disease and/or ipsilateral lymph node metastases.[2,13] Postoperative lung function is dependent on the amount of preserved functioning lung parenchyma after resection of diseased lung.[14] All patients being considered for lung resection surgery should have a physiologic evaluation by a multidisciplinary team to assess ability to survive resection and ability to remain ventilator independent in the postoperative period.[5,15]

Summary of Preoperative Assessment

The preoperative assessment prior to pneumonectomy should include assessment of[5,6,13,15–17]:

1. Cardiovascular risk and possible evaluation by cardiologist based on risk assessment.
2. Respiratory mechanics through spirometry, and most importantly calculation of predicted postoperative forced expiratory volume in 1 second (ppoFEV1).
3. Lung parenchymal function through evaluation of PaO_2 and $PaCO_2$ on arterial blood gas, and most importantly calculation of predicted postoperative diffusion capacity of carbon monoxide (ppoDLCO).
4. Cardiopulmonary interaction using stair climb or shuttle walk test, and/or cardiopulmonary exercise testing if indicated based on findings in Steps 1 to 3.

See Figure 12.2 for an algorithm that summarizes the preoperative assessment.

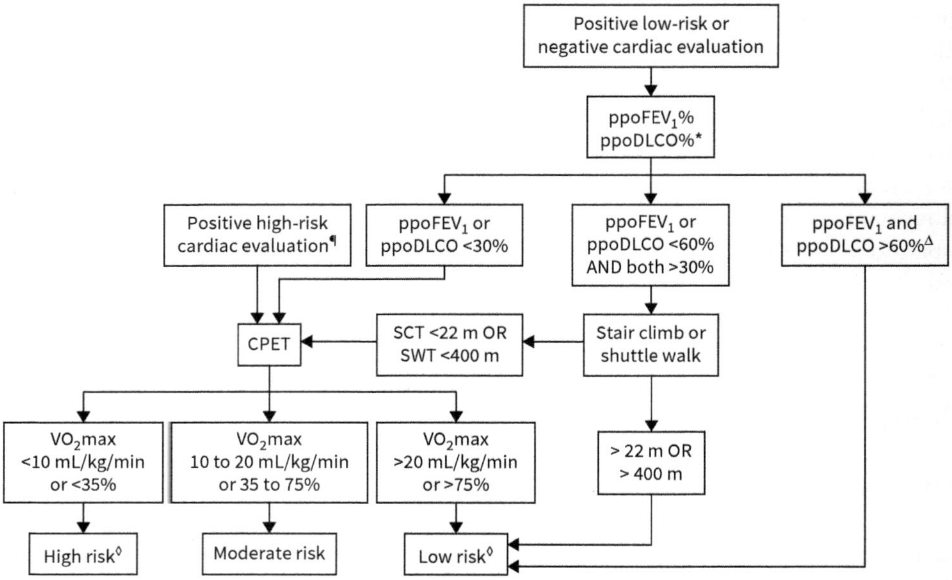

Figure 12.2 Algorithm for pulmonary pre-operative assessment of patients requiring lung resection.

Source: Brunelli A, Kim AW, Berger KI, Addrizzo-Harris DJ. Physiologic evaluation of the patient with lung cancer being considered for resectional surgery: Diagnosis and Management of Lung Cancer, 3rd ed: American College of Chest Physicians evidence-based clinical practice guidelines. *Chest.* 2013;143:e166S. Figure 2 used with the permission of Elsevier Inc. © All rights reserved.

Abbreviations: CPET cardiopulmonary exercise test; DLCO, diffusing capacity of the lungs for carbon monoxide; FEV1, forced expiratory volume in first second; FVC, functional vital capacity; ppo, predicted postoperative; SCT, stair climbing test; SWT, shuttle walk test; VO_2 max, maximal oxygen consumption.

Cardiovascular Risk Assessment and Evaluation

Patients being evaluated for lung resection surgery should undergo preoperative workup including a history, assessment of functional status, physical exam, and baseline electrocardiogram. Patients with audible murmur or unexplained dyspnea should undergo transthoracic echocardiogram.[6] Preoperative transthoracic echocardiogram may also be considered in any patient prior to pneumonectomy as pulmonary hypertension is a relative contraindication due to risks of increased pulmonary vascular resistance (PVR) leading to increased morbidity due to right heart strain.[18,19] This is especially important to consider in the elderly and right-sided pneumonectomy because the remaining left lung has a smaller volume compared to the right lung. The right ventricle becomes increasingly less compliant with age and has increasing difficulty dealing with the increased right ventricle afterload that ensues after resection. Patients with any of the following findings should be referred to see a cardiologist for a formal evaluation[5,6]:

1. Newly diagnosed or active cardiac conditions such as unstable coronary syndrome, decompensated heart failure, significant arrhythmia, or severe valve disease.
2. Poor functional capacity: <4 metabolic equivalents or inability to climb two flights of stairs.
3. High risk of cardiac complication as indicated by Revised Cardiac Risk Index (RCRI) ≥3 or Thoracic RCRI (ThRCRI) ≥2.

Cardiac Risk Calculators

Patients undergoing pneumonectomy have multiple cardiac comorbidities including tobacco dependence, chronic obstructive pulmonary disease (COPD), and underlying coronary artery disease and are at high risk for cardiac complications.[16] There are multiple risk calculations that can be used to predict perioperative cardiac complications and recommendations from different guidelines using these various risk calculators. For completeness, these risk calculators including (i) American College of Surgeons National Surgical Quality Improvement Program surgical risk calculator,[20] (ii) the American College of Surgeons National Surgical Quality Improvement Program Gupta online calculator of perioperative myocardial infarction or cardiac arrest,[21] (iii) Revised Cardiac Risk Index (RCRI),[22] and (iv) Thoracic RCRI[23,24] are described in Figure 12.3.

Respiratory Mechanics

Forced expiratory volume in 1 second (FEV1) can be measured using spirometry and is an independent predictor of respiratory complications, pulmonary morbidity, and cardiovascular complications following lung resection surgery.[5,25] Values obtained from spirometry including FEV1 are expressed as a percentage of predicted volumes that are corrected for age, sex, and height. The preoperative FEV1 is the best measured postbronchodilator value,[5] which must be reproducible without error due to coughing, leaks, hesitation, early termination, or variable efforts. Reproducibility is defined as less than 5% variation between the two highest FEV1 or forced vital capacity values.[15] Predicted postoperative FEV1 (ppoFEV1) has been shown to be associated with increased respiratory morbidity and mortality rates,[5] and can be calculated as follows.

ACS NSQIP surgical risk calculator[20]: Online calculator that predicts the risk of 13 outcomes based on procedure current procedural terminology (CPT) code and multiple patient risk factors. Of the 13 outcomes predicted, one is the risk of major adverse cardiac events (MACE), which include ischemia, infarction, and cardiac arrest (www.riskcalculator.facs.org).

NSQIP 21 factors		
CPT code	Chronic steroid use	Congestive Heart Failure in 30 days prior to surgery
Other potential appropriate treatment options	Ascites within 30 days prior to surgery	Dyspnea
Age	Sepsis within 48 hours prior to surgery	Current Smoker within 1 year
Sex	Ventilator dependent	History of Severe COPD
Fucntional status	Disseminated Cancer	Dialysis
Emergency Case	Diabetes Mellitus	Acute renal failure
ASA Class	Hypertension requiring medication	BMI

ACS NSQIP MICA[21]: Gupta online calculator of perioperative cardiac risk was derived from NSQIP database and calculates risk of Myocardial Infarction or Cardiac Arrest (MICA) based on 5 risk factors (http://www.surgicalriskcalculator.com/miorcardiacarrest)

MICA risk factors
Increased age
Abnormal Creatinine (>/=133micromol/L)
American Society of Anesthesiology (ASA) Class
Preoperative Functional Status
Type of surgery

RCRI[22]: Used to assess risk of major perioperative cardiac complications including myocardial infarction, pulmonary edema, ventricular fibrillation or primary cardiac arrest, and complete heart block using 6 risk factors

Figure 12.3 Cardiac risk calculators.

Anatomical method:

ppoFEV1 = preoperative FEV1 × (1 − subsegments to be removed/total preoperative functional subsegments)

Right Lung		
Lobe	Segments	# of Subsegments
Upper	1. Apical	2
	2. Anterior	2
	3. Posterior	2
Middle	4. Medial	2
	5. Lateral	2
Lower	6. Superior lower	3
	7. Medial basal	2
	8. Anterior basal	2
	9. Lateral basal	2
	10. Posterior basal	3
	Total Subsegments Right Lung	22

Leftt Lung		
Upper	1. Apicoposterior	3
	2. Anterior	3
	3. Superior lingular	2
	4. Inferior lingular	2
Lower	5. Superior lower lobe	3
	6. Anteromedial basal	2
	7. Lateral basal	2
	8. Posterior basal	3
	Total Subsegments Left Lung	20
	Total Subsegments	42

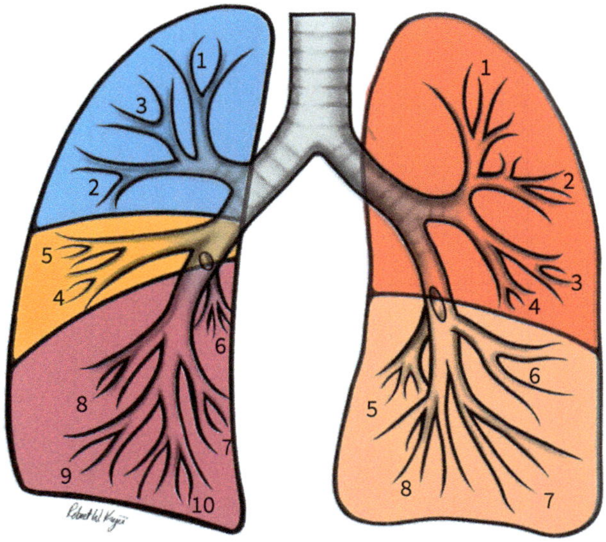

Figure 12.4 The 10 segments on the right and 8 segments of the left lung are labeled. The key indicates the name of the segment and number of subsegments in each segment to account for the 42 subsegments of the lungs.

Perfusion Method:

$$\text{ppoFEV1} = \text{Preoperative FEV1} \times (1 - \%\ \text{of perfusion in lung to be resected})$$

Perfusion method using V/Q lung scanning only accounts for lung parenchyma that is being perfused and is therefore a more accurate predictor than the anatomical method when portions of the resected lung are non-functioning.

Refer to Figure 12.4 for lung segment and subsegment anatomy as used to calculate predicted postoperative values.

Lung Parenchymal Function

PaO_2 <60 and $PaCO_2$ >45 have traditionally been used as cutoff values for pulmonary resection; however, diffusion capacity of carbon monoxide (DLCO) is the most useful test for gas exchange or diffusing capacity of the lung.[13] DLCO correlates with the total functioning surface area of the alveolar–capillary interface and, like FEV1, is also expressed as percentage predicted based on a patients age, sex, and height. This test is performed by having a patient inhale carbon monoxide, breath is held at maximal inspiration for 9 to 11 seconds, and then the exhaled carbon monoxide, or portion that is not absorbed, is measured.[26] One must remember

Table 12.2 Factors That Decrease/Increase DLCO

DLCO is reduced by:	**DLCO is increased by:**
Intrinsic lung disease such as COPD or history of chest irradiation	Conditions that increase lung volumes and expiratory times such as asthma
Conditions that decrease cardiac output such as heart failure	Increased cardiac output such as with exercise or stress
Conditions that increase dead space such as pulmonary embolism	Left to right cardiac shunt
Anemia due to decreased hemoglobin for absorption	Polycythemia due to increased hemoglobin for absorption

Abbreviations: DLCO, diffusing capacity of lung for carbon monoxide; COPD, chronic obstructive pulmonary disease.

that there are many contributing factors that affect DLCO, as shown in Table 12.2. In fact, ppoDLCO correlates with increased risk for pulmonary and cardiac complications. It is independent of ppoFEV1, and is *the single strongest predictor of mortality* following lung resection surgery.[27–29] ppoDLCO can be calculated using the same formulas as used for ppoFEV1.

Anatomic Method

$$\text{ppoDLCO} = \text{preoperative DLCO} \times (1 - \text{segments to be removed/total preoperative functional segments})$$

Perfusion Method

$$\text{ppoDLCO} = \text{Preop DLCO} \times (1 - \%\ \text{of perfusion in lung to be resected})$$

Cardiopulmonary Interaction

Cardiopulmonary Exercise Testing

Formal laboratory cardiopulmonary exercise testing (CPET) is conducted with the patient exercising on a stationary bike or treadmill and records exercise electrocardiogram, heart rate response to exercise, oxygen uptake, and carbon dioxide production.[5,30,31] Of all the information gathered from CPET, the most important is maximum oxygen consumption per unit time (VO_2 max), which is the gold standard for assessment of cardiopulmonary function[2] as it is the *most reproducible indicator of cardiopulmonary fitness.*[31] VO_2 max will change with age, sex, and, height, so values are expressed as absolute values (mL/kg/min) and percentage of predicted values.[30,31]

How VO_2 max is applied to risk assessment for pneumonectomy[2,5,29,32]:

- <10 mL/kg/min—Pneumonectomy is contraindicated.
  - Patients have a high risk of postoperative death.

- 10–15 mL/kg/min—Increased risk for perioperative death.
- >15 mL/kg/min—Good physiologic function.
  - No perioperative mortality in high-risk group (mean preoperative FEV1 of 41% predicted).
- >20 mL/kg/min—Safe for pneumonectomy.

Low Technology Exercise Tests Used to Predict VO_2 max

In addition to formal CEPT, there are three easy-to-perform tests used as adjuncts, and in some cases surrogates, for CPET to predict VO_2 max in patients who have both ppoFEV1 and ppoDLCO between 30% and 60% and are not at high risk for cardiovascular complications.[5] These are the stair climbing test, the shuttle walk test, and the Six-minute walk test.

Stair climbing test. Patient is asked to walk up flights of stairs until they need to stop due symptoms such as dyspnea or fatigue. The duration of climbing, speed of ascent, number of steps per flight, height of each step, and criteria for stopping the test have varied in different studies.[5,29,33]

Correlation between flights climbed and VO_2 max[5,13,29,33]:

<1 flight—correlates with VO_2 max <10 mL/Kg/min
<2 flights—correlates with very high risk
>3 flights (~12–14 m)—correlates with decreased morbidity and mortality following lobectomy
> 22m—correlates with VO_2 max >15 mL/kg/min
>5 flights of stairs—correlates with VO_2 max of >20 mL/Kg/min.

Being able to walk up >22 m of stairs has a positive predictive value of 86% to predict a VO_2 max of 15mL/kg/min and is therefore used as a *cutoff value allowing patients to proceed with pneumonectomy without formal CPET.*[33]

Shuttle walk test. The patient walks back and forth between two markers, 10 meters apart. The walking pace is set by an audio signal and the speed is increased each minute until the patient is no longer able to walk the 10 meters in the allotted time due to dyspnea.[5,29,34]

Correlation between distance walked and VO_2 max[5,29,34]:

- Inability to complete walking 250 meters on two occasions—suggests VO_2 max <10 mL/kg/min
- Walking <400 m—patient needs to undergo cardiopulmonary exercise testing
- Walking > 400 meters correlates with VO_2 max > 15mL/kg/min and indicates patient is appropriate to proceed with pneumonectomy without CPET.

Six-minute walk test. Patient is asked to walk as far as possible in 6 minutes and allowed to regulate their own pace and breaks as needed. This test is not well standardized and is not used in decision-making in the preoperative assessment. However, oxygen desaturation during the 6-minute walk test has been independently associated with the occurrence of major morbidity among patients with elevated risk.[29,35]

Surgical Procedure

Summary of Surgical Procedure

After induction, flexible or rigid bronchoscopy is performed to confirm sufficient length of the bronchus is free of tumor.[2,36] The most common surgical approach is posterolateral thoracotomy at the fourth or fifth intercostal space and occasionally resection of the fifth rib for exposure. The chest can also be accessed via video-assisted thoracoscopy or via an anterior, muscle-sparing approach that does not involve division of the latissimus dorsi or serratus anterior—both of these approaches are associated with decreased postoperative pain.[37,38] Lung is then retracted to expose the anterior hilum, so that pulmonary artery, superior and inferior pulmonary veins, and mainstem bronchus can be evaluated for respectability.[13] If resectable, the superior and inferior pulmonary veins are ligated and divided, followed by the pulmonary artery. The bronchus is then stapled and cut to fully separate the lung from the body. Care must be taken to make sure double-lumen endotracheal tubes (DLTs) or bronchial blockers are not included in the staple line.[2,13] The bronchial stump should be as short as possible to prevent a potential space for fluid collection.[13] Next a leak test is performed by filling the thorax with warm saline and applying positive pressure ventilation via the tracheal lumen while watching to confirm there are no bubbles.[2,13] Some surgeons place thoracostomy tubes while others may not do so to minimize the chances of hemodynamic collapse resulting from suction with a standard underwater-seal system. All patients must have a postoperative chest X-ray to assess the position of the mediastinum.[13]

Types of Pneumonectomy

- Standard pneumonectomy: Pulmonary artery and veins are isolated and ligated without intrapericardial access, and entire lung is removed.
- Intrapericardial pneumonectomy: Pneumonectomy with longitudinal opening of the pericardium posterior to and in parallel with the left phrenic nerve.[39] Needed when right or left main pulmonary arteries are involved or when a pulmonary vein needs to be divided at the level of the left atrium to get clear tumor margins.[2]
- Extrapleural pneumonectomy: Radical resection including excision of the lung, lymph nodes, ipsilateral parietal pleura, hemidiaphragm, hemopericardium with patch reconstruction, and chest wall.[2,13,40] Performed for selective malignant pleural mesotheliomas in conjunction with high-dose radiotherapy in the postoperative period.[13]
- Completion pneumonectomy: Excision of remaining lung tissue after previous resection.
- Tracheal sleeve pneumonectomy/carinal pneumonectomy: Excision of the lung and carina with reconstruction of the trachea and bronchus with tracheobronchial anastomosis.[4] Performed for tumors of the proximal portions of mainstem bronchus, carina, and distal 3 to 4 cm of the trachea.[3,13,41] The carina is more easily accessible through a right thoracotomy.[2,41] Right sleeve pneumonectomy can generally be completed through right-sided thoracotomy; posterior thoracotomy is most common, but anterior approach is also possible.[41] The left mainstem bronchus is longer and more challenging to expose through a right thoracotomy due to its subaortic location (see Figure 12.5); therefore, left sleeve

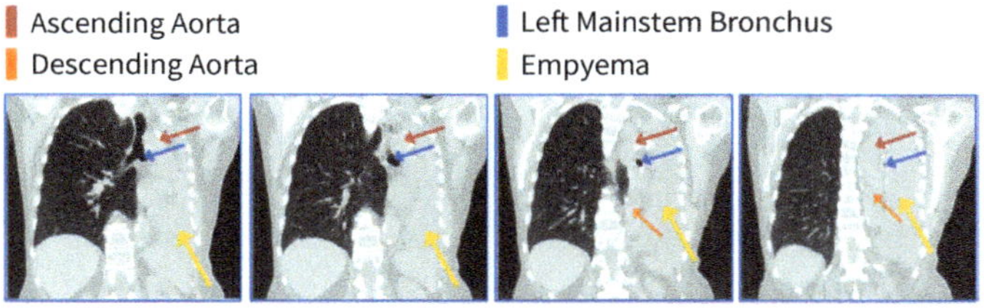

Figure 12.5 Demonstrates the subaortic position of the left mainstem bronchus in a patient who presented with large left-sided empyema after previous left sided pneumonectomy.

pneumonectomies are commonly performed via (i) median sternotomy, where the procedure may or may not be started using video-assisted thoracoscopic surgery to transect the pulmonary artery and veins prior to sternotomy; (ii) hemi-clamshell; or (iii) in two stages: left pneumonectomy followed by right thoracotomy for carinal excision.[41]

Anesthetic Management

Preoperative Planning and Review

Prior to taking the patient to the operating room (OR), a thorough history and physical exam are performed, and all labs, studies, and imaging must be reviewed. Close attention must be paid to baseline arterial blood gas, starting hemoglobin and platelet count, type and cross, electrolyte abnormalities, results of special tests for associated paraneoplastic syndromes, spirometry, cardiac studies, chest X-ray, chest CT, bronchoscopy reports, and all other imaging.[14,16] Prior to entering the OR, the anesthesiologist should ensure the appropriate blood products are readily available. Imaging is reviewed to assess for vascular and airway invasion or obstruction by tumor as well as overall anatomy and condition of the lungs, which can help to guide decisions such as most appropriate intubation technique, appropriateness for one-lung ventilation (OLV), most suitable modality for OLV, and give insight to risk for airway and hemodynamic collapse after induction of anesthesia. With significant risk for airway or hemodynamic collapse, such as with an anterior mediastinal mass, one must consider need for prone or lateral positioning, ENT consult for rigid bronchoscopy to pass obstruction, preoperative cannulation for extracorporeal membrane oxygenation, or need for emergent median sternotomy to manually lift chest contents and relieve obstruction.[42]

Monitors and Lines

Intraoperatively, standard American Society of Anesthesiologists monitors are applied, and patients undergoing pneumonectomy should have a large bore peripheral intravenous line for transfusion of fluids and blood products, an arterial line for monitoring and blood sampling, urinary catheter for accurate measurement of urine output, and frequently a central venous catheter to guide intravascular fluid management and for vasopressor administration.[2,13,16] Pulmonary artery catheters (PACs) and transesophageal echocardiograms (TEEs) are also reasonable, but not used in all cases.[16] Arterial line can be placed preinduction or postinduction of anesthesia depending on patient factors and provider preferences.

Lung Isolation

After induction of anesthesia and placement of lines and monitors, bronchoscopy is performed using flexible bronchoscopy through single lumen endotracheal tube or rigid bronchoscopy can be performed with the use of intravenous anesthesia. Next, lung isolation is achieved using, in order of most to least common: a DLT, a bronchial blocker, or a single-lumen endotracheal tube advanced into the nonoperative mainstem bronchus. DLTs are considered the gold standard.[16] In general, left-sided DLTs are easier to place and preferred for lung isolation in thoracic surgeries due to the short length of the right mainstem bronchus and early takeoff of the right mainstem bronchus (see Figure 12.6). Options for lung isolation for left and right pneumonectomy can be seen in Figure 12.7. Left-sided DLT for left pneumonectomy and all bronchial blockers must be withdrawn prior to stapling to avoid incorporation into staple line and nidus for inflammation and/or infection causing tissue breakdown and impaired wound healing of the ligated bronchus, which can lead to development of bronchopleural fistula.[2,13,41] Following lung isolation and confirmation of ability to perform OLV, the patient is placed in lateral decubitus position, and eyes, pressure points, and neck position are confirmed to be satisfactory.[2] Once positioning is complete, a fiberoptic scope is used to recheck for optimal positioning of DLT, bronchial blocker, or endotracheal tube.[2,16]

OLV Recommendations

1. Tidal volume of 4 to 6 mL/kg ideal body weight.
2. Peak airway pressure <35 cmH_2O.

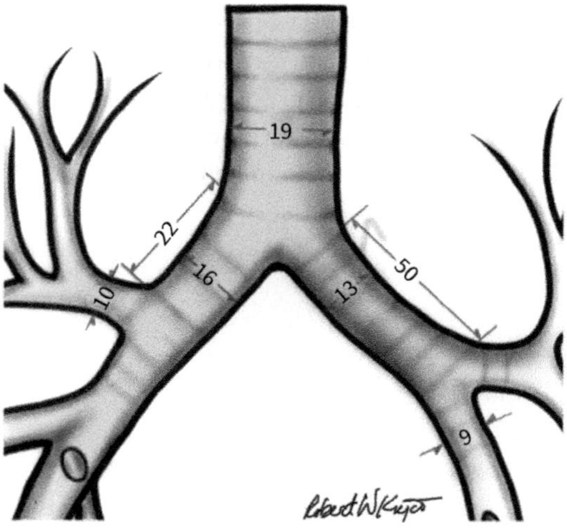

Figure 12.6 Bronchus dimensions.

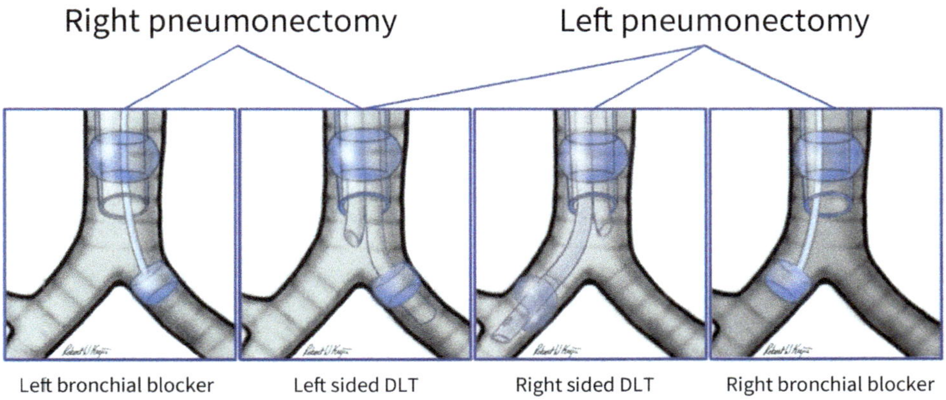

Figure 12.7 Options for lung isolation. Right pneumonectomy lung isolation options: right-sided bronchial blocker or left-sided double-lumen endotracheal tube (DLT). Left pneumonectomy lung isolation options: left-sided bronchial blocker, right-sided DLT with correct alignment of Murphy's eye with the right upper lobe or left sided DLT.

3. Plateau airway pressure < 25 cmH_2O.
4. Positive end expiratory pressure of 5 to 10.
5. Maintain normocarbia by increasing respiratory rate.
6. Avoid hyperoxia—titrate FiO_2 to maintain O_2 saturations of 94% to 98%.
7. Minimize surgical time and OLV time.
8. Pressure control is a good mode of ventilation for patients at risk for lung injury such as patients undergoing pneumonectomy or with bullae.[2,13,16,38,43,44]

Hemodynamic Management and Clamping of the Pulmonary Artery

Awareness of the surgical field, understanding what is taking place, anticipating the next step, and strong communication between surgeon and anesthesiologist are essential throughout the procedure. For example, hypotension and arrhythmias may occur when hilar structures or pericardium are retracted.[36] Communication between surgeon and anesthesia is also crucial when clamping the pulmonary artery to maintain stable cardiac output with the entire pulmonary circulating volume beginning to pass through only one lung. Significant elevation in the central venous pressure (CVP) and hemodynamic perturbations indicate insufficient compliance of the right ventricle and is concerning for cardiovascular collapse and postoperative cardiac complications with high mortality.[2] The resulting increase in PVR can start a self-perpetuating chain reaction leading to both right and left heart failure (See Figure 12.8).

Postoperative mortality increases with increasing age and right-sided pneumonectomy[2,13] for reasons previously discussed in the Cardiovascular Risk Assessment and Evaluation section. Surgical compression of the heart must be ruled out as a possible cause of poor hemodynamic response to pulmonary artery clamping. If there is no hemodynamic tolerance for pulmonary artery clamping, even after addressing all possible reversible causes, then the surgical and anesthesia team need to decide if it is appropriate[2] to proceed versus resorting to

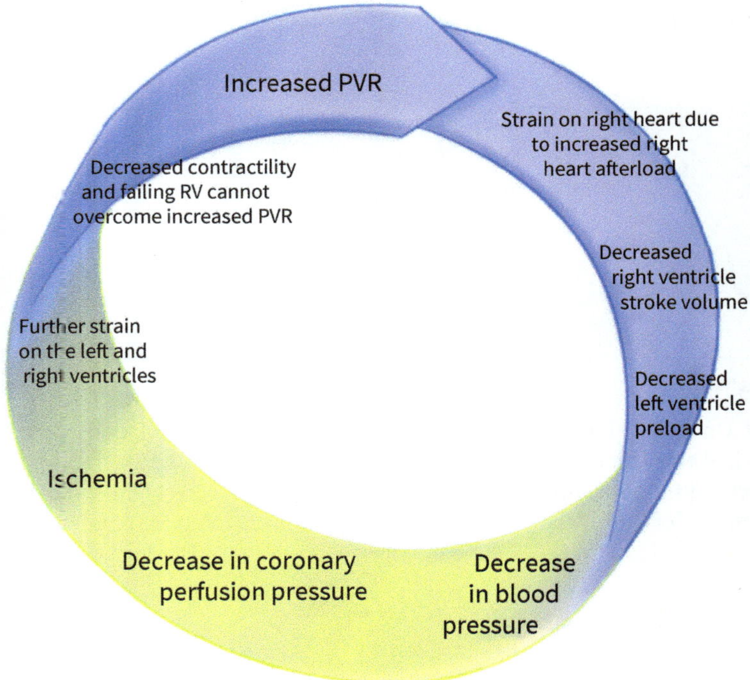

Figure 12.8 Physiologic consequences of increased pulmonary vascular resistance and the development of left and right heart failure.
PVR, pulmonary vascular resistance.

nonsurgical options such as radiotherapy, stereotactic radiotherapy, or radiofrequency ablation.[29] These nonsurgical options should be discussed with patients during the preoperative evaluation. However, with appropriate preoperative workup and patient selection, it is rare to come to this point.[2]

Supplemental Studies

In the case of increased CVP, pulmonary hypertension, and signs of right heart failure, following pulmonary artery clamping, efforts are made to decrease PVR (increase FiO_2, normocapnea or slightly hypocapnic, treat acidosis, normothermia, inhaled nitric oxide 10 to 40 ppm or prostacyclin 50 ng/kg/min) and additional monitors such as PAC and TEE may be employed.[16] PACs are used to monitor right atrium, right ventricle, and pulmonary artery pressures and cardiac output and guide treatment of pulmonary hypertension.[16] TEE transgastric short axis view can be used to visually confirm right heart failure due to increased PVR through demonstration of right ventricle enlargement, flattening of the interventricular septum or D-shape of the left ventricle, and paradoxical motion with bulging of the right ventricle into the left ventricle, which is most pronounced during systole (see Figure 12.9).[45,46] More advanced techniques such as calculation of pulmonary artery pressure using Bernoulli equation (see Figure 12.10), or evaluation of right ventricular function using modalities such as tricuspid annular plane systolic excursion or right ventricle strain through techniques such as 2D speckle tracking can also be used by providers trained in TEE.[45–48]

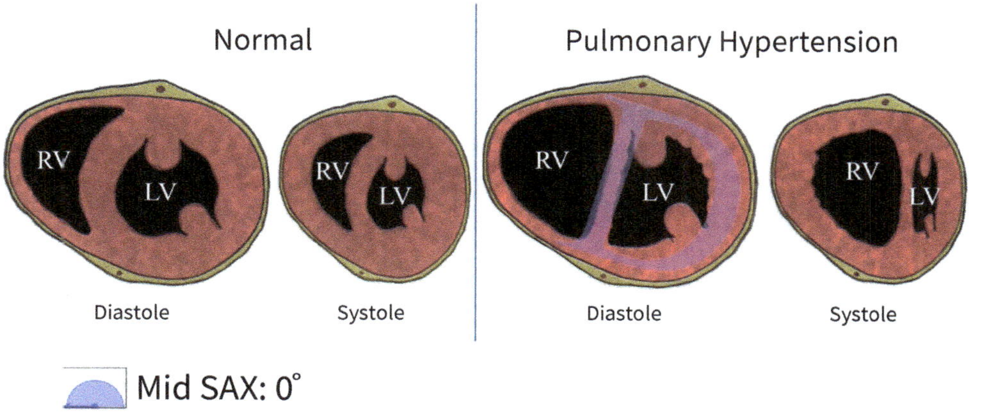

Figure 12.9 Transgastric mid papillary short axis view. Normal appearance of the left and right ventricles during diastole and systole on left. Left and right ventricles in diastole and systole in a patient with pulmonary hypertension on right–right ventricle enlargement, flattening of the interventricular septum or D shape of the left ventricle, and paradoxical motion with bulging of the right ventricle into the left ventricle, which is most pronounced during systole.
Abbreviations: LV, left ventricle; RV, right ventricle.

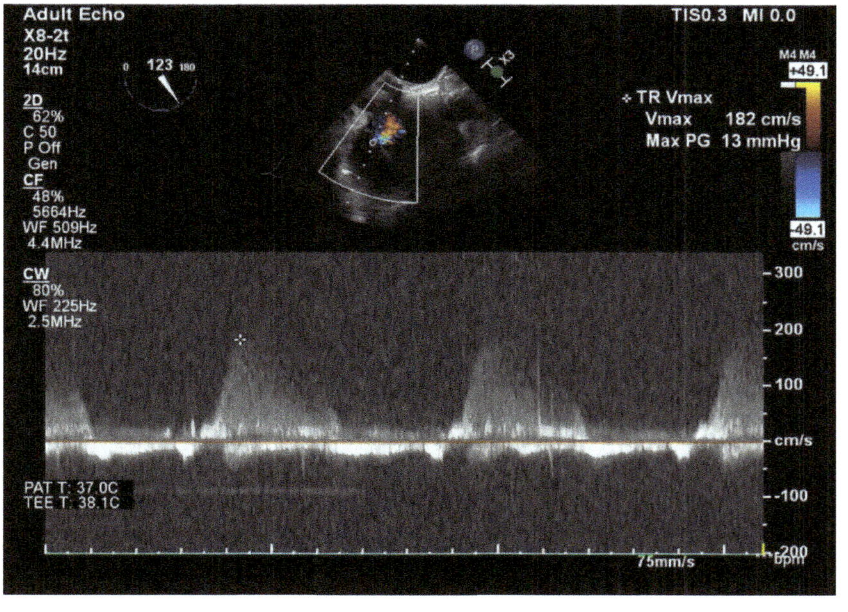

Figure 12.10 Systolic pulmonary artery pressure can be determined with transesophageal echocardiography by using continuous wave Doppler to obtain the peak velocity of the tricuspid regurgitant as seen in figure and Bernoulli equation to calculate the pressure gradient between the right atrium and right ventricle.

Intraoperative Fluid Management

Risk factors for postpneumonectomy pulmonary edema or acute lung injury include pneumonectomy itself, right-sided pneumonectomy, excessive perioperative intravenous fluid administration, high urine output in the intraoperative and postoperative period, high intraoperative ventilatory pressure index (combined airway pressure and time), and preoperative alcohol abuse.[13,49,50] Greater than 3 L in first 24 hours is an independent risk factor for acute lung injury.[50] Fluid administration is carefully managed and goals include less than 20 mL/kg total positive fluid balance in the first 24 hours, less than 3 L of crystalloids administered in the first 24 hours, no fluid administration for third space fluid losses, and fluids should be adjusted so urine output does not exceed 0.5 mL/kg/hr.[13] Infusion of fluids at a rate of 2 to 3 mL/kg/hour is not associated with acute kidney injury in lung resection patients.[38] It is important to avoid hypovolemia and acute kidney injury, while also limiting intravenous fluid administration, so vasopressors are frequently utilized to maintain mean arterial pressure and compensate for autonomic effects of neuraxial blockade.[2,13,16,38] Hemorrhage must be excluded with persistent hypotension,[2] and invasive monitors and vasopressors are used both intraoperatively and postoperatively in efforts to increase tissue perfusion.[13,16,38]

Special Considerations

Extrapleural Pneumonectomy

- Associated with significant blood loss due to involvement of chest wall vessels.
- Venous return to the heart can be compromised by blood loss, compression of SVC by tumor, or surgical causes.
- Cardiac herniation of hemodynamic instability can occur when patient is moved from lateral decubitus to supine position.
- Patients typically remain intubated due to the extended duration of surgery and large fluid shifts.
- If using a DLT, it is typically exchanged to a single-lumen endotracheal tube at the end of the procedure.
- Perioperative morbidity of 0% to 82.6% and mortality of 0% to 11.8%.
- 5-year survival 0% to 78%
- Complications include: acute respiratory distress syndrome, pericardial tamponade, cardiac herniation, pulmonary embolism, respiratory infections, respiratory failure, atrial arrhythmia, and myocardial infarction.[13,40]

Tracheal Sleeve Pneumonectomy/Carinal Pneumonectomy

- Ventilation during tracheobronchial resection and anastomosis can be achieved with
  1. Cross-field ventilation—a long single-lumen sterile endobronchial tube is advanced through the surgical field and into the left mainstem bronchus, or
  2. High-frequency jet ventilation.
- Intermittent apnea is used during placement of anastomotic sutures.
- Occasionally performed with cardiopulmonary bypass or extracorporeal membrane oxygenation.

- Flexible bronchoscopy is performed prior to extubation, to check anastomosis and clear endobronchial secretions.
- The morbidity rate (11%–50%) and mortality rate (3%–20%) are higher, and 5-year survival (20%) is lower than other pulmonary resections.
- Postpneumonectomy pulmonary edema is a common complication after right sleeve pneumonectomy.
- Acute respiratory distress syndrome in up to 20% of patients and has a mortality rate of 50% to 100%.[13,41]

Extubation

Extubation in the OR versus the intensive care unit will be determined on a case-by-case basis depending on multiple factors such as fluid balance, intraoperative course, and patient comorbidities. The following are general recommendations that can be used to guide decision-making[13]:

- ppoFEV1 >40%—extubate in OR when alert, warm, and comfortable.
- ppoFEV1 > 30% to 40%.
  - Good exercise tolerance and lung parenchymal function—extubating in OR is possible.
  - Poor exercise tolerance and lung parenchymal function high—Most appropriate to wean from mechanical ventilation so the effect of increased O2 consumption from spontaneous ventilation can be assessed.
- ppoFEV1 20% to 30%—Can be considered for early extubation if favorable exercise tolerance and lung parenchymal function and thoracic epidural analgesia (TEA) is used.

Pain Management

Adequate analgesia is essential to allow patients the ability to cough and clear secretions. A thoracic epidural catheter or paravertebral catheter (PVC) should be placed preoperatively for both intraoperative and postoperative pain control unless contraindicated.[16,38,51,52] Benefits of TEA include but are not limited to improved perioperative analgesia compared to systemic opioids, decreased pulmonary complications, decreased duration of mechanical ventilation, and decreased postoperative protein catabolism.[51] TEA has also been shown to decrease complications in the high-risk group of patients undergoing pulmonary resection,[53] so is therefore most commonly used and considered the gold standard for pain management for thoracic surgery.[16,38,52] Although TEA is still considered the gold standard, recent studies have shown that PVCs may provide comparable analgesia and a better short-term side effect profile as TEA can cause urinary retention, hypotension, nausea and vomiting, and pulmonary complications.[54] TEA have shown to decrease the incidence of chronic postthoracotomy pain syndrome,[55] but PVCs have the benefit of being unilateral without depression of respiratory function or sympathectomy on the contralateral side.[16,52,56] PVCs have been proven to be beneficial in limiting the amount of fluids administered during pneumonectomy and may decrease risk of major complications including arrhythmias, hemodynamic instability, respiratory complications, intensive care unit admissions, additional surgery, or 30-day mortality.[52] It is not clear at this time whether these perceived advantages of PVCs may be due to factors such as more complicated or sicker patients receiving epidural analgesia. Other regional techniques such as serratus plane blocks and erector spinae blocks are also proving to be beneficial adjuncts in thoracic surgery.[16,38,57,58] Surgical technique with intercostal nerve-sparing techniques with creation of intercostal muscle flap protects the intercostal nerve from crush injury due to compression by surgical retraction and decreases pain.[38]

Postoperative Monitoring and Complications

Postoperatively patients are monitored for hemorrhage, postpneumonectomy pulmonary edema, retained secretions, airway plugging within the contralateral lung, and cardiac arrhythmias. Postoperative chest drains can be used to monitor for hemorrhage, but it is very important to be cautious as to not cause mediastinal shift.

Cardiac Arrhythmias

Postoperative cardiac arrhythmias include atrial fibrillation (AF), atrial flutter, and supraventricular tachycardia.[2,59] AF is the most common postoperative cardiac arrhythmia, and it has been shown that up to 40% of patients will develop postoperative AF,[60] which is associated with increased hospital stay and mortality.[61] See Figure 12.11, which demonstrates how AF can lead to adverse cardiac consequences and left ventricle dysfunction.[62] Risk factors for postoperative AF include, but are not limited to, increased age, male sex, preoperative heart disease, hypovolemia, intraoperative hypotension, anemia, sympathetic activity, catecholamine release, metabolic disturbances (hypoglycemia, hypokalemia, hypomagnesemia), pulmonary arterial vasoconstriction, and excessive fluid shifts.[59,61,63] Potentially modifiable risk factors for AF following lung resection surgery include preoperative alcohol consumption, red cell transfusion, open surgery, and use of inotropes.[64] Increased age is considered the most important risk factor for developing AF.[65] Prevention of postoperative AF includes recognition of increased risk and avoidance of aforementioned triggers. Amiodarone, beta-blockers, and statins have been shown to decrease the incidence of perioperative AF.[66] Management includes prompt investigation of underlying cause, correction of acid/base and electrolyte abnormalities, and pharmacologic treatment with beta-blockers, non-dihydropyridine calcium channel blockers, amiodarone, or digoxin—each with their own pros and cons.[59,63] Prophylactic amiodarone is reasonable and beta blockers may be considered; however, there are no definitive recommendations for prophylaxis, and it is decided on a case by case basis.[2,63]

Stroke

Patients undergoing pneumonectomy have an increased risk of stroke due to thrombosis of the pulmonary vein stumps. The left upper pulmonary vein is believed to be the most likely source of thrombi due to its longer length and slower blood flow as detected by ultrasound.[67]

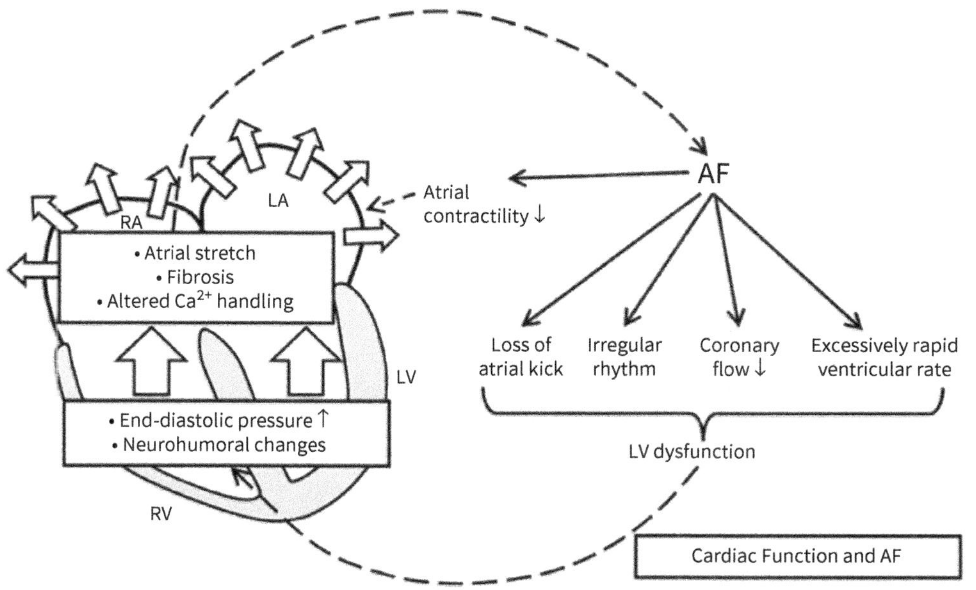

Figure 12.11 Interaction between atrial fibrillation and cardiac function.

Source: Iwasaki Y, Nishida K, Kato T, Nattel S. Atrial Fibrillation pathophysiology: implications for management. *Circulation*. 2011;124(20):2264–2274. doi:10.1161/CIRCULATIONAHA.111.019893. Used with the permission of Elsevier Inc. © All rights reserved.

Abbreviations: AF, atrial fibrillation; LA, left atrium; LV, left ventricle; RA, right atrium; RV, right ventricle.

Perioperative Pulmonary Complications and Postpneumonectomy Pulmonary Edema

Perioperative pulmonary complications including postoperative respiratory failure, pneumonia, atelectasis, bronchospasm, and pulmonary edema occur in 3.9% to 37.5% of patients after lung cancer surgery,[63,68–70] and postpneumonectomy pulmonary edema occurs in 2% to 5%[2,13,16,23,71] of patients after lung resection surgery and has a mortality of up to 50%.[2,13] Risk factors for postpneumonectomy pulmonary edema can be found in the previous discussion of intraoperative fluid management. Postpneumonectomy pulmonary edema typically has a biphasic presentation. Early presentation occurs within the first 72 hours and is due to leaky capillary beds in remaining lung resulting in respiratory distress and hypoxemia.[2] Late presentation occurs greater than 72 hours after pneumonectomy and is usually associated with aspiration, bronchopulmonary fistula, or surgical complications. Treatment includes fluid restriction, diuretics, low ventilatory pressures if patient is mechanically ventilated, and employing measures to decrease PVR.[13]

Bronchopleural Fistula

Bronchopleural fistula (BPF) is a sinus tract with communication between the bronchus and pleural space. Incidence and mortality of BPF are as high as 2.9% to 20% and 18% to 67%, respectively after pneumonectomy.[12,72] Patients present with cough, chest drains with continued air leaks or falling fluid levels, and/or new air fluid levels on chest X-ray.[2] Risk factors for the development of BPF include induction therapy, active smoking, alcohol abuse/dependence, MRC Dyspnea Scale score of 2 or higher, right-sided pneumonectomy, increased operative times, prolonged postoperative ventilation, residual tumor in the stump, and large diameter stumps.[2,12] BPF can be prevented by achieving a healthy anastomosis covered with viable tissue.[41] Due to the left bronchial stump's subaortic location (see Figure 12.5), it is usually protected by tissues within the mediastinum. The right bronchial stump is more exposed and needs to be protected by covering with a well-vascularized tissue flap such as an intercostal muscle.[2,38] Right pneumonectomy has a greater risk of developing BPF due to its location, as well as its single blood supply from one bronchial artery, compared to the left with two bronchial arteries.[2] Patients should ideally be medically managed and stabilized prior to surgical repair, but occasionally patients need to be emergently taken to the OR for surgical re-exploration and may even require carinal resection due to BPF following pneumonectomy.[41] These patients are exceptionally challenging to manage as they can have sepsis, hypoxia, respiratory failure, and cardiac collapse.[2] It is best to maintain spontaneous ventilation prior to intubation and BPF is an absolute indication for OLV.[44] Rapid lung isolation is needed to avoid overspill from the BPF to the remaining lung and to prevent positive pressure ventilation from being delivered to the stump as it can worsen the leak and even lead to a tension pneumothorax.[44,73] Late presentation of BPF is associated with more nonspecific signs and are often associated with empyema. If associated with empyema, patient is treated with draining the fluid, antibiotics, and surgical repair of the fistula (see Figure 12.5, demonstrating a large empyema).[2]

Cardiac Herniation

Cardiac herniation is a deadly complication with greater than 50% mortality.[2,13] The heart herniates through a defect in pericardium into the postpneumonectomy space due to pressure difference between the two hemithoraces. This usually occurs within the first 24 hours after surgery, when the pericardium is incompletely closed or the closure breaks down. Cardiac herniation after right pneumonectomy leads to an impedance of venous return and presents with increased CVP, tachycardia, hypotension, shock, and torsion of the heart can cause an acute superior vena cava syndrome.[74] With cardiac herniation after left sided pneumonectomy compression of the myocardium can lead to myocardial ischemia, arrhythmias, and ventricular outflow obstruction.[13] Cardiac herniation can rapidly lead to cardiac arrest, and if the diagnosis is suspected, the patient should be placed in lateral decubitus position with the operative side up and taken to the OR for surgical repair.[2,13] Due to the emergent nature, a single-lumen endotracheal tube is normally used.[13]

Acknowledgment

We would like to thank Robert Krejci for designing figures and providing illustrations in this chapter.

References

1. Fell SC. A history of pneumonectomy. *Chest Surg Clin N Am*. 1999;9(2):267–290, ix.
2. Hackett S, Jones R, Kapila R. Anaesthesia for pneumonectomy. *BJA Educ*. 2019;19(9):297–304. doi:10.1016/j.bjae.2019.04.004
3. Quint LE. Lung cancer: assessing resectability. *Cancer Imaging*. 2003;4(1):15–18. doi:10.1102/1470-7330.2003.0028
4. Shapiro M, Swanson SJ, Wright CD, et al. Predictors of major morbidity and mortality after pneumonectomy utilizing the Society for Thoracic Surgeons General Thoracic Surgery Database. *Ann Thorac Surg*. 2010;90(3):927–935. doi:10.1016/j.athoracsur.2010.05.041
5. Brunelli A, Kim AW, Berger KI, Addrizzo-Harris DJ. physiologic evaluation of the patient with lung cancer being considered for resectional surgery. *Chest*. 2013;143(5):e166S–e190S. doi:10.1378/chest.12-2395
6. Lim E, Baldwin D, Beckles M, et al. Guidelines on the radical management of patients with lung cancer. *Thorax*. 2010;65(Suppl 3):iii1–iii27. doi:10.1136/thx.2010.145938
7. Bray F, Ferlay J, Soerjomataram I, Siegel RL, Torre LA, Jemal A. Global cancer statistics 2018: GLOBOCAN estimates of incidence and mortality worldwide for 36 cancers in 185 countries. *CA Cancer J Clin*. 2018;68(6):394–424. doi:10.3322/caac.21492
8. Siegel RL, Miller KD, Jemal A. Cancer statistics, 2019. *CA Cancer J Clin*. 2019;69(1):7–34. doi:10.3322/caac.21551
9. Goldstraw P, Chansky K, Crowley J, et al. The IASLC lung cancer staging project: proposals for revision of the TNM stage groupings in the forthcoming (eighth) edition of the TNM Classification for Lung Cancer. *J Thorac Oncol*. 2016;11(1):39–51. doi:10.1016/j.jtho.2015.09.009
10. British Thoracic Society. Guidelines on the selection of patients with lung cancer for surgery. *Thorax*. 2001;56(2):89–108. doi:10.1136/thorax.56.2.89
11. Miller RD, ed. *Miller's Anesthesia*. 7th ed. Philadelphia, PA: Churchill Livingstone/Elsevier; 2010.
12. Thomas PA, Berbis J, Baste J-M, et al. Pneumonectomy for lung cancer: Contemporary national early morbidity and mortality outcomes. *J Thorac Cardiovasc Surg*. 2015;149(1):73–83. doi:10.1016/j.jtcvs.2014.09.063
13. Slinger P. Update on anesthetic management for pneumonectomy: *Curr Opin Anaesthesiol*. 2009;22(1):31–37. doi:10.1097/ACO.0b013e32831a4394
14. Slinger P, Darling G. Preanesthetic Assessment for Thoracic Surgery. In: Slinger P, ed. *Principles and Practice of Anesthesia for Thoracic Surgery*. New York, NY: Springer New York; 2011:11–34. doi:10.1007/978-1-4419-0184-2_2
15. Roy PM. Preoperative pulmonary evaluation for lung resection. *J Anaesthesia Clin Pharmacol*. 2018;34(3):296–300.
16. Lederman D, Easwar J, Feldman J, Shapiro V. Anesthetic considerations for lung resection: preoperative assessment, intraoperative challenges and postoperative analgesia. *Ann Transl Med*. 2019;7(15):356–356. doi:10.21037/atm.2019.03.67
17. Della Rocca G, Vetrugno L, Coccia C, et al. Preoperative evaluation of patients undergoing lung resection surgery: defining the role of the anesthesiologist on a multidisciplinary team. *J Cardiothorac Vasc Anesth*. 2016;30(2):530–538. doi:10.1053/j.jvca.2015.11.018
18. Wilkinson JN, Pennefather SH, McCahon RA. *Thoracic Anaesthesia*. Oxford, UK: Oxford University Press; 2011.
19. Ramakrishna G, Sprung J, Ravi BS, Chandrasekaran K, McGoon MD. Impact of pulmonary hypertension on the outcomes of noncardiac surgery: predictors of perioperative morbidity and mortality. *J Am Coll Cardiol*. 2005;45(10):1691–1699. doi:10.1016/j.jacc.2005.02.055
20. Cohen ME, Ko CY, Bilimoria KY, et al. Optimizing ACS NSQIP modeling for evaluation of surgical quality and risk: patient risk adjustment, procedure mix adjustment, shrinkage adjustment, and surgical focus. *J Am Coll Surg*. 2013;217(2):336–346.e1. doi:10.1016/j.jamcollsurg.2013.02.027
21. Gupta PK, Gupta H, Sundaram A, et al. Development and validation of a risk calculator for prediction of cardiac risk after surgery. *Circulation*. 2011;124(4):381–387. doi:10.1161/CIRCULATIONAHA.110.015701

22. Ford MK, Beattie WS, Wijeysundera DN. Systematic review: prediction of perioperative cardiac complications and mortality by the revised cardiac risk index. *Ann Intern Med*. 2010;152(1):26–35. doi:10.7326/0003-4819-152-1-201001050-00007
23. Brunelli A, Varela G, Salati M, et al. Recalibration of the Revised Cardiac Risk Index in Lung Resection Candidates. *Ann Thorac Surg*. 2010;90(1):199–203. doi:10.1016/j.athoracsur.2010.03.042
24. Thomas DC, Blasberg JD, Arnold BN, et al. Validating the Thoracic Revised Cardiac Risk Index Following Lung Resection. *Ann Thorac Surg*. 2017;104(2):389–394. doi:10.1016/j.athoracsur.2017.02.006
25. Ferguson MK, Siddique J, Karrison T. Modeling major lung resection outcomes using classification trees and multiple imputation techniques. *Eur J Cardio-Thorac Surg*. 2008;34(5):1085–1089. doi:10.1016/j.ejcts.2008.07.037
26. DeCato TW, Hegewald MJ. Breathing red: physiology of an elevated single-breath diffusing capacity of carbon monoxide. *Ann Am Thorac Soc*. 2016;13(11):2087–2092. doi:10.1513/AnnalsATS.201605-355CC
27. Ferguson MK, Vigneswaran WT. Diffusing capacity predicts morbidity after lung resection in patients without obstructive lung disease. *Ann Thorac Surg*. 2008;85(4):1158–1165. doi:10.1016/j.athoracsur.2007.12.071
28. Ferguson MK, Reeder LB, Mick R. Optimizing selection of patients for major lung resection. *J Thorac Cardiovasc Surg*. 1995;109(2):275–281; discussion 281–283. doi:10.1016/S0022-5223(95)70389-6
29. Beckles MA, Spiro SG, Colice GL, Rudd RM; American College of Chest Physicians. The physiologic evaluation of patients with lung cancer being considered for resectional surgery. *Chest*. 2003;123(1 Suppl):105S–114S. doi:10.1378/chest.123.1_suppl.105s
30. Albouaini K, Egred M, Alahmar A, Wright DJ. Cardiopulmonary exercise testing and its application. *Postgrad Med J*. 2007;83(985):675–682. doi:10.1136/hrt.2007.121558
31. Milani RV, Lavie CJ, Mehra MR, Ventura HO. Understanding the basics of cardiopulmonary exercise testing. *Mayo Clin Proc*. 2006;81(12):1603–1611. doi:10.4065/81.12.1603
32. Walsh GL, Morice RC, Putnam JB, et al. Resection of lung cancer is justified in high-risk patients selected by exercise oxygen consumption. *Ann Thorac Surg*. 1994;58(3):704–710, discussion 711. doi:10.1016/0003-4975(94)90731-5
33. Brunelli A, Xiumé F, Refai M, et al. Peak oxygen consumption measured during the stair-climbing test in lung resection candidates. *Respiration*. 2010;80(3):207–211. doi:10.1159/000279331
34. Win T. Comparison of shuttle walk with measured peak oxygen consumption in patients with operable lung cancer. *Thorax*. 2005;61(1):57–60. doi:10.1136/thx.2005.043547
35. Towe CW, Wu K, Khil A, et al. Desaturation during six-minute walk testing predicts major morbidity following anatomic lung resection among patients with COPD. *Healthc Basel Switz*. 2019;7(1). doi:10.3390/healthcare7010016
36. Jaffe RA. *Anesthesiologist's Manual of Surgical Procedures*. 5th ed. Philadelphia, PA: Wolters Kluwer; 2014
37. Batchelor TJP, Ljungqvist O. A surgical perspective of ERAS guidelines in thoracic surgery. *Curr Opin Anaesthesiol*. 2019;32(1):17–22. doi:10.1097/ACO.0000000000000685
38. Batchelor TJP, Rasburn NJ, Abdelnour-Berchtold E, et al. Guidelines for enhanced recovery after lung surgery: recommendations of the Enhanced Recovery After Surgery (ERAS®) Society and the European Society of Thoracic Surgeons (ESTS). *Eur J Cardiothorac Surg*. 2019;55(1):91–115. doi:10.1093/ejcts/ezy301
39. Rendina EA, Venuta F, Ibrahim M. Intrapericardial pneumonectomy. *Multimed Man Cardiothorac Surg MMCTS*. 2006;2006(109):mmcts.2004.000091. doi:10.1510/mmcts.2004.000091
40. Duranti L, Pardolesi A, Bertolaccini L, et al. Extra-pleural pneumonectomy. *J Thorac Dis*. 2019;11(3):1022–1030. doi:10.21037/jtd.2019.02.61
41. Weder W, Inci I. Carinal resection and sleeve pneumonectomy. *J Thorac Dis*. 2016;8(S11):S882–S888. doi:10.21037/jtd.2016.08.47
42. Ku CM. Anesthesia for Patients with Mediastinal Masses. In: Slinger P, ed. *Principles and Practice of Anesthesia for Thoracic Surgery*. New York, NY: Springer; 2011:201–210. doi:10.1007/978-1-4419-0184-2_14

43. Ferrando C, Mugarra A, Gutierrez A, et al. Setting individualized positive end-expiratory pressure level with a positive end-expiratory pressure decrement trial after a recruitment maneuver improves oxygenation and lung mechanics during one-lung ventilation. *Anesth Analg*. 2014;118(3):657–665. doi:10.1213/ANE.0000000000000105
44. Ashok V, Francis J. A practical approach to adult one-lung ventilation. *BJA Educ*. 2018;18(3):69–74. doi:10.1016/j.bjae.2017.11.007
45. Rudski LG, Lai WW, Afilalo J, et al. Guidelines for the echocardiographic assessment of the right heart in adults: a report from the American Society of Echocardiography. *J Am Soc Echocardiogr*. 2010;23(7):685–713. doi:10.1016/j.echo.2010.05.010
46. Vegas A. *Perioperative Two-Dimensional Transesophageal Echocardiography: A Practical Handbook*. New York, NY: Springer; 2012.
47. Tousignant C, Desmet M, Bowry R, Harrington AM, Cruz JD, Mazer CD. Speckle tracking for the intraoperative assessment of right ventricular function: a feasibility study. *J Cardiothorac Vasc Anesth*. 2010;24(2):275–279. doi:10.1053/j.jvca.2009.10.022
48. Savage RM, Aronson S, eds. *Basic Perioperative Transesophageal Echocardiography: A Multimedia Review*. 1st ed. Philadelphia: Wolters Kluwer/Lippincott Williams & Wilkins Health; 2013.
49. Zeldin RA, Normandin D, Landtwing D, Peters RM. Postpneumonectomy pulmonary edema. *J Thorac Cardiovasc Surg*. 1984;87(3):359–365.
50. Licker M, de Perrot M, Spiliopoulos A, et al. Risk factors for acute lung injury after thoracic surgery for lung cancer: *Anesth Analg*. 2003;97(6):1558–1565. doi:10.1213/01.ANE.0000087799.85495.8A
51. Manion SC, Brennan TJ. Thoracic epidural analgesia and acute pain management. *Anesthesiology*. 2011;115(1):181–188. doi:10.1097/ALN.0b013e318220847c
52. Powell ES, Cook D, Pearce AC, et al. A prospective, multicentre, observational cohort study of analgesia and outcome after pneumonectomy. *Br J Anaesth*. 2011;106(3):364–370. doi:10.1093/bja/aeq379
53. Cerfolio RJ, Allen MS, Trastek VF, Deschamps C, Scanlon PD, Pairolero PC. Lung resection in patients with compromised pulmonary function. *Ann Thorac Surg*. 1996;62(2):348–351.
54. Davies RG, Myles PS, Graham JM. A comparison of the analgesic efficacy and side-effects of paravertebral vs epidural blockade for thoracotomy: a systematic review and meta-analysis of randomized trials. *Br J Anaesth*. 2006;96(4):418–426. doi:10.1093/bja/ael020
55. Khoronenko V, Baskakov D, Leone M, et al. Influence of regional anesthesia on the rate of chronic postthoracotomy pain syndrome in lung cancer patients. *Ann Thorac Cardiovasc Surg*. 2018;24(4):180–186. doi:10.5761/atcs.oa.18-00044
56. Daly DJ, Myles PS. Update on the role of paravertebral blocks for thoracic surgery: are they worth it? *Curr Opin Anaesthesiol*. 2009;22(1):38–43. doi:10.1097/ACO.0b013e32831a4074
57. Lee J, Kim S. The effects of ultrasound-guided serratus plane block, in combination with general anesthesia, on intraoperative opioid consumption, emergence time, and hemodynamic stability during video-assisted thoracoscopic lobectomy: a randomized prospective study. *Medicine (Baltimore)*. 2019;98(18):e15385. doi:10.1097/MD.0000000000015385
58. Bang S, Chung K, Chung J, Yoo S, Baek S, Lee SM. The erector spinae plane block for effective analgesia after lung lobectomy: three cases report. *Medicine (Baltimore)*. 2019;98(29):e16262. doi:10.1097/MD.0000000000016262
59. Fleisher LA, Fleischmann KE, Auerbach AD, et al. 2014 ACC/AHA guideline on perioperative cardiovascular evaluation and management of patients undergoing noncardiac surgery. *J Am Coll Cardiol*. 2014;64(22):e77–e137. doi:10.1016/j.jacc.2014.07.944
60. De Decker K, Jorens PG, Van Schil P. Cardiac complications after noncardiac thoracic surgery: an evidence-based current review. *Ann Thorac Surg*. 2003;75(4):1340–1348. doi:10.1016/S0003-4975(02)04824-5
61. Roselli EE, Murthy SC, Rice TW, et al. Atrial fibrillation complicating lung cancer resection. *J Thorac Cardiovasc Surg*. 2005;130(2):438.e1–438.e9. doi:10.1016/j.jtcvs.2005.02.010
62. Iwasaki Y, Nishida K, Kato T, Nattel S. Atrial fibrillation pathophysiology: implications for management. *Circulation*. 2011;124(20):2264–2274. doi:10.1161/CIRCULATIONAHA.111.019893

63. Karamchandani K, Khanna AK, Bose S, Fernando RJ, Walkey AJ. Atrial fibrillation: current evidence and management strategies during the perioperative period. *Anesth Analg.* 2020;130(1):2–13. doi:10.1213/ANE.0000000000004474
64. Lee SH, Ahn HJ, Yeon SM, et al. Potentially modifiable risk factors for atrial fibrillation following lung resection surgery: a retrospective cohort study. *Anaesthesia.* 2016;71(12):1424–1430. doi:10.1111/anae.13644
65. Amar D. Older age is the strongest predictor of postoperative atrial fibrillation. 2002;96(2):5.
66. Oesterle A, Weber B, Tung R, Choudhry NK, Singh JP, Upadhyay GA. Preventing postoperative atrial fibrillation after noncardiac surgery: a meta-analysis. *Am J Med.* 2018;131(7):795–804.e5. doi:10.1016/j.amjmed.2018.01.032
67. Riddersholm S, Tayal B, Kragholm K, et al. Incidence of stroke after pneumonectomy and lobectomy: a nationwide, register-based study. *Stroke.* 2019;50(5):1052–1059. doi:10.1161/STROKEAHA.118.024496
68. Reeve JC, Nicol K, Stiller K, et al. Does physiotherapy reduce the incidence of postoperative pulmonary complications following pulmonary resection via open thoracotomy? A preliminary randomised single-blind clinical trial. *Eur J Cardio-Thorac Surg Off J Eur Assoc Cardio-Thorac Surg.* 2010;37(5):1158–1166. doi:10.1016/j.ejcts.2009.12.011
69. Rodriguez-Larrad A, Vellosillo-Ortega JM, Ruiz-Muneta C, Abecia-Inchaurregui LC, Seco J. Postoperative respiratory exercises reduce the risk of developing pulmonary complications in patients undergoing lobectomy. *Arch Bronconeumol.* 2016;52(7):347–353. doi:10.1016/j.arbres.2015.11.017
70. de la Gala F, Piñeiro P, Reyes A, et al. Postoperative pulmonary complications, pulmonary and systemic inflammatory responses after lung resection surgery with prolonged one-lung ventilation: randomized controlled trial comparing intravenous and inhalational anaesthesia. *Br J Anaesth.* 2017;119(4):655–663. doi:10.1093/bja/aex230
71. Dulu A, Pastores SM, Park B, Riedel E, Rusch V, Halpern NA. Prevalence and mortality of acute lung injury and ARDS after lung resection. *Chest.* 2006;130(1):73–78. doi:10.1378/chest.130.1.73
72. Sarkar P, Chandak T, Shah R, Talwar A. Diagnosis and management bronchopleural fistula. *Indian J Chest Dis Allied Sci.* 2010;52(2):97–104.
73. Khurana JS, Sharma VN. Bronchopleural fistula management during anaesthesia. *Br J Anaesth.* 1964;36:302–306. doi:10.1093/bja/36.5.302
74. Mehanna MJ, Israel GM, Katigbak M, Rubinowitz AN. Cardiac herniation after right pneumonectomy: case report and review of the literature. *J Thorac Imaging.* 2007;22(3):280–282. doi:10.1097/RTI.0b013e31803bb451

13
Anesthesia for Pleural Space Procedures

Harendra Arora and Alan Smeltz

Introduction

The pleural space is located between the visceral pleura, lining the surface of each lung, and the parietal pleura, lining the interior chest wall. These structures function to transmit changes in intrathoracic pressure generated by the diaphragm and chest wall to the lungs and permit lung sliding during respiratory movement. The pleural linings are intimately apposed and create a potential space with pressure that is slightly more negative than atmospheric pressure.

There are many types of pleural diseases. These include conditions such as inflammation (pleurisy), hemothorax, chylothorax, pneumothorax, pleural effusion, and empyema as well as pleural tumors. Pleural tumors can either arise from the pleura itself (e.g., mesothelioma) or can spread to the pleura (metastatic) from another site. These conditions typically present with nonspecific cardiopulmonary symptoms such as dyspnea, cough, pleuritic chest pain, and hypotension, but there might also be features that indicate a particular etiology. As a group, pleural diseases are common and frequently managed surgically. This chapter will focus on the conditions that are most likely to require surgical management. Although pleural pathology is generally situated more peripherally from vital mediastinal structures than other categories of thoracic pathology, they have their own risks and set of challenges for the thoracic anesthesiologist.

Surgical Considerations for Specific Pleural Diseases

Pleural Effusion

Pleural effusion is excessive collection of fluid in the pleural space (Figure 13.1). The collection can either be a transudate or an exudate, based on Light's criteria (Table 13.1).[1,2] A transductive collection occurs when there is either a net increase in hydrostatic pressure or decrease in oncotic pressure across the intact capillary beds, as is seen in patients with congestive heart failure or liver cirrhosis. An exudative collection occurs when there is either decreased lymphatic drainage or increased capillary permeability that results in fluid leakage into the pleural space, as seen in pneumonia, malignant pleural disease, or pulmonary embolism. The most common malignant etiologies are lung cancer (37.5%), breast cancer (16.8%), lymphoma (11.5%), and genitourinary cancer (9.4%).[3] As fluid accumulates

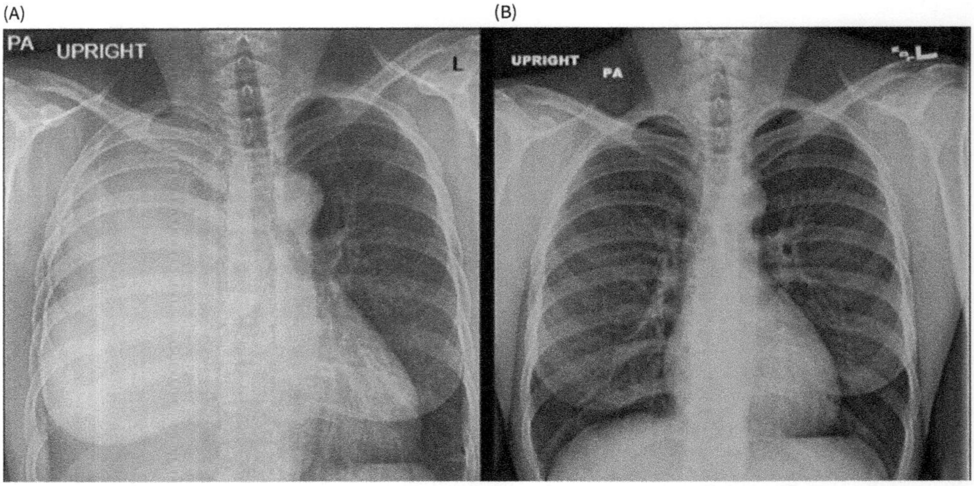

Figure 13.1 Pleural effusion. (A) Postero-anterior chest X-ray showing a large right-sided pleural effusion with a complete white-out. (B) Chest X-ray of the same patient a month later with complete resolution of the pleural effusion.

Table 13.1 Etiologies of Pleural Effusions

	Transudate	Exudate
Light's criteria		
Protein, pleural:serum	≤0.5	>0.5
LDH, pleural:serum	≤0.6	>0.6
	or	*or*
	pleural LDH ≤2/3 upper limit normal for serum LDH	pleural LDH >2/3 upper limit normal for serum LDH
Mechanisms	↑serum hydrostatic pressure	↑capillary permeability
	↓serum oncotic pressure	↓pleural lymphatic drainage
Etiologies	Congestive heart failure	Pneumonia
	Atelectasis	Malignancy
	Nephrotic syndrome	Pulmonary embolism
	Hypoalbuminemia	Chylothorax
	Hepatic hydrothorax	Empyema
	Urinothorax	Constrictive pericarditis
	Peritoneal dialysis	Trapped lung
	Pulmonary embolism	Superior vena cava obstruction
		Sarcoidosis

Sources: Adapted from Light RW, Macgregor MI, Luchsinger PC, Ball WC, Jr, Pleural effusions: the diagnostic separation of transudates and exudates, *Ann Intern Med.* 1972;77(4):507–513, and Light RW, Clinical practice, pleural effusion, *N Engl J Med.* 2002;346(25):1971–1977.

Abbreviation: LDH, lactate dehydrogenase

in the pleural space, the external mass effect limits lung expansion, leading to ineffective ventilation, increased work of breathing, atelectasis, and hypoxemic shunting.

Thoracentesis to drain pleural effusion, either diagnostic or therapeutic, is generally safe but can lead to some degree of pneumothorax in as many as 39% of cases.[4] Other more common complications include hemothorax, solid organ puncture, and ineffective aspiration of fluid. To minimize the risk of complications, ultrasound should be used to guide access. Large volume drainage can be performed to alleviate symptoms and/or assess the lung for re-expandability, if pleurodesis is being considered. One method to assess re-expandability is to measure the change in pleural pressure after removing 500 mL of fluid and calculate the elastance of the pleural space. Less than a 19 cmH_2O decrease suggests the lung will re-expand.[5] Removal of a volume >1.5 L, however, increases the risk of re-expansion pulmonary edema. Patients with lung entrapment (non–re-expandable lungs) are at increased risk of this complication due to the introduction of extreme negative pleural pressure that accompanies large volume thoracentesis. Although uncommon (incidence <1%), re-expansion pulmonary edema can manifest with sudden worsening of respiratory distress. Treatment is usually supportive, although returning fluid to the pleural space has also been associated with rapid resolution of symptoms.[6]

If the lung is re-expandable, the insertion of an indwelling pleural drainage catheter and/or pleurodesis, the induced adherence of visceral and parietal pleura through scarification, is recommended. Although sclerosing chemical, and not abrasive mechanical, pleurodesis is specifically mentioned in the 2013 American Thoracic Society/Society of Thoracic Surgeons/Society of Thoracic Radiology practice guideline,[4] there is conflicting evidence regarding which method is more efficacious.[7,8] Talc is the most effective and commonly used agent for chemical pleurodesis, although it is associated with a greater incidence of pleuritic chest pain, pneumonitis, and acute respiratory distress syndrome, as compared to other agents like tetracyclines or bleomycin (Table 13.2 and Box 13.1).[3,9] Talc can be administered either through the indwelling pleural catheter in slurry form (powder mixed with saline) or in its powder form through direct thoracoscopic application. Pleural catheters should remain clamped for at least an hour following the administration of talc slurry. However, if the lung is not re-expandable (as occurs in 30% of cases), placement of an indwelling catheter alone is preferred over attempting pleurodesis. Lysis of adhesions and loculations can be attempted by either the administration of a fibrinolytic agent into the catheter or by thoracoscopic mechanical disruption and clearance. Surgical pleurodesis has a reported success rate of 90%, as compared to chemical injection into the pleural catheter of 60%.[3] This difference may be due to more thorough liberation of loculations and therefore increased lung mobilization.

For patients dealing with chronic malignant pleural effusion that are either refractory to pleurodesis or have lung entrapment, another palliative option is pleuroperitoneal shunting. This approach helps patients minimize fluid accumulation in their thorax as one-way valves permit drainage into the peritoneal cavity. One important risk of this procedure is the possibility of malignant cells seeding into the abdomen.

Chylothorax

The thoracic duct transports around 4 L of chyle, a mixture of lymphatic fluid and gut-absorbed fats, cephalad through the posteromedial thorax, terminally draining into the venous system

Table 13.2 Common Sclerosing Agents Used for Pleurodesis and Their Associated Success Rate

Sclerosing Agent	Success Rate (%)
Talc	70–100
Tetracycline	50–92
Bleomycin	58–85
Cisplatin	65–83
Doxycycline	60–89
Taxol	85–93
Erythromycin	85–88

Source: Adapted from Zarogoulidis K, Zarogoulidis P, Darwiche K, et al. Malignant pleural effusion and algorithm management. *J Thorac Dis*. 2013;5(Suppl 4):S413–419.

at the juncture of the left subclavian and internal jugular veins. Either congenital, neoplastic, or traumatic processes can lead to thoracic duct injury, resulting in the intrathoracic leakage of chyle, also known as chylothorax. Traumatic injury of the duct can occur in up to 2.6% of patients after video-assisted thoracoscopic lung resections and 10.5% after esophageal surgery.[10] The degree of chyle leak can be classified as low (<500 mL over 24 hours) or high volume (>1000 mL over 24 hours).[11] High volume chylous losses can increase the risk of malnutrition, immunosuppression, infection, and respiratory disorders. If left untreated, chylothorax is associated with a 30% risk of mortality.[10] If the leak remains high volume after 5 to 7 days of dietary fat restriction, surgical management is indicated. Options include pleurodesis, thoracic duct ligation, and non-invasive intravascular thoracic duct embolization.

Empyema

Empyema is an exudative collection of purulent fluid that results from infection within the pleural space (Figure 13.2). There are three stages of development: Stage I, the exudative

Box 13.1 Adverse Effects Related to Pleurodesis With Talc

- Fever
- Chest pain
- Dyspnea
- Atelectasis
- Subcutaneous emphysema
- Prolonged air leak
- Empyema

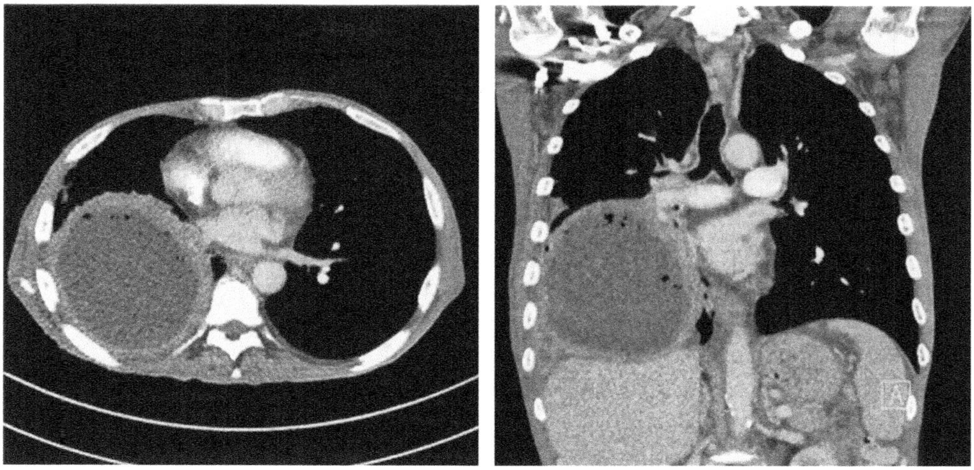

Figure 13.2 Empyema. (A) A transverse chest computed tomography scan (with contrast) showing a large posteriorly located right-sided empyema. (B) Coronal section of the chest computed tomography demonstrating the extent of the empyema.

phase, where fluid can be easily drained and the affected lung remains fully re-expandable; Stage II, the fibropurulent phase, where the exudate thickens and fibrin deposits, forming loculations; and Stage III, the chronic organizing phase, where granulation tissue forms followed by scarring that leads to contraction of the hemithorax and ipsilateral shifting of the mediastinum.[12] In addition to appropriate antibiotic medications and therapeutic drainage of the effusion, surgical intervention is often indicated. A meta-analysis of eight randomized controlled trials demonstrated patients with earlier stage empyema (Stages I and II) had a similar rate of mortality whether managed with or without surgery.[13] However, patients that underwent surgery had shorter hospital lengths of stay. One factor that has been attributed to the success of patients undergoing nonsurgical management has been the administration of fibrinolytic agents into the thoracostomy drainage tube.[14]

For patients undergoing surgery, thoracoscopic deloculation and decortication may be performed, and depending on the stage of development, entrapped lung segments may require resection as well. If there are larger segments of non–re-expandable lung, the pleural space may then be obliterated to prevent empyema re-accumulation. This can be accomplished by the insertion of muscle flaps or silicone implants so as to obliterate the newly voided pleural space (Figure 13.3).[15] For patients with comorbid conditions that might compromise their survivability after one of these interventions, establishing a temporary open-window thoracotomy can be attempted to enable drainage of the infected material.

Hemothorax

Blood can accumulate in the pleural space as a result of blunt or penetrating chest trauma, surgery, coagulopathy, vascular disease, or vascular-invasive or angioproliferative neoplastic processes or from a variety of other less common etiologies.[16] Hemothorax occurs in up to

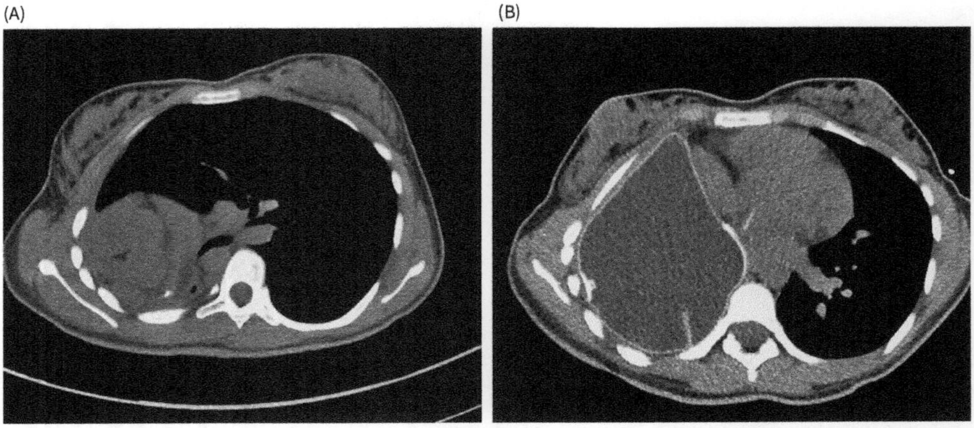

Figure 13.3 Postpneumonectomy syndrome. (A) A transverse chest computed tomography scan demonstrating rightward shift of the mediastinal structures following right pneumonectomy. (B) A transverse chest computed tomography scan of the same patient following insertion of a saline-filled silicone implant. Obliteration of the pleural space in this manner can also be used to prevent re-accumulation of material, such as empyema.

60% of multitrauma patients and is responsible for up to 25% of deaths in this patient population.[17] Initial management of hemothorax involves the placement of a thoracostomy drain. Factors that suggest further surgical intervention include initial release of 1500 mL or more of bloody fluid, the sustained release of 200 mL or more over 4 hours, and unstable hemodynamics that are refractory to nonsurgical management. Bloody exudate may become retained (i.e., failed evacuation despite the presence of a thoracostomy tube) if either blood has clotted or if loculations develop. Retained blood may serve as a nidus for pleural infection and empyema. Once the source of pleural hemorrhage has been identified, additional disease-specific therapy may then be warranted.

Pneumothorax

There are many ways gas can enter the pleural space, causing a pneumothorax (Figure 13.4). Mechanisms include spontaneous pneumothorax, both in the presence or absence of an underlying lung pathology, traumatic chest wall injury, and iatrogenic procedural complication. Conditions resulting from chest wall defects may require specific early intervention to close the defect. However, in general, whether or not to primarily manage medically or place a thoracostomy drain tube is based on the presence of concurrent lung disease, a pleural-to-chest wall distance >2 cm on coronary chest radiograph and the degree of associated respiratory insufficiency.[18] For prolonged pleural leaks that do not abate within 3 to 5 days, surgical intervention is warranted. For patients unable or unwilling to undergo surgery, nonoperative chemical pleurodesis injection into the thoracostomy drain may be attempted. Surgical options include pleurodesis and resection of associated diseased lung segments.[19,20]

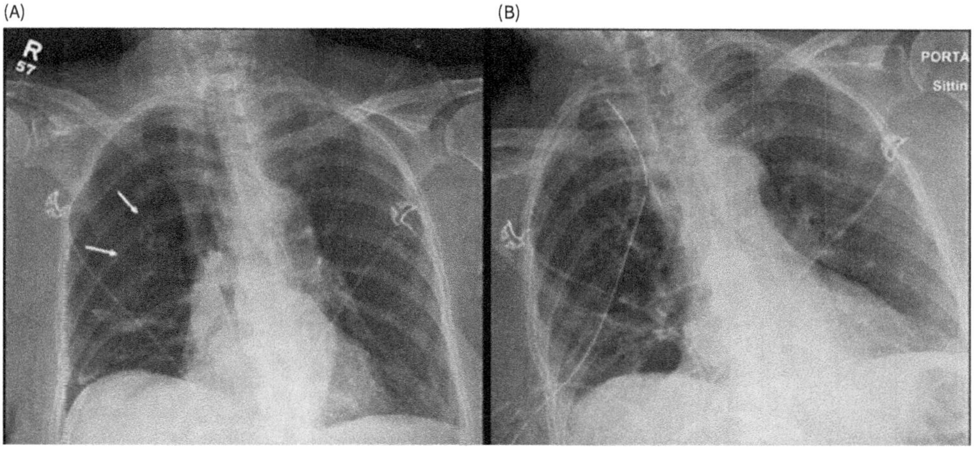

Figure 13.4 Pneumothorax. (A) Anteroposterior chest X-ray showing a large right-sided pneumothorax with arrows pointing to the collapsed lung border. (B) An anteroposterior chest X-ray showing expansion of the lung following chest tube placement.

Malignant Mesothelioma

Malignant mesothelioma is a highly aggressive cancer that can involve mesothelial tissues, including the pleura (Figure 13.5). The cancer is highly invasive locally and produces malignant pleural effusion. Median survival is 4.5 months with best medical management and 14.5 months with surgery.[21] Treatment usually involves chemotherapy along with radiation therapy, and surgical debridement is often performed for palliation. The infiltrative spread of the cancer renders any surgical option technically challenging and high risk. Surgical management options include talc pleurodesis, pleurectomy with or without decortication, and extrapleural pneumonectomy. Pleurectomy is the removal of diseased pleura, and with decortication, the thickened cancerous rind is peeled away from the pleural space. Extrapleural pneumonectomy is the *en bloc* resection of cancer-infiltrated lung, pleura, pericardium, and hemidiaphragm, with subsequent repair of pericardium and hemidiaphragm with patches, as necessary.

In the Mesothelioma and Radical Surgery multicenter trial, patients were randomized to either have extrapleural pneumonectomy or not (medical management with or without pleurectomy).[21] This study demonstrated that patients who underwent extrapleural pneumonectomy suffered harm, with decreased survival at 1 year and no increase in quality of life. A subsequent retrospective study that specifically compared patients having undergone extrapleural pneumonectomy with those having had pleurectomy with decortication demonstrated the former was associated with increased morbidity and mortality.[22] Later, in the MesoVATS multicenter randomized controlled trial, patients undergoing video-assisted thoracoscopic surgery either underwent talc pleurodesis or pleurectomy. Both groups had equivalent 1-year survival, but patients having had talc pleurodesis had fewer respiratory complications and shorter hospital length of stay.[23] Unfortunately, this study did not discern whether or not pleurectomy had any benefit in patients with lung entrapment. As

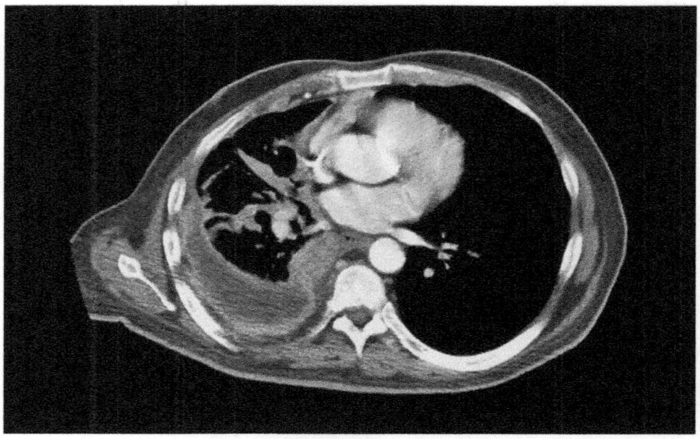

Figure 13.5 Mesothelioma. A transverse chest computed tomography scan showing a large mesothelioma located in the right chest.

a result of these findings, many recommend against performing extrapleural pneumonectomy, and the utility of pleurectomy with decortication over talc pleurodesis is still somewhat controversial.[24]

Bronchopleural or Alveolopleural Fistula

Bronchopleural fistulas are communications between either a mainstem, lobar, or segmental bronchus and the pleural space, whereas alveolopleural fistulas connect the pleural space to airway that is distal to the segmental bronchus (Figure 13.6). Bronchopleural fistulas occur in as many as 4% to 5% of patients after pneumonectomy and are associated with an increased risk of mortality.[25] Alveolopleural fistulas are more likely to occur across staple line defects after performing pulmonary wedge resections. Management of airway fistulas is based on the severity of the leak and the likelihood of recovery with nonsurgical care. The severity of air leak can be graded into four classes, ranging from air leak only with forced expiration to continuous air leak (see Table 13.3).[26,27] Prolonged air leak (>5 days) and more central sources of leak are more likely to require surgical correction. In general, bronchopleural fistulas often require surgical intervention, whereas alveolopleural fistulas are more amenable to spontaneous recovery.[25]

Anesthetic Considerations

Preanesthetic Evaluation

In addition to standard preanesthetic evaluation, as recommended by the American Society of Anesthsiologists,[28] patients undergoing thoracoscopic surgery may require additional pulmonary and/or cardiac functional assessment. For example, there should be a lower threshold to pursue additional testing for even milder cases of dyspnea or decreased functional capacity. In these patients, pulmonary function tests and transthoracic echocardiography can

(A) (B)

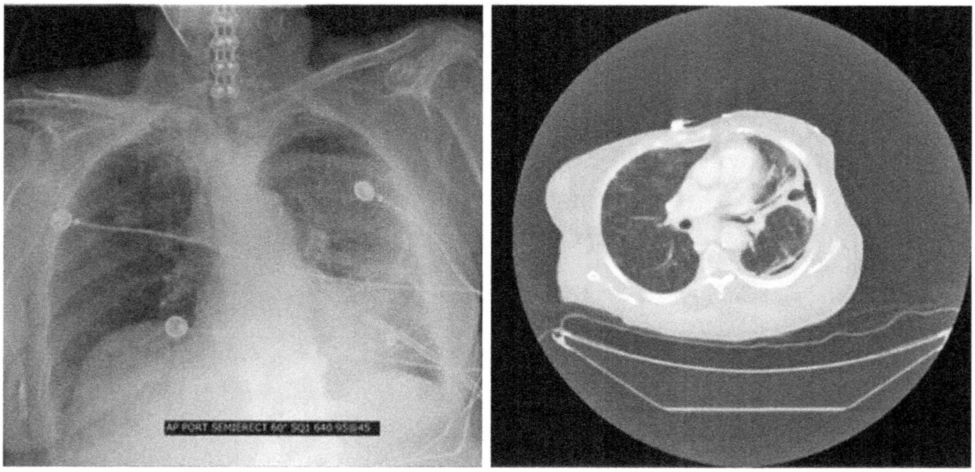

Figure 13.6 Bronchopleural fistula. (A) An anteroposterior chest X-ray of a patient with left-sided bronchopleural fistula. (B) A transverse chest computed tomography scan of the same patient showing the bronchopleural fistula as well as a small pneumothorax on the left side.

help predict how well a patient might tolerate the temporary iatrogenic shunt and elevated right ventricular afterload associated with one-lung ventilation.[29]

For patients with symptoms of either reactive airway disease or hypervolemia, preoperative pulmonary optimization, such as administration of nebulized bronchodilators or diuretics, should be considered. Patients with bronchopleural fistula or empyema may present with septicemia in which case antibiotic therapy should ideally be optimized prior to elective surgery. Patients with large volume chylous drainage are likely to be hypovolemic and malnourished. Whenever possible, nutritional therapy should be optimized prior to elective surgery for these patients. For selected procedures where anticipated blood loss is likely to be significant, such as with extensive pulmonary decortication, it is advisable to crossmatch 2 to 4 units of packed red blood cells.

In patients with a large pleural effusion, the induction of general anesthesia and positive pressure ventilation can be especially treacherous. Patients with poor pulmonary reserve may benefit from a therapeutic thoracentesis prior to induction of anesthesia. Due to the limiting effect of the effusion on lung expansion, increased inspiratory pressures are generally

Table 13.3 The Cerfolio Classification of Air Leakage Severity

Class 1	Air leak only during forced expiration.
Class 2	Air leak only during normal spontaneous expiration.
Class 3	Air leak only during normal spontaneous inspiration.
Class 4	Continuous air leak throughout respiratory cycle with normal spontaneous ventilation.

Source: Adapted from Cerfolio RJ. Recent advances in the treatment of air leaks. *Curr Opin Pulm Med.* 2005;11(4):319–323.

required to achieve adequate tidal volumes. For patients with underlying pulmonary disease, such as emphysematous blebs or recent pulmonary resection, increased airway pressures could conceivably lead to barotrauma and/or rupture, airway fistula formation and pneumothorax. Further, large pleural effusions have also been reported to compress the mediastinum, inducing cardiac tamponade physiology.[30] Therefore, conversion to positive pressure ventilation can conceivably lead to catastrophic hemodynamic collapse for a patient with a large pleural effusion and borderline elevated mediastinal pressure. If the risk of fulminant cardiac tamponade physiology is high (e.g., arterial waveform with pulsus paradoxus), consideration should be given to placing a preinduction arterial line, maintaining spontaneous ventilation, and targeting a state of higher heart rate, systemic vascular resistance and intravascular volume.[31]

In patients with suspected tension pneumothorax, emergent decompressive needle thoracostomy, followed by chest tube thoracostomy, should be performed as soon as possible. This condition should be suspected with the development of chest hyperresonance, contralateral tracheal deviation, distended neck veins, hemodynamic collapse, and increased airway pressures.[32]

Intraoperative Management

The conventional approach to pleural-based surgery has been general anesthesia followed by oral endotracheal intubation using either a double-lumen endotracheal tube or a single-lumen tube with a bronchial blocker for lung isolation. Lung isolation can optimize surgical visualization and workspace within the hemithorax. For patients with bronchopleural fistulas, lung isolation is also beneficial to prevent air flow across the defect. The decision of whether or not to perform a rapid sequence induction should weigh both the patient's likelihood of aspirating gastric contents and pulmonary risk, if aspiration were to occur. In particular, for patients undergoing repair for chylothorax, it is common practice to administer a solution of high lipid content though a nasogastric tube prior to surgery. This increases the production of chyle and thereby facilitates identification of the source of the leak. It does, however, increase gastric content volume and possibly also the risk of aspiration during anesthesia.

Over the last several decades, however, these procedures have also been successfully performed under nonintubated, "awake" conditions.[33,34] The rationale for attempting this has been to avoid the risks of intubation and mechanical ventilation on one lung and to expedite recovery. For patients with bronchopleural fistulas, avoidance of positive pressure ventilation can also help minimize the risk of developing a tension pneumothorax. To carry out a nonintubated technique, complete nerve blockade and patient cooperation is required, as pain, coughing, and other movement can make the procedure more technically challenging. To help blunt the coughing reflex, a stellate ganglion block can be performed.[35] However, this block may, on rare occasion, precipitate a coughing attack and should therefore be reserved as a rescue technique.[36] Intravenous sedation should also be titrated to provide patient comfort while preserving spontaneous ventilation. Reported reasons to convert to general anesthesia include inadequate block, cardiac arrest, azygous vein injury, carbon dioxide retention, extensive adhesions, and uncontrollable coughing.[35] To lower the risk of requiring emergent conversion to general anesthesia in the middle of the operation, it is advisable to abstain from performing awake thoracoscopic procedures in patients with an American Society of Anesthesiology classification of 3 or more, left ventricular ejection fraction <40%, body mass index >25 kg/m^2, poorly controlled reactive airway disease, hemodynamic instability, hypovolemia, coagulopathy, or local contrast allergy.[37] With appropriate patient selection, however, awake video-assisted thoracoscopic surgery has been associated with decreased operative time, hospital length of stay, and total cost. For patients undergoing talc pleurodesis randomized to be either awake with thoracic epidural analgesia or intubated under general anesthesia, the awake group had a shorter hospital stay with no difference in operative time or patient satisfaction.[34]

Unless patients otherwise have specific comorbidities, most pleural procedures themselves do not require additional monitoring beyond the basic standards outlined by the American Society of Anesthesiology. The exception to this is when patients are undergoing pleurectomy, extrapleural pneumonectomy, decortication of chronic empyema, and/or extensive manipulation of central cardiovascular structures. For these cases, the risk of major hemorrhage is high, and a central venous catheter, arterial cannulation and pre-emptive blood product preparation should be considered.[24] For patients undergoing extensive resections, a nasogastric tube can be placed to minimize gastric compression on the diaphragm. Further, in patients with distorted anatomy due to pleural disease, placement of a palpable esophageal bougie can aid the surgical team in identification of the esophagus and thereby avoid injury.

For most pleural procedures, general anesthesia can be safely maintained with either inhaled or intravenous agents. For patients with airway fistulas, however, total intravenous anesthesia can ensure more reliable delivery of medications and prevent operating room contamination by gases. Nitrous oxide should be avoided in patients with fistulas as well to prevent the risk of operative fire with the concurrent use of electrocautery equipment.

Perioperative Analgesia

As with other types of thoracic surgery, adequate perioperative analgesia and avoidance of lingering sedative effects are critical for patients undergoing surgery for pleural disease (see Table 13.4). This enables patients to take full breaths that are not limited by pain or decreased ventilatory drive. Thoracic epidural analgesia, paravertebral nerve blocks, intercostal blocks, myofascial plane blocks, surgical site injection of local anesthetics, and systemic medications have all been shown to be effective in decreasing pain during and after thoracic surgery.[38,39] Combinations of various analgesic options can achieve an effective multimodal regimen as part of a well-orchestrated enhanced recovery program. Such programs have been shown to minimize postoperative complications and expedite patient discharge from the hospital.[40]

There are some factors, however, that might provide compelling reason to choose one analgesic strategy over another. For example, thoracic epidural analgesia and paravertebral blockade have the greatest opioid-sparing analgesic effect,[38] but they require adherence to guidelines for safe practice when also using anticoagulation.[41] When pleurectomy is performed, it is recommended to avoid performing either a postsurgical paravertebral block or preprocedural paravertebral catheter.[24] This is because the pleura forms the anterolateral border of the paravertebral space and removal of the pleura would result in noncontainment,

Table 13.4 Perioperative Opioid-Sparing Options for Patients Undergoing Surgery for Pleural Disease

Type of Analgesia	Comment
Thoracic epidural	• High efficacy • Single procedure works bilaterally • Requires adherence to ASRA guidelines if also anticoagulated
Paravertebral block	• High efficacy • Requires adherence to ASRA guidelines if also anticoagulated • Lacks efficacy if posteromedial pleura removed
Intercostal block or local infiltration	• Can be performed by surgeon
Myofascial plane block	• Retrolaminar or erector spinae blocks
Oral or intravenous medications	• Acetaminophen, gabapentin, pregabalin, nonsteroidal anti-inflammatory drugs, ketamine, dexmedetomidine, intravenous lidocaine and magnesium infusions

Abbreviation: ASR, American Society of Regional Anesthesia and Pain Medicine.

and therefore decreased efficacy, of medications injected into this space (Figure 13.7). Nonsteroidal anti-inflammatory drugs have traditionally been avoided for patients undergoing pleurodesis due to the theoretical concern that a reduction in inflammation would minimize the effectiveness of pleural cohesion. However, when patients undergoing pleurodesis were randomized to either receive opioids or nonsteroidal anti-inflammatory drugs, there was no difference in procedural efficacy.[42]

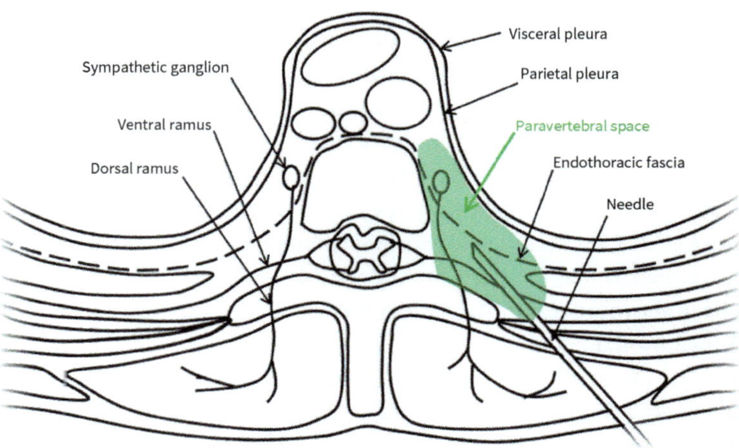

Figure 13.7 A transverse schematic of the posterior chest wall demonstrating the anatomic relationship of the paravertebral space to the pleura.

Postoperative Management

Except for patients with severe preoperative respiratory limitations, most patients undergoing surgery for pleural disease can be extubated prior to leaving the operating room. Early termination of positive pressure ventilation is particularly beneficial in minimizing air leak in patients with airway to pleural fistulas. For patients who do not adequately meet extubation criteria and have a double-lumen endotracheal tube, the airway should be exchanged for a single-lumen endotracheal tube prior to being transported to recover in an intensive care unit. Elevated position of the head of the bed, a combination of opioid-sparing analgesia, and avoidance of residual neuromuscular blockade or sedation are advisable to optimize respiratory mechanics throughout the recovery period.

Acknowledgments

We want to thank Drs. Clayton Commander and Benjamin Haithcock for providing us the figures.

References

1. Light RW, Macgregor MI, Luchsinger PC, Ball WC, Jr. Pleural effusions: the diagnostic separation of transudates and exudates. *Ann Intern Med.* 1972;77(4):507–513.
2. Light RW. Clinical practice: pleural effusion. *N Engl J Med.* 2002;346(25):1971–1977.
3. Antunes G, Neville E, Duffy J, Ali N; Pleural Diseases Group SoCCBTS. BTS guidelines for the management of malignant pleural effusions. *Thorax.* 2003;58(Suppl 2):ii29–ii38.
4. Feller-Kopman DJ, Reddy CB, DeCamp MM, et al; Management of Malignant Pleural Effusions. An official ATS/STS/STR clinical practice guideline. *Am J Respir Crit Care Med.* 2018;198(7):839–849.
5. Lan RS, Lo SK, Chuang ML, Yang CT, Tsao TC, Lee CH. Elastance of the pleural space: a predictor for the outcome of pleurodesis in patients with malignant pleural effusion. *Ann Intern Med.* 1997;126(10):768–774.
6. Sunderland N, Maweni R, Akunuri S, Karnovitch E. Re-expansion pulmonary oedema: a novel emergency therapeutic option. *BMJ Case Rep.* 2016 Apr 27;2016:bcr2016215076.
7. Hojski A, Leitgeb M, Crnjac A. Release of growth factors after mechanical and chemical pleurodesis for treatment of malignant pleural effusion: a randomized control study. *Radiol Oncol.* 2015;49(4):386–394.
8. Sepehripour AH, Nasir A, Shah R. Does mechanical pleurodesis result in better outcomes than chemical pleurodesis for recurrent primary spontaneous pneumothorax? *Interact Cardiovasc Thorac Surg.* 2012;14(3):307–311.
9. Zarogoulidis K, Zarogoulidis P, Darwiche K, et al. Malignant pleural effusion and algorithm management. *J Thorac Dis.* 2013;5(Suppl 4):S413–419.
10. Martucci N, Tracey M, Rocco G. Postoperative Chylothorax. *Thorac Surg Clin.* 2015;25(4):523–528.
11. Morabito J, Bell MT, Montenij LJ, et al. Perioperative considerations for chylothorax. *J Cardiothorac Vasc Anesth.* 2017;31(6):2277–2281.
12. Shiraishi Y. Surgical treatment of chronic empyema. *Gen Thorac Cardiovasc Surg.* 2010;58(7):311–316.
13. Redden MD, Chin TY, van Driel ML. Surgical versus non-surgical management for pleural empyema. *Cochrane Database Syst Rev.* 2017;3:CD010651.

14. Samancilar C, Akcam TI, Kaya SO, Ozturk O, Akcay O, Ceylan KC. The efficacy of VATS and intrapleural fibrinolytic therapy in parapneumonic empyema treatment. *Ann Thorac Cardiovasc Surg.* 2018;24(1):19–24.
15. Khan H, Woo E, Alzetani A. Modified thoracoplasty using a breast implant to obliterate an infected pleural space: an alternative to traditional thoracoplasty. *Ann Thorac Surg.* 2015;99(4):1418–1420.
16. Patrini D, Panagiotopoulos N, Pararajasingham J, Gvinianidze L, Iqbal Y, Lawrence DR. Etiology and management of spontaneous haemothorax. *J Thorac Dis.* 2015;7(3):520–526.
17. Broderick SR. Hemothorax: etiology, diagnosis, and management. *Thorac Surg Clin.* 2013;23(1):89–96, vi–vii.
18. MacDuff A, Arnold A, Harvey J; BTS Pleural Disease Guideline Group. Management of spontaneous pneumothorax: British Thoracic Society Pleural Disease Guideline 2010. *Thorax.* 2010;65(Suppl 2):ii18–ii31.
19. Min X, Huang Y, Yang Y, et al. Mechanical pleurodesis does not reduce recurrence of spontaneous pneumothorax: a randomized trial. *Ann Thorac Surg.* 2014;98(5):1790–1796; discussion 1796.
20. Goto T, Kadota Y, Mori T, et al. Video-assisted thoracic surgery for pneumothorax: republication of a systematic review and a proposal by the guideline committee of the Japanese association for chest surgery 2014. *Gen Thorac Cardiovasc Surg.* 2015;63(1):8–13.
21. Treasure T, Lang-Lazdunski L, Waller D, et al. Extra-pleural pneumonectomy versus no extra-pleural pneumonectomy for patients with malignant pleural mesothelioma: clinical outcomes of the Mesothelioma and Radical Surgery (MARS) randomised feasibility study. *Lancet Oncol.* 2011;12(8):763–772.
22. Burt BM, Cameron RB, Mollberg NM, et al. Malignant pleural mesothelioma and the Society of Thoracic Surgeons Database: an analysis of surgical morbidity and mortality. *J Thorac Cardiovasc Surg.* 2014;148(1):30–35.
23. Rintoul RC, Ritchie AJ, Edwards JG, et al. Efficacy and cost of video-assisted thoracoscopic partial pleurectomy versus talc pleurodesis in patients with malignant pleural mesothelioma (MesoVATS): an open-label, randomised, controlled trial. *Lancet.* 2014;384(9948):1118–1127.
24. Woolhouse I, Maskell NA. Introducing the new BTS guideline: the investigation and management of pleural malignant mesothelioma. *Thorax.* 2018;73(3):210–212.
25. Poulin V, Vaillancourt R, Somma J, Gagné N, Bussières JS. High frequency ventilation combined with spontaneous breathing during bronchopleural fistula repair: a case report. *Can J Anesth* 2008;56(1):52–56.
26. Singh N, Agarwal R. Bronchopleural fistula or alveolopleural fistula? Not just semantics. *Chest.* 2006;130(6):1948; author reply 1948–1949.
27. Cerfolio RJ. Recent advances in the treatment of air leaks. *Curr Opin Pulm Med.* 2005;11(4):319–323.
28. Apfelbaum JL, Connis RT, Nickinovich DG, et al; Committee on Standards and Practice Parameters, American Society of Anesthesiologists Task Force on Preanesthesia Evaluation. Practice advisory for preanesthesia evaluation: an updated report by the American Society of Anesthesiologists Task Force on Preanesthesia Evaluation. *Anesthesiology.* 2012;116(3):522–538.
29. Karzai W, Schwarzkopf K. Hypoxemia during one-lung ventilation: prediction, prevention, and treatment. *Anesthesiology.* 2009;110(6):1402–1411.
30. Werlang ME, Pimentel MR, Diaz-Gomez JL. Thoracentesis-reverting cardiac tamponade physiology in a patient with myxedema coma and large pleural effusion. *Proc (Bayl Univ Med Cent).* 2017;30(3):295–297.
31. Aye T, Milne B. Ketamine anesthesia for pericardial window in a patient with pericardial tamponade and severe COPD. *Can J Anaesth.* 2002;49(3):283–286.
32. Galvagno SM Jr., Nahmias JT, Young DA. Advanced Trauma Life Support® update 2019: management and applications for adults and special populations. *Anesthesiol Clin.* 2019;37(1):13–32.
33. Pompeo E, Tacconi F, Mineo D, Mineo TC. The role of awake video-assisted thoracoscopic surgery in spontaneous pneumothorax. *J Thorac Cardiovasc Surg.* 2007;133(3):786–790.
34. Pompeo E, Dauri M; Awake Thoracic Surgery Research Group. Is there any benefit in using awake anesthesia with thoracic epidural in thoracoscopic talc pleurodesis? *J Thorac Cardiovasc Surg.* 2013;146(2):495–497.e1.

35. Al-Abdullatief M, Wahood A, Al-Shirawi N, et al. Awake anaesthesia for major thoracic surgical procedures: an observational study. *Eur J Cardiothorac Surg.* 2007;32(2):346–350.
36. Atici S, Akoz K. Transient cough attacks after right stellate ganglion block. *Reg Anesth Pain Med.* 2010;35(3):318–319.
37. Caronia FP, Loizzi D, Nicolosi T, Castorina S, Fiorelli A. Tubeless tracheal resection and reconstruction for management of benign stenosis. *Head Neck.* 2017;39(12):e114–e117.
38. Joshi GP, Bonnet F, Shah R, et al. A systematic review of randomized trials evaluating regional techniques for postthoracotomy analgesia. *Anesth Analg.* 2008;107(3):1026–1040.
39. Forero M, Rajarathinam M, Adhikary S, Chin KJ. Erector spinae plane (ESP) block in the management of post thoracotomy pain syndrome: a case series. *Scand J Pain.* 2017;17:325–329.
40. Teeter EG, Kolarczyk LM, Popescu WM. Examination of the enhanced recovery guidelines in thoracic surgery. *Curr Opin Anaesthesiol.* 2019;32(1):10–16.
41. Horlocker TT, Vandermeuelen E, Kopp SL, Gogarten W, Leffert LR, Benzon HT. Regional Anesthesia in the Patient Receiving Antithrombotic or Thrombolytic Therapy: American Society of Regional Anesthesia and Pain Medicine Evidence-Based Guidelines (Fourth Edition). *Reg Anesth Pain Med.* 2018;43(3):263–309.
42. Rahman NM, Pepperell J, Rehal S, et al. Effect of opioids vs NSAIDs and larger vs smaller chest tube size on pain control and pleurodesis efficacy among patients with malignant pleural effusion: the TIME1 randomized clinical trial. *JAMA.* 2015;314(24):2641–2653.

14
Surgical Airway Management

Zipei Feng, Mengjie Wu, Melissa Nikolaidis, and Yi Deng

Introduction

Airway surgery generally can be separated into two distinct categories: endoscopic and open. It can be used to address various disease of the larynx such as stenosis, benign or malignant tumors, and voice disorders, as well as gain access to the infraglottic airway either in a planned or emergent fashion. The chapter will discuss both endoscopic and external approaches in surgical airway management for both pediatric and adult patients.

Anatomy

Thorough knowledge of the larynx anatomy is critical in performing airway surgery in a safe and efficient manner. The larynx is comprised from cranial to caudal four palpable landmarks—hyoid bone, thyroid cartilage, cricoid cartilage, and sternal notch (Figure 14.1). The hyoid bone is a palpable bony prominence inferior to the mandible. Its position can affect pharyngeal airway opening and can be an important contributor to obstructive sleep apnea. The thyroid cartilage consists of two broad laminae that are fused anteriosuperiorly into a prominence known as the laryngeal prominence. Inferior to the thyroid cartilage is the cricoid cartilage. It is the only complete cartilaginous ring and as a result usually represents the narrowest part of the airway especially in pediatric population. It serves as the attachment of the muscles, cartilage, and ligaments for phonation and airway opening. Cricoid pressure can be applied during intubation to posteriorly displace the larynx for improved view as well as close the esophageal opening which may reduce reflux during rapid sequence intubation known as Sellick maneuver.

In patients with thin necks, the cricothyroid ligament can be palpated between the thyroid and cricoid cartilages. The median part of this ligament comprises of a fibroconnective tissue that links anteroinferior thyroid cartilage with anterosuperior cricoid cartilage, while the lateral component extends from the superolateral borders of the cricoid cartilage terminating as the vocal ligaments.

The most inferiorly palpable landmark in airway surgery is the sternal notch, which serves as the inferior limit of the cervical trachea.

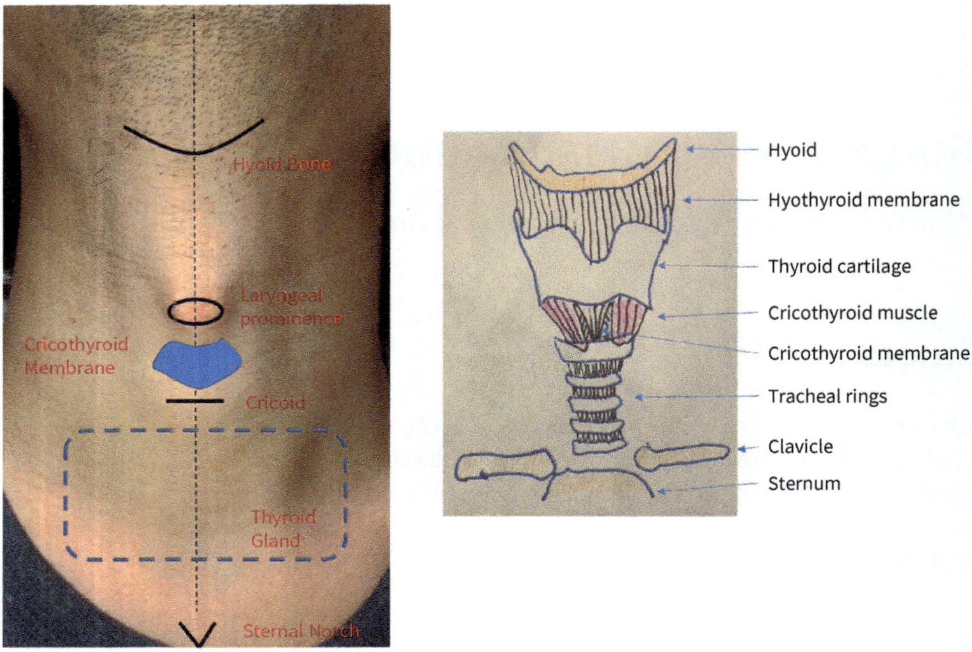

Figure 14.1 Surface anatomic landmarks.

Procedures

The following is an overview of common procedures performed for planned or emergency airway management.

Direct Laryngoscopy, Bronchoscopy With Interventions

Indication

This is a common procedure performed in both pediatric and adult population for diagnosis, biopsy, airway foreign body retrieval, airway dilation, stent placement, or obstructive sleep apnea.

Instruments

For setup, rigid laryngoscope is required. For pediatric population, either a Parsons, Phillips, or Miller laryngoscope is preferred for initial visualization. Compared to Miller, Phillips has a more rounded tip and can be advanced both in the vallecula as well as under the epiglottis.

In the rare instances when the view is inadequate secondary to conditions such as Pierre Robin sequence, a Hollinger anterior commissure scope can be used improve visualization. For adults, either a Lindholm, Dedo, or Miller laryngoscope may be used for initial visualization. If the view is inadequate, a Hollinger or anterior shelf laryngoscope may be required. Included in the setup should also be a rigid telescope with camera (Figure 14.2), suspension equipment, and bronchoscopes. If difficult airway is anticipated, a 4.0 or 4.5 Pedi rigid bronchoscope should be set up (Figure 14.3). A 6.0 endotracheal tube can fit

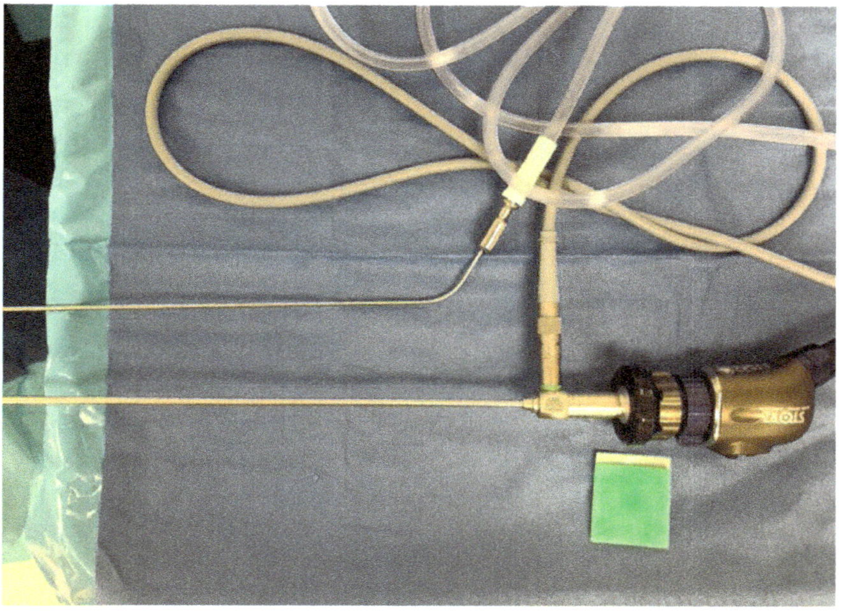

Figure 14.2 Camera and telescope setup.

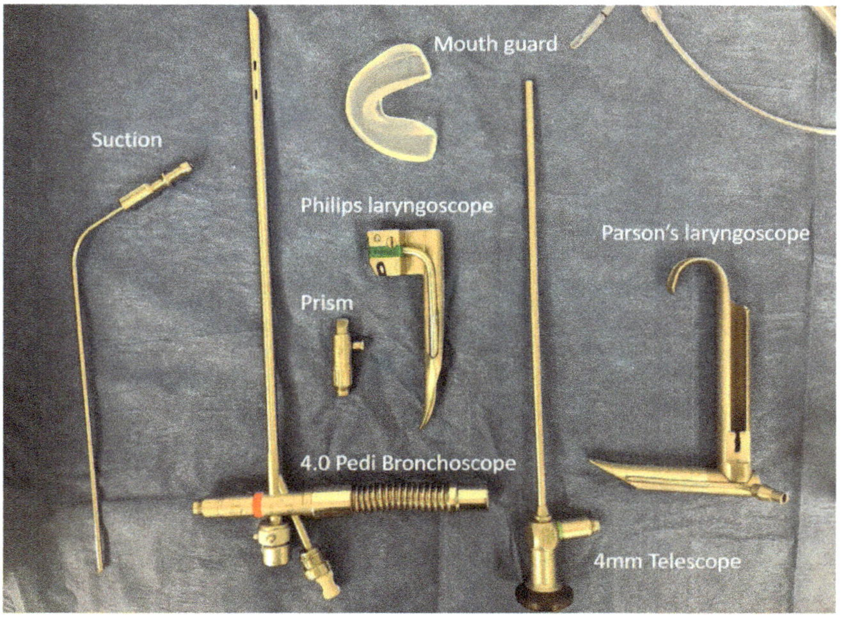

Figure 14.3 Direct laryngoscopy instruments.

through a 4.5 rigid bronchoscope and be used to establish a difficult airway via Seldinger method especially when there is significant glossoptosis. Surgical instruments such as optical forceps, endoscopic scissors, lasers, and balloons may be set up depending on the procedure.

Ventilation Considerations

Ventilation methods should be discussed with the surgeon prior to the induction of anesthesia. Spontaneous ventilation is preferred for endoscopic airway procedures especially in pediatric population. Jet ventilation can sometimes be considered in adults; however, it is associated with high rate of pneumothorax in pediatric population. Other techniques such as intermittent apnea with either endotracheal tube or bronchoscope, or intubation with small endotracheal tube for supraglottic procedures can be performed to maintain oxygenation during the procedure. Newer techniques such as STRIVE Hi can be used in selected patient population to maintain saturation without the need for repeated intubation and extubation. SponTaneous Respiration using IntraVEnous Anesthesia and Hi flow nasal oxygen (STRIVE Hi) is a relatively new tubeless airway management technique during airway surgeries utilizing high-flow nasal oxygen for preoxygenation and increasing to 70 LPM with deepening planes of anesthesia. STRIVE Hi permits uninterrupted access to the air way, decreases risk of barotrauma (compared to jet ventilation), decreases risk of airway fire, and facilitates respiratory mechanics while providing equal or better oxygenation and ventilation than traditional inhalation inductions. This method is especially useful in patients with anticipated difficult airway or ventilations (laryngotracheal stenosis, obesity, chronic obstructive pulmonary disease, pregnancy). An extension to STRIVE-Hi for patient unable to maintain spontaneous respiration is transnasal humified rapid-insufflation ventilatory exchange (THRIVE). This is a novel advanced oxygenation technique allows to prolonged periods of apnea while maintaining oxygenations by reducing airway pressure, generated positive airway pressure, flushes of anatomic dead space to reduce hypercarbia, and permit gas exchange by passive oxygenation.

THRIVE has successfully extended apnea time during hypopharyngeal and laryngotracheal surgeries by delivering transnasal high-flow humidified oxygenation at 70 LPM with occasional jaw-thrust to maintain upper airway patency. Recently, this method has also been used in patients requiring emergent surgical airways to prevent "cannot intubate, cannot ventilate" scenarios.

Procedure in Detail

1. Position the patient supine on the operating table and induce anesthesia.
2. Place a mouthguard and perform direct laryngoscopy to visualize the larynx.
3. Spray plain topical 2% lidocaine into the glottis. In pediatric population, lidocaine toxicity should be calculated prior to the case. A maximum of 4 mg/kg lidocaine can be administered per case.
4. Mask the patient again and perform direct laryngoscopy. Visualize the supraglottis, glottis, subglottis, trachea, carina, and mainstem bronchi with rigid telescope. Take photodocumentation.

5. Gently suspend patient and perform indicated airway procedures. These include removing lesions of the supraglottis, glottis, or subglottis, and dilation of the airway. Depending on the ventilation technique, bronchoscope, endotracheal tube, or jet ventilator may be used to maintain oxygenation. If laser is used, laser safety precautions should be taken into consideration at the beginning of the case. These include laser-safe endotracheal tube with water-filled cuff, eye and face protection for patient and for staff, and low FiO_2 concentration.

Cricothyroidotomy

Indication and Contraindication

Cricothyroidotomy should be performed in an emergent setting for establishment of a surgical airway in a patient that cannot be intubated from above secondary to trauma, edema, hemorrhage, radiation, or anatomic limitations. Absolute contraindication includes known tracheal stenosis or discontinuity. Relative contraindications include inability to identify surface landmarks, obesity, cervical trauma, coagulopathic patients, and patients with laryngeal cancer.

Instruments

Cricothyroidotomy kits can be utilized when available. However, in emergent situation a 15- or 11-blade, blunt dissection instruments such as mosquito, small endotracheal tube (typically 6.0), and suction can be used to establish the airway. Other useful equipment includes tracheal dilator, cricoid hook, and silk suture.

Ventilation Consideration

Maintain spontaneous ventilation as much as possible. Proper bag-masking techniques should be maintained to avoid emergent need for airway establishment. A laryngeal masking device should be attempted if able. If the patient is bag-maskable or can be ventilated through a laryngeal mask airway (LMA), formal tracheostomy may be considered instead.

Procedure in Detail

1. Position the patient supine and place shoulder roll to extend neck whenever possible.
2. Palpate and mark surface landmarks (Figure 14.1).
3. Prep and drape patient in a sterile fashion if time allows.
4. Infiltrate the area between cricoid and thyroid cartilage with 1% lidocaine with 1:100,000 epinephrine for hemostasis.
5. Make a horizontal stab incision between the thyroid and cricoid cartilage on the inferior edge of cricothyroid membrane.
6. If surface landmark cannot be easily palpated, make a vertical midline incision and dissect with finger until both cricoid and thyroid cartilages can be felt and then make a horizontal incision between the two cartilages on the inferior aspect of the cricothyroid membrane.
7. Once the airway is entered, using blunt instruments such as mosquito to dilate the airway, suction any blood in the field.
8. Place cuffed tracheostomy tube or small endotracheal tube into the airway, confirm ventilation, and secure to the skin with 2-0 silk sutures.

9. Although some literature suggests that patient following cricothyroidotomy can be safely decannulated with good long-term follow-up, there has been limited research on whether patient should be converted to formal tracheostomy. This should be assessed in a case-by-case basis, if there is concern about airway trauma during emergency cricothyroidotomy, patient should be taken to operating room as soon as possible for a second look with or without conversion to formal tracheostomy.

Comments

1. Percutaneous cricothyroidotomy via a Seldinger method can also be performed in emergent situations. See instructions from each kit for assembly and procedure in detail. Overall, anatomic considerations are similar; however, percutaneous methods is discouraged in patients with history of extensive radiation as dilation can be very difficult, and a higher chance of false-passage rate exists.
2. During the procedure, it is important to stabilize the larynx with one hand, especially in patients with thick neck. Check for landmarks periodically during dissection to ensure airway entry at the correct position.
3. If time allows, local anesthesia with epinephrine can improve visualization of the field by inducing vasoconstriction. Suction can be used to improve visualization, help retract, and dissect bluntly.

Tracheostomy

Indication and Contraindication

Planned tracheostomy is generally indicated for (i) prolonged intubation, which is typically more than 1 week, and (ii) failure to extubate due to neurological or respiratory compromise. Compared to endotracheal tube, tracheostomy can allow for decreased sedation requirement and improved pulmonary hygiene and rehabilitation, and reports have shown that early tracheostomy decreases the length of intensive care unit stay. Tracheostomy can also be performed either in planned or emergent fashion for acute respiratory failure with inability to intubate from above secondary to hemorrhage, mass, or trauma. Relative contraindications include anticoagulation, high vent settings, multiple pressors, thyroid goiter, or inability to extend cervical neck.

Instruments

Standard tracheostomy set is available (Figure 14.4). In emergent situations, the requirement is similar to that of cricothyroidotomy. A 15- or 11-blade, blunt dissection instruments such as mosquito, small endotracheal tube (typically 6.0), and suction can be used to establish the airway.

Ventilation Consideration

Maintain spontaneous ventilation as much as possible. In patient with supraglottic mass preventing intubation, awake tracheostomy is performed with local anesthesia. In emergent situation, proper bag-masking techniques or placement of an LMA is important to buy time for an urgent tracheostomy as opposed to emergent (slash) tracheostomy.

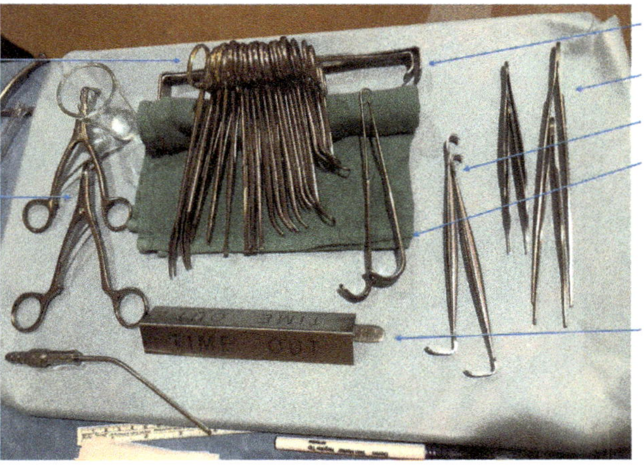

Figure 14.4 Standard tracheostomyset.

Procedure in Detail

For planned tracheostomy

1. Position the patient supine, preoxygenate the patient, and place shoulder roll to extend neck.
2. Palpate and mark surface landmarks (Figure 14.1).
3. Prep and drape patient in a sterile fashion.
4. Mark a 3 cm incision line about one-finger breadth inferior to the cricoid cartilage, allow for two-finger breath above the sternal notch. In patients with short neck, the incision may need to be moved to just inferior to the inferior edge of the cricoid cartilage.
5. Infiltrate the area with 1% lidocaine with 1:100,000 epinephrine.
6. Make a horizontal incision with the knife through the epidermis and dermis (Figure 14.5A).
7. Use electrocautery to control bleeding and dissect through platysma (Figure 14.5A).
8. Use finger to bluntly create small subplatysmal flaps superiorly and inferiorly. Be careful not to extend subplatysmal flaps too far inferiorly as this may increase the chance of false passage during tracheostomy tube exchange.
9. Palpate for airway, use electrocautery to score the midline, and use mosquito to dissect through the midline raphe (Figure 14.5B).
10. Elevate the strap muscles in a layered fashion and place Army–Navy retractors underneath the strap muscles until thyroid is reached (Figure 14.5C).
11. Palpate for the cricoid cartilage, dissect slowly using electrocautery onto the cricoid cartilage until the pretracheal fascia is reached. Drop the inspired oxygen to 40% or lower during this process and use care to not inadvertently enter the airway.
12. Use a mosquito forceps (type of hemostatic forcepts) to dissect along the pretracheal fascia and divide the thyroid isthmus slowly with electrocautery to maintain hemostasis.
13. Elevate the thyroid isthmus off the tracheal laterally with electrocautery. Do not elevate past the anterior 180 degrees of the trachea to not inadvertently injury the recurrent laryngeal nerve.

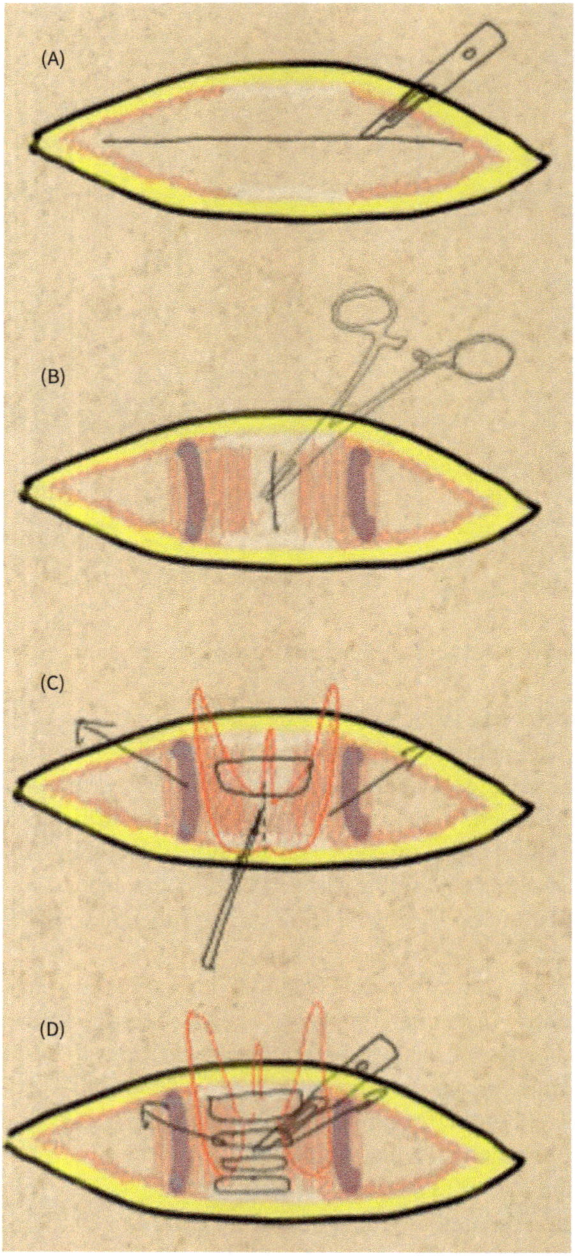

Figure 14.5 Simple schematic on tracheostomy. (A) Skin incision is made sharply through the epidermis and dermis (black), subcutaneous tissue (yellow), platysma (red). (B) Midline raphe is established and dissected with a mosquito clamp. Care should be taken to avoid injury to anterior jugular veins (blue). (C) The straps are retracted laterally until thyroid gland is visible. Bovie electrocautery is used to divide thyroid isthmus. (D) Tracheal rings is visible once thyroid isthmus s divided and retracted laterally. Incision is made between first and second tracheal rings.

14. With thyroid isthmus retracted, the airway is now in clear visualization (Figure 14.5D). Confirm hemostasis. Score the space between the first and second tracheal ring with electrocautery. At this point, the patient can be turned back to 100% FiO_2.
15. Confirm all equipment is ready and properly tested. This includes a 15-blade, mosquito forceps, curved Mayo scissors, 2-0 silk stay suture, tracheal dilator, and tracheostomy tube with cuff tested and deflated and obturator inserted.
16. Place stay suture through the skin and bend the needle slightly. Keep the needle loaded but protected.
17. Deflate the balloon, advance the endotracheal tube as far as possible, and reinflate the balloon.
18. Make the incision with 15-blade between the first and second tracheal rings; be care not to damage the cuff of the endotracheal tube (Figure 14.5D). Once the airway is entered, use a mosquito to further expand the opening.
19. Make lateral incisions or create Bjork flaps with curved Mayo scissors. Dilate with tracheal spreader and place stay suture through the inferior ring.
20. Disconnect the circuit, deflate the cuff, and slowly withdraw the endotracheal tube until the tip is just superior to the tracheal opening.
21. Suction the trachea for any blood and place tracheostomy tube through the opening. Confirm ventilation.
22. Tie the stay suture and secure the tracheostomy tube with 2-0 silk sutures and a tracheostomy tube tie.

For emergent tracheostomy:

1. Position the patient in supine position and place shoulder roll.
2. Palpate for landmarks.
3. Infiltrate the area inferior to the cricoid with local anesthesia if time allows.
4. With one hand stabilizing the larynx, make a vertical midline incision along the airway.
5. Palpate for the airway and dissect bluntly with finger; use suction to help improve visualization and retract.
6. Make a vertical incision on the airway. Use suction to remove blood and visualize the airway opening.
7. Place endotracheal tube in the airway and secure with sutures.
8. Take patient to the operating room as soon as possible for revision tracheostomy.

Comments

1. In patients with high cricoid cartilage and large thyroid, the incision can be two-finger breadths above the sternal notch to avoid dividing the thyroid isthmus.
2. In planned tracheostomy it is always a good idea to palpate for high-riding innominate artery and avoid inadvertent injury.
3. Always suction any blood out of the trachea during the placement of tracheostomy.
4. In patients who are highly coagulopathic, having a bipolar setup can be helpful, and topical hemostatic agents may be placed at the end of the case for hemostasis.

Concluding Remarks

Surgical intervention of the airway is important in treating diseases that affect voice and breathing, as well as establishment of a secured airway in patient with respiratory distress or failure. Emergency airway surgery can usually be avoided with proper noninvasive airway management include spontaneous ventilation, bag-masking, placement of LMA, and video-assisted intubation techniques. However, in situations when emergency airway surgery is required, proper identification of anatomic landmarks can increase safety, efficiency, and reduce complication rates. For procedures that involve utilization of a kit, it is important to become familiar with the instruments and set up ahead of time to increase efficiency and safety during a true airway emergency.

Further Reading

Arkin N. Surviving and THRIVE-ing the difficult airway: gaining calm, control, and time during an emergent tracheostomy. *J Head Neck Anesth*. 2017;2(2):23–28.

Booth AQ, Vidhani K. The SponTaneous Respiration using IntraVEnouse anesthesia and High flow nasal oxygen (STRIVE Hi) approach to endoscopic airway surgery. *J Head Neck Anesth*. 2017;2(2):11–13.

Booth AWG, Vidhani K, Lee PK, Thomsett C-M. Spontaneous Respiration Using Intravenous Anaesthesia and Hi-Flow Nasal Oxygen (Strive Hi) maintains oxygenation and airway patency during management of the obstructed airway: an observational study. *Br J Anaesth* 2017;118(3):444–451.

Cheung NH, Napolitano LM. Tracheostomy: epidemiology, indications, timing, technique, and outcomes. *Respir Care*. 2014;59(6):895–919.

Cortinez LI, De la Fuente N, Eleveld DJ. Performance of propofol target-controlled infusion models in the obese: pharmacokinetic and pharmacodynamic analysis. *Anesth Analg*. 2014;119(2):302–310.

Gibbs MA, Mick NW (2013). Surgical airway. In: Hagberg CA, ed. *Benumof and Hagberg's Airway Management*. 3rd ed. Philadelphia, PA: Elsevier/Saunders, 2013: 640–656.e2. doi:10.1016/b978-1-4377-2764-7.00031-2

Graham DB, Eastman AL, Aldy KN, Carroll EA, Minei JP, Brakenridge SC, Phelan HA. Outcomes and long term follow-up after emergent cricothyroidotomy: is routine conversion to tracheostomy necessary? *Am Surg*. 2011;77(12):1707–1711.

Koji H, Masaji N, Moritoki E, Jean-Louis V. Timing of tracheotomy in ICU patients: a systematic review of randomized controlled trials. *Crit Care*. 2015;19:424. doi:10.1186/s13054-015-1138-8

Koufman JA, Fortson JK, Strong MS. Predictive factors of cricoid ring size in adults in relation to acquired subglottic stenosis. *Otolaryngol Head Neck Surg*. 1983;91:177–182.

Patel A, Nouraei SA. Transnasal humidified rapid-insufflation ventilatory exchange (Thrive): a physiological method of increasing apnoea time in patients with difficult airways. *Anaesthesia*. 2015;70(3):323–329.

Thurairatnam R, Arora A, Mir F. Use of THRIVE to maintain oxygenation during the management of an anticipated difficult airway and emergency tracheostomy. *J Head Neck Anesth*. 2017;2(2):19–22.

15
Bronchopleural Fistula

Jose C. Humanez, Saurin Shah, Thimothy Graham, Kishan Patel, and Paul Mongan

Introduction

Bronchopleural fistula (BPF) is a pathological communication between the bronchial tree and pleural space.[1] BPF is a relatively rare but feared complication of several pulmonary conditions and procedures. The incidence of BPF has been reported as low as 1% for nonsurgical etiologies and as high as 30% following pulmonary procedures. The etiologies are varied with postoperative complication after pulmonary resection being the most common cause, followed by chronic necrotizing pneumonia, radiotherapy, cyst/bulla rupture, and trauma.[2] Incidence has been reported anywhere from 4.5% to 20% after pneumonectomy and 0.5% to 1% post lobectomy—with right-sided procedures carrying the highest incidence.[2] BPFs carry a high morbidity and mortality; some reports suggest mortality rates as high as 70%, regardless of etiology.[3,4] Because of the high morbidity and mortality associated with BPFs, it is important to identify high-risk patients and apply applicable preventative measures to reduce occurrence. Once a BPF has developed, early recognition and treatment are critical.[2]

Causes

Etiologies are varied and the occurrence of BPFs are multifactorial, with postsurgical etiologies carrying the highest incidence and potentially worst prognosis. Box 15.1 lists the most common postoperative and non-postoperative causes of BPFs.

BPFs most commonly arise as a postoperative complication following failure of the bronchial/surgical stump to heal. Failure to heal may be from improper initial closure, vascular insufficiency, infection or residual malignancy at the surgical site, or prolonged postoperative ventilator support. Nonsurgical causes such as necrotizing pneumonia, lung malignancy, blunt/penetrating trauma, or minimally invasive procedures (chest tube placement, thoracentesis, and radiation therapy) are less prevalent causes of BPFs. As with other disease states, incidence and severity are multifactorial; factors such as diabetes mellitus, cirrhosis, and chronic steroid intake may contribute to a higher risk of BPFs in this patient population.

Clinical Presentation

The clinical presentation is variable and can be divided into acute, subacute, and chronic forms. Acute forms is usually due to postoperative complication related to inadequate closure or breakdown of the stump anastomosis. Subacute and chronic forms are usually secondary

Box 15.1 Classification of Bronchopleural Fistula

Postoperative
- Associated with resection
  - Malignancy
  - Trauma
  - Infectious (i.e., removal of pneumatocele, tuberculosis, abscess, fungus ball)
- Associated with pleuroparenchymal disease
  - Emphysema
  - Thoracic trauma
  - Other infections (i.e., *Pneumocystis carinii*, liver abscess opening into the chest)
- Others
  - Tracheal or esophageal perforation repairs
  - Gastroesophageal reflux disease
  - Boerhaave syndrome

Non-postoperative
- After procedures (i.e., line placement, pleural biopsy, bronchoscopy, lung biopsy)
- Idiopathic
- Infections
- Persistent spontaneous pneumothorax
- Thoracic trauma
- Necrotizing lung disease associated with radiation or chemotherapy
- Acute respiratory distress syndrome

Adapted from, Lois M, Noppen M. Bronchopleural fistulas: an overview of the problem with special focus on endoscopic management. *Chest*. 2005;128(6):3955–3965.

to nonoperative etiologies such as infections. The timing of presentation, severity of symptoms, and underlying etiology are important in determining the best treatment options.

Acute BPF usually presents within the first few postoperative days and is characterized by the sudden onset of the following symptoms: (i) dyspnea, (ii) hypotension, (iii) subcutaneous emphysema, (iv) purulent cough, (v) tracheal/mediastinal shift, (vi) persistent air leak, and (vii) loss of pleural effusion. Acute BPFs may be life-threatening and require immediate intervention. Subacute and chronic forms of BPF may present over days to weeks with a myriad of symptoms including but not limited to (i) malaise, (ii) fever, (iii) minimally productive cough, and (iv) dyspnea. Regardless of the onset and severity of symptoms, BPFs require early detection and prompt treatment as they are associated with a high morbidity and mortality.

Diagnosis

The diagnosis of BPF is often obvious from the clinical presentation.[3] Definitive diagnosis is made based on the entire clinical picture in conjunction with appropriate laboratory, radiographic, and procedural tests. Elevated white blood cell count and abnormal arterial blood gas samples may be found in the setting of a BPF. Plain radiograph findings such as

(i) increase in intrapleural space, (ii) new or increasing air-fluid level, (iii) tension pneumothorax, and (iv) drop or disappearance of pleural fluid (in the absence of a chest tube) may be suggestive of BPFs in the setting of the aforementioned symptoms. Computed tomography may demonstrate pneumothorax and/or pneumomediastinum in addition to any underlying pre-existing pathology (Figure 15.1); evidence of fistulous communications may be difficult to see via computed tomography and other radiographic modalities.

Selective injection of methylene blue via the bronchoscope at a suspected BPF site with chest tube drainage can also aid in identifying and localizing a BPF. When bronchography does not provide a definitive diagnosis, bronchoscopic balloon occlusion may be used in select airways to decrease the air leak and help localize the BPF. Additionally, the use of capnography through the bronchoscope has been used to assist in localizing a BPF.

Other techniques, outside of bronchoscopy, have been used to confirm the diagnosis of BPF or localize it. Ventilation scintigraphy utilizes radioactive gases to assist in the diagnosis. However, this test requires patient cooperation, substantial time, and offers no clear diagnostic advantage over bronchoscopy and/or diagnostic surgical procedures.

Management of Bronchopleural Fistulas

There is a lack of consensus on the optimal therapy of patients with BPF. In the case of postoperative BFP, the best way for management is prevention at the time of pulmonary resection by avoiding disruption of the bronchial blood supply, rough handling of the bronchial mucosa, excessive suture tension, and steroid administration.[4] Management of BPF involves

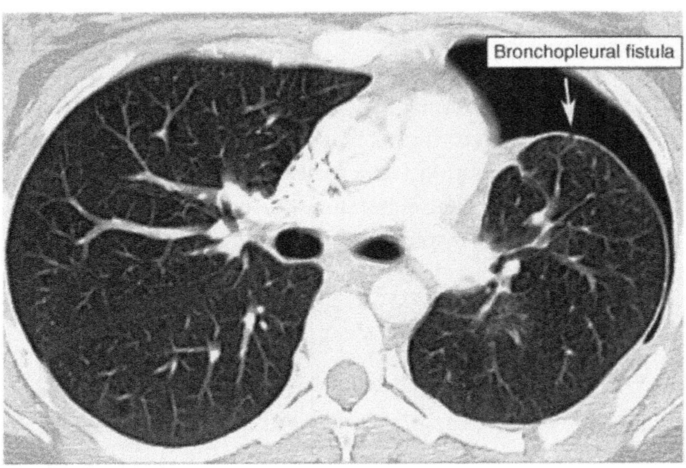

Figure 15.1 Computed tomography scan identifying a peripheral bronchopleural fistula (BPF) in a patient 2 weeks after a left lower lobectomy.[a] Fiberoptic bronchoscopy can be used to confirm and sometimes localize the BPF through variety of different procedures. Direct visualization may be possible in select cases, whereas the presences of continuous bubbles with bronchial lavage may also be suggestive of BPF and help to localize the defect.

Source: Truong A, Truong D-T, Thakar D, Riedel B. Bronchopleural fistula: anesthetic management. In: Barbeito A, Shaw AD, Grichnik K, eds. Thoracic Anesthesia. New York, NY: McGraw-Hill Medical. https://doctorlib.info/anesthesiology/thoracic/19.html

[a]See Sarkar P, Chandak T, Shah R, Talwar A. Diagnosis and management bronchopleural fistula. *Indian J Chest Dis Allied Sci.* 2010;52(2):97–104.

a combination of surgical procedures, medical therapy, and bronchoscopy with the use of different glues, coils, and sealants. Initial nonoperative management focuses on decreasing the gradient between airway pressures and the pleural space by minimizing mean airway pressure and suction on pleural tubes.[2] A stepwise evaluation and management of patients with BPF was described by Cooper and Miller.[5] It consists of an initial control of any life-threatening conditions (Table 15.1). Small (<3–5 mm) air leaks following pulmonary resection may be treated conservatively, with trial of drainage, antibiotics, and serial diagnostic or even interventional bronchoscopy (with application of sealants). The presence of major bronchial stump dehiscence requires immediate re-suturing and reinforcement. Protection against soilage of remaining lung tissue, respiratory and ventilator support, early diagnostic bronchoscopy, and minimizing tension and air flow through the fistula are basic principle in the management of these patients. Delayed postpneumonectomy BPFs are usually associated with an empyema. Due to their underlying conditions, these patients are often debilitated, and therefore it is important to aggressively manage underlying comorbidities and conditions that led to the BPF. Empyema must be treated with closed and/or open drainage procedure. Proper nutrition either by enteral or parental route is required. Successful treatment of chronic BPF requires aggressive control of infections, adequate drainage of the chest cavity, closure of the fistula with vascularized tissue, and obliteration of the chest cavity once infection is well controlled.

Chest Tube

The goal is to drain the pleural space and, in the case of postlobectomy BPF, to promote the re-expansion of ipsilateral lung.

The use of chest tube in patients with BPF has benefits but also has complications. Box 15.2 describes different complications associated with chest tube in BPF patients.

Indication for chest tube include high-flow BPF, pneumothorax, and drainage of empyema. In addition, in patients receiving mechanical ventilation, the chest tube could be used to decrease air leak during expiration (thus maintaining positive end-expiratory pressure [PEEP]) by adding positive intrapleural pressure during the expiratory phase. Chest tubes also can decrease BPF flow during inspiration by occluding it in the inspiratory phase.[6] Chest tube should be of sufficient diameter to allow drainage of the air leak and can be used to apply sclerosing agents to promote pleurodesis (talc, bleomycin).

Table 15.1 Life-Threatening Conditions and Suggested Treatment

Condition	Treatment
Tension pneumothorax	Emergent drainage with chest tube
Pulmonary flooding	Airway control Postural drainage positioning affected lung down
Bronchial stump dehiscence	Immediate re-suture and reinforcement
Empyema	Drainage Proper antimicrobial therapy

Box 15.2 Negative Effects of Chest Tube on Patients With Bronchopleural Fistula

Tidal volume loss in mechanically ventilated patients
Abnormal gas exchange
Appearance of ventilator cycling
Potential increase in flow through fistulous tract due to negative pressure to the chest tube
Interfere with closure and healing
Predisposition to infection both at the insertion site and in the pleural space

Suction is contraindicated in the early post-pneumonectomy patient since it could result in mediastinal shift, hemodynamic compromise, or even cardiac herniation (after right pneumonectomy with pericardial defect).

Mechanical Ventilation

In some patients, mechanical ventilation may be required. In postsurgical patients and in patients with chronic obstructive pulmonary disease or acute respiratory distress syndrome, the use of mechanical ventilation is an independent risk factor for the development of BPF. The air escaping through the BPF not only delays healing of the fistulous tract, but because this is an area of low resistance, it also accounts for a significant loss of tidal volume, affecting minute ventilation and oxygenation. To reduce fistula flow and loss of tidal volume, maneuvers that reduce airway pressure and promote healing of the BPF are needed. These maneuvers include limitation of the amount of PEEP used during ventilation, limiting the effective tidal volume, shortening the inspiratory time, and reducing the respiratory rate.[7,8] Others maneuvers include the use of selective intubation of the unaffected lung, the use of double-lumen intubation with differential lung ventilation, or the use of independent lung ventilation (using two ventilators) and patient positioning.[7–10] High frequency ventilation has also been used in patients with massive air leak that is difficult to manage with conventional mechanical ventilation.[11]

Surgery

The success rate of surgical closure of BPF has been reported between 80% and 95%[2,7] but is associated with the risk of open thoracotomy. Surgical closure includes chronic open drainage, direct stump closure with intercostal muscle reinforcement, omental flap, transsternal bronchial closure, and thoracoplasty with or without extrathoracic chest wall muscle transposition. Video-assisted thoracoscopy also has been used to treat BPF. A staged closure of complicated BPF has been recommended. In the first stage, the patients undergo an Eloesser or a Clagett procedure for chest cavity drainage consisting of a muscle flap operation; once the patient is optimized, it is followed by a chest cavity obliteration with an omental flap. All patients with a postlobectomy and sleeve resection BPF necessitate additional surgery: the BPF is additionally covered with a vascularized flap (Figure 15.2).[5] If patient functional status is not optimal, then interventional bronchoscopy is needed.

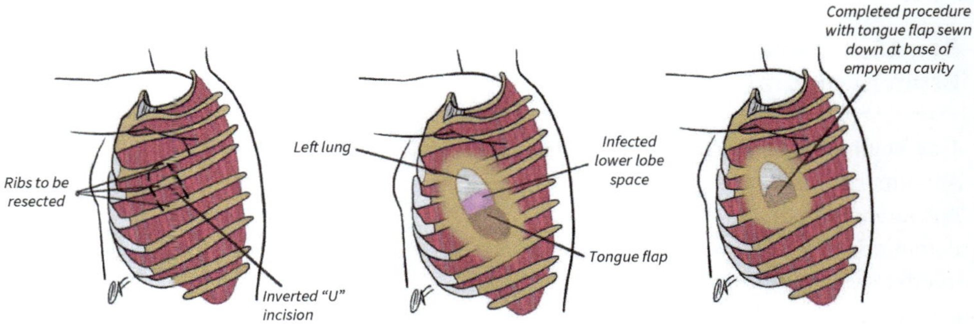

Figure 15.2 Clagett procedure. It is a technique for the management of postpneumonectomy empyema. It is a 2 stage procedure that require an open pleural drainage for control of septic cavity and closure of BPF and then obliteration of the pleural cavity with antibiotic solution.
Source: Pairolero PC, Arnold PG, Bronchopleural fistula:treatment by transposition of pectoralis major muscle. *J Thorac Cardiovasc Surg.* 1980;79:142–145.

Bronchoscopy

Bronchoscopy is usually the first step in the surgical management of BPF. BPF associated with pneumonectomy or lobectomy can be directly visualized, while distal BPF require the use of balloons to systematically occlude the bronchial segments to locate the one leading to the fistula (Figure 15.3).[2] To successfully manage a BPF with bronchoscopic techniques, the fistula must be directly visualized or prove that occlusion significantly decreases or stops the air leak. Multiple sealing compounds have been applied directly to the fistula through the bronchoscope. The potential success of this approach is that most of the leaks are peripheral or alveolar, rather than at the large airways. In addition, this offers an alternative to patients who are otherwise poor surgical candidates unable to tolerate a major thoracic procedure. Once

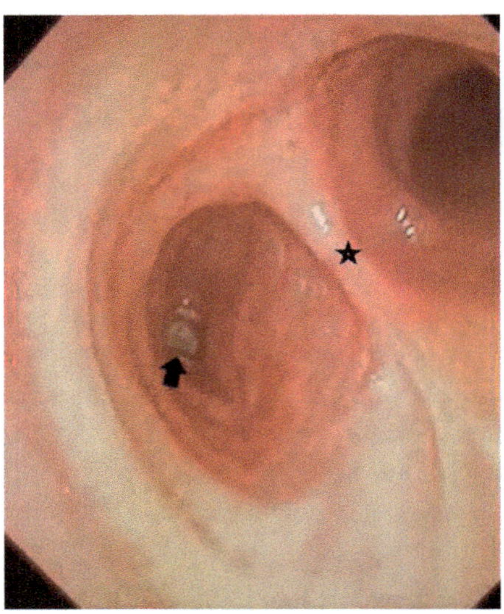

Figure 15.3 Healthy looking left upper lobe bronchial stump showing return of continuous bubbles on bronchial washing raising suspicion of bronchopleural fistula.
Source: Puskas J, Mathisen D, Grillo H, et al. Treatment strategies for bronchopleural fistula. *J Thorac Cardiovasc Surg.* 1995;109(5):989–995.

Table 15.2 Sealants Used in the Treatment of BFP Bronchoscopically

Sealant	Comment
Polyethylene glycol: FocalSeal-L (Focal; Lexington, MA)	Water-soluble polyethylene glycol-based gel xomes as a polymer and sealant activated by a xenon-generated light in the spectrum of 440 to 550 nm
Ethanol	Takaoka et al[a] recommended injecting absolute ethanol directly into the submucosal layer of a fistula as a first-line therapy for patients with a postoperative central BPF with an orifice 3 mm in diameter.
Lead shots	One of the first sealant used
Cyanoacrylate glue	One of the most common sealant compounds along with fibrin. Seal by acting as a plug and later by inducing an inflammatory response that leads to fibrosis and mucosal proliferation, permanently sealing the defect. Cyanoacrylate glues polymerize into solid material on contact with body fluids or tissue.
Fibrin glue	Closure of small postresection BPFs can be accomplished with selective bronchography and placement of fibrin sealant through the flexible fiberoptic bronchoscope. Fibrin clot forms over the fistula, sealing the leak. Fibrin glue is eventually reabsorbed, preventing foreign body reaction.
Blood clot	Blood clot is based on a principle similar to that above
Albumin-Glutaraldehyde Tissue Adhesive	BioGlue (Cryolife; Kennesaw, GA) applied during surgery BioGlue proved to be safe and effective in the sealing of lung lacerations and in preventing air leakage from suture or staple lines in emphysematous lungs. Successful in sealing BPFs when applied either intrabronchially through the rigid bronchoscope or during thoracotomy.68
Cellulose	Surgicel (Ethicon; Piscataway, NJ): It has successful been used in the management of BPF.
Gel foam	Theoretical advantages of availability and being totally reabsorbed. Cut in small strips, moistened with normal saline solution, and flushed through the working channel of the bronchoscope into the affected area (or instilled directly through the rigid scope).
Coils	Coils have been used alone or in conjunction with other sealants to treat BPF
Balloon Catheter Occlusion	Method of choice to detect the site of air leak and place the sealant substance.
Silver nitrate	Has been used through the rigid scope to seal stump leaks.75
Calf bone	Has been used along with fibrin glue to seal a BPF. Bone is shaped to the form of the fistula and sprayed with fibrin after insertion.
Stents	Extensively used mostly for the management of esophageal-to-airway fistulas, with malignancy being more common than the congenital or other acquired forms. Indicated for the sealing of stump fistulas after pneumonectomy and dehiscence after bronchoplastic operations. Goal of the stent is to provide as tight seal in the airway as possible to prevent aspiration and pneumonias.

[a]Takaoka K, Inoue S, Ohira S, Central bronchopleural fistulas closed by bronchoscopic injection of absolute ethanol, *Chest.*. 2002;122(1):374–378. doi:10.1378/chest.122.1.374.

the site is located, the application of sealants substances into the fistula have been tried. These include ethanol silver nitrate, cyanoacrylate compounds, coils, lead plugs, balloons, fibrin or tissue glue, antibiotics, gel foam, spigots, and autologous blood patch. Table 15.2 provides a list of different sealants used in the treatment of BFP bronchoscopically.

Anesthetic Considerations and Management

Postneumonectomy BPF is usually associated with an empyema; thus, it requires the creation of an open-window thoracotomy (Clagett vs. Eloesser procedure) to debride and clean the chest cavity and promote growth of granulation tissue. During this phase, the cavity is irrigated with an antibiotic solution and then an antibiotic solution is placed in the cavity to fill the entire space.

Also during this phase, the main anesthetic goal is to avoid contamination of the unaffected lung. This is achieved by proper lung isolation intubating the unaffected bronchus either with a double-lumen tube or endobronchial tube. Lung isolation and intubation should be done under direct fiberoptic guidance to have an accurate placement and to prevent further damage to the bronchial stump. As previously mentioned, failure of proper lung isolation could lead to spillage of purulent material into the unaffected lung and to difficulties with ventilation and other complications.

Intubation can be done using an awake fiberoptic technique with topicalization of the airway with a local anesthetic (with or without sedation) or in an anesthetized but spontaneously breathing patient (avoiding positive pressure ventilation). The use of bronchial blocker has been described but requires that the location of the BPF is distal enough from the carina.

Once patient is intubated, ventilation is achieved by using lung protective single-lung ventilation techniques (see previous discussion on mechanical ventilation). Suctioning of purulent material from tracheal lumen should be done frequently and prior to deflating the bronchial cuff at the end of the case. Patients are generally extubated at the end of surgery to avoid positive pressure on the stump.

Other preoperative considerations include the following. Patients are usually septic and debilitated, requiring systemic antibiotic therapy and intravenous hydration. The patient may also need nutritional and metabolic support. The presence of bacteremia may prevent the placement of thoracic epidural due to the risk of hematogenous seeding of the catheter.

As mentioned before, surgical treatment of BFP is a staged procedure. Once open, drainage of infection is performed, infection is controlled, healing has started, and the patient is medically optimized definitive fistula closure with obliteration of the cavity with a muscle flap (latissimus dorsi, serratus anterior, pectoralis major), omentum or thoracoplasty is performed. Anesthetic considerations for this stage are similar to those for open drainage, except that infection and cross-contamination are less concerning.

Ventilation goal during this stage is to minimize airflow across fistula while maintaining oxygenation by using one or a combination of techniques described previously. Also, a strategy of coordinating ventilation with chest tube suction can improve ventilation while minimizing fistula air flow (9). The use of high frequency jet ventilation has been described during this stage as well. Advantages include adequate gas exchange at lower peak airway pressure and improved recruitment and expansion of the residual lung. Drawbacks include the need for special, unfamiliar equipment; inability to monitor end-tidal CO_2; and the risk for barotrauma (11).

Prognosis

After major pulmonary surgery, the development of a BPF is relatively uncommon, around 2.6% to 8% in some studies, but can have devastating consequences. One study indicated a mortality rate of 40% in patients who developed BPF after major lung surgery. Another study showed the all-cause mortality from lobectomy or pneumonectomy reaching 6.4%, and BPF contributing to 54% of the total mortality (12).

Prevention

It has been shown that in the setting of unilateral total pneumonectomy, a right-sided pneumonectomy is an independent risk factor for increased development of BPFs (12). Although most authors indicate the cause to be multifactorial, anatomical considerations are important, including that the right bronchial stump is more exposed to the pleural space and less likely to be naturally buffered by mediastinal soft tissues than the left. The size of the bronchial stump has been shown to also be an independent risk factor for BPF formation. Other risk factors include preoperative chemotherapy with or without concurrent radiotherapy. In larger studies, no statistically significant relation between tumor size, metastatic adenopathy, extent of lymph node dissection, residual malignant cells in the bronchial stump, and diabetes mellitus was seen in the development of BPFs (12,13).

After lobectomy or pneumonectomy, the standard of care is to perform pressure testing of the anastomosis in the intraoperative setting. This is accomplished by endobronchial intubation of the affected bronchus and insufflating to a pressure of 30 cmH_2O. Any air leak present at that time could be primarily repaired in the operating room. Small fistulas that are missed during primary closure of the bronchus are often found by persistent air leak via chest tube in the immediate postoperative setting. Delayed discovery usually results in contamination of the chest cavity, empyema, or sepsis.

When the decision is made to attempt a secondary repair, selective endobronchial intubation is imperative to aid in operative repair and prevent spillover of fluid from the pleural cavity into the normal lung, loss of gases through the fistula into the pleural cavity or exterior, or possible tension pneumothorax should the pleural cavity lack external drainage or the fistula behave in a ball–valve fashion. During the operation, care must be taken during ventilation, as the employment of one-lung ventilation and the decubitus positioning required for the operation pose significant challenges. Alveolar recruitment techniques are used to help prevent atelectasis, but elevated PEEP has also been shown to impair oxygenation, especially important in one-lung ventilation.

References

1. Batihan G, Ceylan KC. Bronchopleural fistula: causes, diagnosis and management. In: Stojšić J, ed. *Diseases of Pleura*. London, UK: IntechOpen; 2020.
2. Lois M, Noppen M. Bronchopleural fistulas: an overview of the problem with special focus on endoscopic management. *Chest*. 2005;128(6):3955–3965.
3. Sarkar P, Chandak T, Shah R, Talwar A. Diagnosis and management bronchopleural fistula. *Indian J Chest Dis Allied Sci*. 2010;52(2):97–104.

4. Puskas J, Mathisen D, Grillo H, et al. Treatment strategies for bronchopleural fistula. *J Thorac Cardiovasc Surg.* 1995;109(5):989–995.
5. Cooper WA, Miller JI. Management of bronchopleural fistula after lobectomy. *Semin Thorac Cardiovasc Surg.* 2001;13:8–12.
6. Blanch PB, Koens JC Jr, Layon AJ. A new device that allows synchronous intermittent inspiratory chest tube occlusion with any mechanical ventilator. *Chest.* 1990;97:1426–1430.
7. Downs JB, Chapman RL. Treatment of bronchopleural fistulas during continuous positive pressure ventilation. *Chest.* 1976;69:363–366.
8. Zimmerman JE, Colgan DL, Mills M. Management of bronchopleural fistula complicating therapy with positive end expiratory pressure (PEEP). *Chest.* 1973;64:526–529.
9. Bauman MH, Sahn SA. Medical management and therapy of bronchopleural fistulas in the mechanically ventilated patient. *Chest.* 1990;97:721–728.
10. Carvalho P, Thompson WH, Riggs R, et al. Management of bronchopleural fistula with a variable-resistance valve and a single ventilator. *Chest.* 1997;111:1452–1454.
11. Shen NH, Lu FL, Wu HW, et al. Management of tension pneumatocele with high-frequency oscillatory ventilation. *Chest.* 2002;121:184.
12. Darling G, Abdurahman A, Qi-Long Yi, et al. Risk of a right pneumonectomy: role of bronchopleural fistula. *Ann Thorac Surg.* 2005;79:433–437.
13. Lawrence GH, Ristroph R, Wood J, Starr A. Methods for avoiding a dire surgical complication: bronchopleural fistula after pulmonary resection. *Am J Surg.* 1983;144:136–140.

16 Esophagectomy

Tiffany D. Perry, Tricia Desvarieux, and Kevin Sidoran

Introduction

Elective partial or total esophagectomy is most commonly performed as potentially curative or palliative treatment of esophageal cancers (Figure 16.1). Esophagectomy for benign disease is uncommon. However, it may be considered for esophageal disorders that have failed multiple attempts at more conservative management (Figure 16.2). Examples include motility disorders such as achalasia or spasm, scleroderma, and intractable gastroesophageal reflux disease (GERD) with stricture [1]. Emergent esophagectomy may be necessary in the setting of acute esophageal perforation or severe caustic injury.

The esophagus traverses three body regions—the neck, thorax, and abdomen—and lies in close proximity to major vital organs and vessels, thus presenting challenges from a surgical and anesthetic perspective [2]. Although overall mortality from esophagectomy has declined over the last 30 years to 8% to 11%, morbidity rates may still be as high as 40% to 50% [3–5]. The procedure generally involves the resection of the esophagus (partial or total) and a portion of the stomach as well as lymph nodes. The stomach is almost always used as the conduit to replace the esophagus, although less commonly, the colon or jejunum may be used (Figures 16.3 and 16.4) [6]. Multiple surgical approaches are employed for esophageal resection and the choice of approach depends on esophageal pathology including tumor location if applicable, surgeon experience/preference, as well as patient factors (prior surgical history, age, pulmonary function) (Figure 16.5) [6].

Common surgical approaches for the procedure are described in Table 16.1 [7]. The Ivor Lewis approach is a two-incision procedure utilizing a laparotomy and right thoracotomy with a thoracic esophagogastric anastomosis. The trans-hiatal approach (Orringer) involves a midline laparotomy and a left neck incision for a cervical esophagogastric anastomosis (Figure 16.6). The three-incision approach (McKeown) includes an abdominal incision, a right thoracotomy, and a neck incision for cervical anastomosis [8]. The less commonly employed left thoracoabdominal approach provides wide surgical exposure via a single, long incision [9]. Minimally invasive techniques utilizing laparoscopy, thoracoscopy, and robotic assistance are increasingly prevalent [6] (Figures 16.7A and 16.7B).

Preoperative Assessment and Management

A thorough preoperative evaluation should be performed. Patients presenting for esophagectomy often have significant comorbidities such as chronic obstructive pulmonary disease, cardiovascular disease, and gastrointestinal reflux disease, which should be assessed and

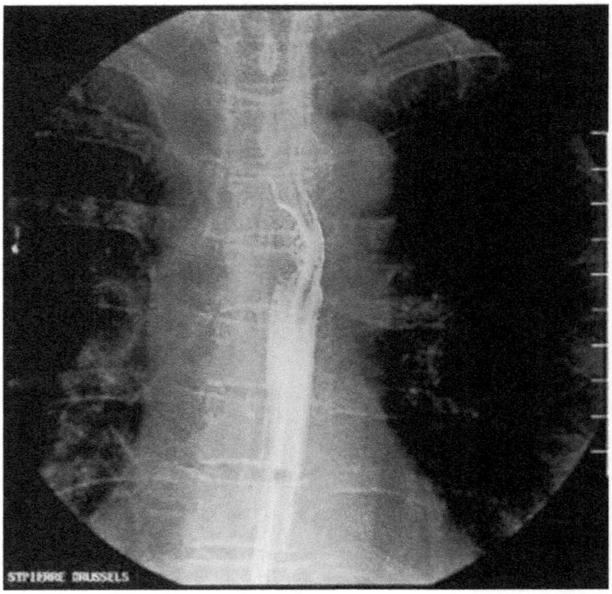

Figure 16.1 Barium swallow demonstrating a malignant tumor of the midesophagus.
From Khatri V. *Atlas of Advanced Operative Surgery*. Philadelphia, PA: Elsevier, 2012.

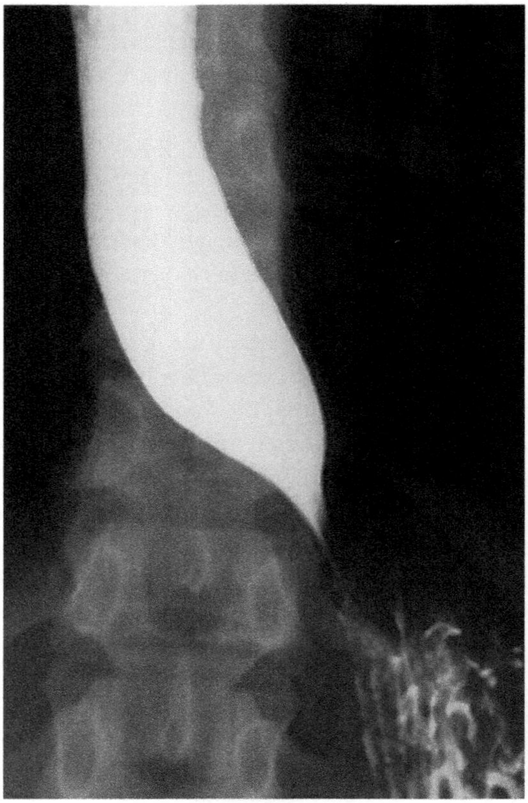

Figure 16.2 Barium swallowing demonstrating achalasia.
From Khatri V. *Atlas of Advanced Operative Surgery*. Philadelphia, PA: Elsevier, 2012.

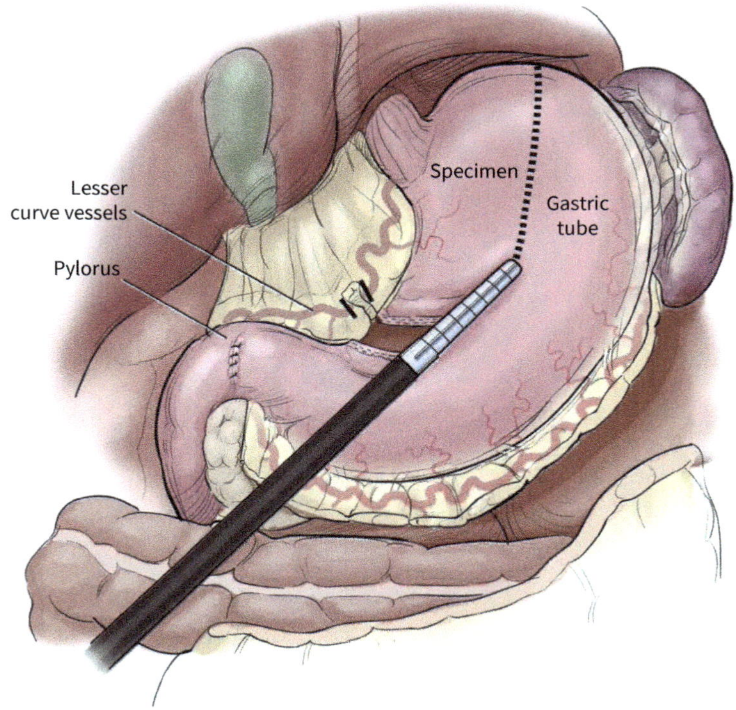

Figure 16.3 Separation of specimen and gastric tube preparation.
From Khatri V. *Atlas of Advanced Operative Surgery*. Philadelphia, PA: Elsevier, 2012.

optimized preoperatively [10]. Additionally, alcohol and tobacco abuse are common risk factors for esophageal cancer, and consideration should be given to potential physiologic consequences. Possible complications from neoadjuvant radiation and chemotherapy should be considered including pulmonary fibrosis, dilated cardiomyopathy, thrombocytopenia, and anemia [11,12].

Preoperative pulmonary evaluation should consider if one-lung ventilation (OLV) will be necessary for the procedure as well as assess risk factors for challenges with oxygenation, ventilation or weaning from mechanical ventilation. The American College of Cardiology/ American Heart Association guidelines should be used for preoperative cardiovascular evaluation management [13]. The airway should be carefully assessed in patients who have received preoperative radiation. Prophylactic medications to increase gastric pH and decrease gastric volume such as H_2 receptor antagonists and proton pump inhibitors should be considered in patients with severe GERD. Finally, patient preoperative optimization must be balanced with the risk of delayed resection of malignant tumors.

Monitoring

Standard American Society of Anesthesiologists monitors should be used with careful attention to electrocardiogram placement of leads II and V5 as cardiac arrhythmias and ischemia

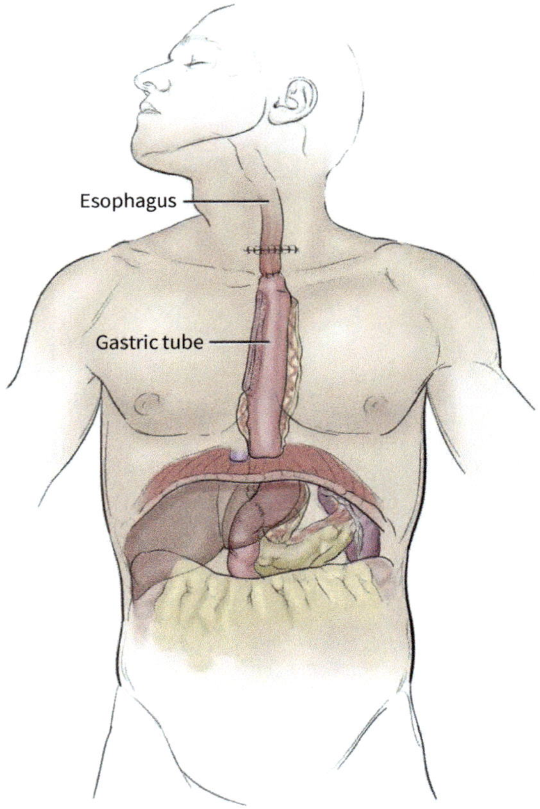

Figure 16.4 Gastric conduit with cervical esophagogastric anastomosis.
From Khatri V. *Atlas of Advanced Operative Surgery*. Philadelphia, PA: Elsevier, 2012.

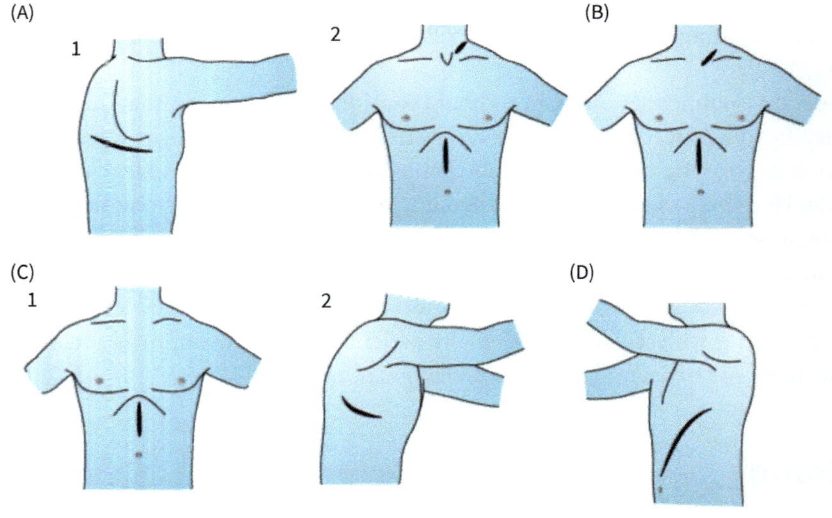

Figure 16.5 Common surgical approaches for esophagectomy. (A) Three incision (McKeown). (B) Transhiatal (Orringer). (C) Ivor Lewis. (D) Left thoracoabdominal.
From Barbeito A., Grichnik K., Shaw AD. *Thoracic Anesthesia*. New York: McGraw-Hill Medical, 2012.

Table 16.1 Surgical Techniques for Esophagectomy

Surgical Technique	Surgical Incisions/Positioning	Special Considerations
Ivor Lewis	*Surgical incisions*: 2 Midline laparotomy, right thoracotomy *Position:* Supine to left lateral decubitus	One-lung ventilation necessary Pain control
Transhiatal (Orringer)	*Surgical incisions*: 2 Midline laparotomy, left neck *Position:* Supine	Hemodynamic instability secondary to blunt intrathoracic dissection Potential for trachealbronchial tree perforation during blunt dissection No vascular access in left neck Pain control
Three-incision (McKeown)	*Surgical incisions:* 3 Right thoracotomy, midline laparotomy, left neck *Position:* Left lateral decubitus to supine	One-lung ventilation necessary No vascular access in left neck Pain control
Left thoracoabdominal	*Surgical incisions*: 1 Left thoracotomy with extension to left upper lateral abdominal wall *Position:* Right lateral decubitus	One lung ventilation necessary Pain control
Minimally invasive (laparoscopic, thoracoscopic and/ or robotic)	*Surgical incisions:* Multiple Combination of small abdominal and right thoracoscopic incisions Possible left neck incision at end of procedure *Position:* Supine, left lateral decubitus and/or prone	One-lung ventilation necessary Potential for extended surgery duration

Adapted from Slinger P, Campos JH, Anesthesia for thoracic surgery, in Miller RD, Cohen NH, eds., *Miller's Anesthesia*. Philadelphia, PA: Elsevier/Saunders; 2015.

are possible during mediastinal manipulation [14]. Invasive arterial monitoring is also indicated for close hemodynamic monitoring as well as for arterial blood gas sampling during OLV. Large-bore intravenous access is necessary. A central venous catheter can be considered in patients with poor peripheral venous access or for patients who are likely to require vasopressor or inotropic support. If a central venous catheter is placed, it should be placed on the right side if the surgical technique includes a cervical esophagogastric anastomosis.

Induction

Minimizing pulmonary aspiration risk is of critical importance during induction for patients undergoing esophagectomy surgery. Given the increased aspiration risk, a rapid sequence induction or an awake endotracheal intubation should be performed with the head of the bed elevated. The airway should be secured with a cuffed single-lumen or double-lumen endotracheal tube (DLT) depending on the surgical approach and ventilation strategy.

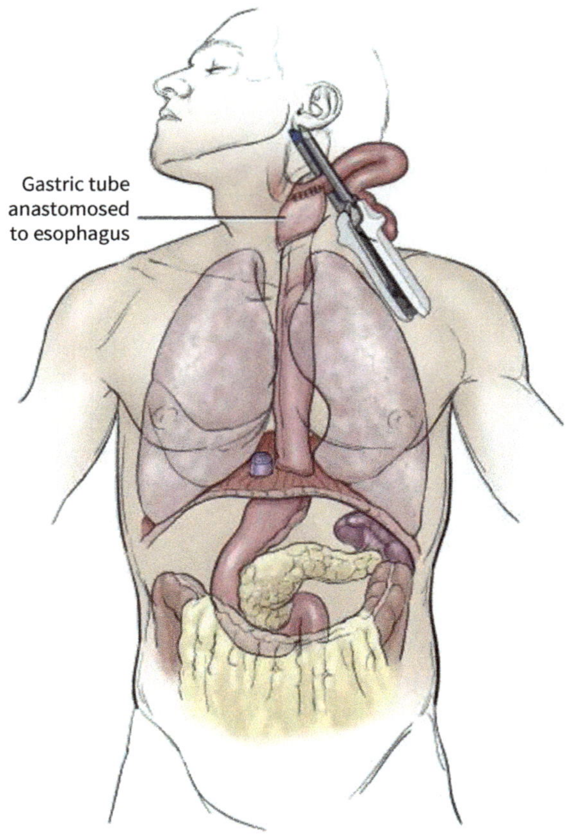

Figure 16.6 Left neck incision with cervical esophagogastric anastomosis.
From Khatri V. *Atlas of Advanced Operative Surgery*. Philadelphia, PA: Elsevier, 2012.

A nasogastric (NG) tube should be placed for gastric decompression after the airway is secured. The NG tube additionally provides digital feedback to the surgeon during dissection and will need to be withdrawn and advanced at various stages in the procedure. Once the NG tube is in its final position, it should be carefully secured in place to avoid dislodgement during extubation or patient transfer.

Ventilation

With the exception of the trans-hiatal approach, surgical approaches for esophagectomy require lung isolation and OLV. DLTs and bronchial blockers are most commonly utilized to achieve OLV. DLT placement provides reliable lung isolation and large lumens facilitate suctioning of blood or secretions. Bronchial blockers may be preferred in patients with difficult airways or anatomic abnormalities that may make placement of a DLT challenging (e.g., subglottic stenosis, external compression of the trachea or mainstem bronchus). Bronchial

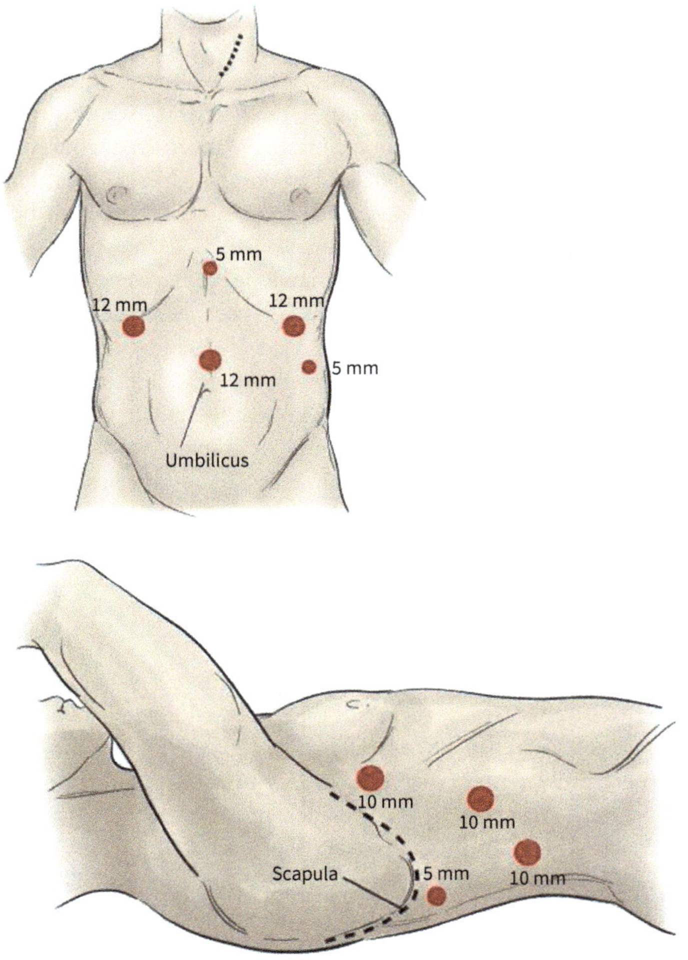

Figure 16.7 Minimally invasive esophagectomy. (A) Port sites for laparoscopic abdominal surgical phase. (B) Port sites for thoracic surgical phase.
From Khatri V. *Atlas of Advanced Operative Surgery*. Philadelphia, PA: Elsevier, 2012.

blockers have received lung collapse scores equivalent to DLTs, although they may require more time for final positioning and may require more repositioning throughout the surgery [15]. The need to secure the airway rapidly to reduce aspiration risk should be considered when selecting a lung isolation technique.

Esophagectomy surgery is associated with a large proinflammatory response that may contribute to the development of acute lung injury. OLV is associated with an inflammatory response and protective ventilatory strategies should be employed. Tidal volumes of 5 mL/kg with positive end expiratory pressure of 5 cmH_2O to the dependent lung have been demonstrated to decrease the inflammatory response during OLV [5].

Pain Management

Postoperative pain following esophagectomy can be challenging to manage, particularly for surgical approaches involving a thoracotomy and laparotomy. Pain management following the procedure plays a crucial role in facilitating recovery, reducing complications and decreasing hospital length of stay [16]. Thoracic epidural analgesia (TEA) has been the gold standard for pain management for open surgical approaches with a large body of evidence supporting its superiority over systemic opioids [17,18]. TEA has been shown to provide superior analgesia and a reduction in postoperative pulmonary complications as well as a reduction in postthoracotomy pain [19]. TEA has also been associated with a decreased incidence of anastomotic leak and may additionally exert favorable immunomodulatory effects [20,21]. Recent studies have shown that paravertebral blockade provides comparable analgesia to TEA as well as a comparable reduction in postoperative pulmonary complications with a lower side effect profile [16,22,23]. Truncal blocks (e.g., transversus abdominis plane, rectus sheath) may also be considered for esophagectomy approaches requiring laparotomy in patients where neuraxial is contraindicated or technically challenging [24].

Fluid Management

Appropriate fluid administration is an important component of anesthetic planning and management during esophagectomy surgery. Preoperative fluid deficits must be considered, particularly if advanced esophageal disease has contributed to limited intake. Additionally, the surgical approach and length of surgery will heavily impact fluid requirements. An ideal strategy must balance the need for adequate perfusion pressure and oxygen delivery to vital organs and the anastomotic site with the avoidance of excessive fluid accumulation. Multiple studies have linked fluid overload to impaired wound healing, pulmonary edema and acute lung injury, and impaired cardiac function [25,26]. Additionally, restrictive fluid management has been linked with successful early extubation [5,27]. Most current literature recommends a fluid restrictive or goal-directed management strategy although the lack of a standard definition for volume restriction complicates analysis [28–31]. Furthermore, position changes, changes in intrathoracic pressure and OLV limit the usefulness and accuracy of several parameters traditionally used in goal-directed therapy such as stroke volume variation and pulse pressure variation [32,33]. Additional research is needed to further elucidate optimal fluid administration protocols.

Vasopressor Use

Vasopressor use in esophagectomy surgery has been cautioned given concerns for vasoconstriction and resulting anastomotic ischemia [5,34,35]. However, systemic hypotension is also problematic for anastomotic perfusion [5,36]. If hypovolemia as the cause of hypotension has been excluded, recent studies indicate vasopressors can be safely used to improve gastric conduit perfusion [5,36–38]. It should additionally be noted that total avoidance of vasopressors can lead to fluid overload in an attempt to treat hypotension, which can also compromise anastomotic perfusion. Close communication with the surgical team is recommended regarding intraoperative vasopressor use.

Intraoperative Complications

Hypotension is a common intraoperative complication of esophagectomy surgery and may result from compression and manipulation of the heart and major vascular structures during dissection, hypovolemia, the use of neuraxial analgesia, or cardiac arrhythmias [10,14]. Cardiac arrhythmias may occur in as many as 65% of patients during esophagectomy surgery and are particularly common during trans-hiatal procedures [2,39]. Hypoxemia may present an additional challenge during esophagectomy particularly if OLV is utilized [10]. Mechanisms include atelectasis, shunt flow if OLV is employed, surgical trauma or pulmonary edema. Major bleeding during esophagectomy, although uncommon, may occur as the esophagus lies in close proximity to the aorta, azygous vein, and pulmonary vessels [40]. Damage to a large vessel and may necessitate the conversion from a minimally invasive technique to an open technique. Tracheal injury is quite rare (0.2%–2% incidence) [14], and most injuries are small lesions. Injuries are typically detected by the smell of anesthetic gas in the surgical field and rarely, large lesions may a cause a pressure drop in the anesthetic circuit and a loss of volume. In the event of tracheal injury, the endotracheal tube will need to be advanced beyond the tracheal injury often with surgeon guidance. Surgical repair via a right thoracotomy may be necessary for larger lesions.

Emergence and Intensive Care Unit Transfer

Traditionally, early extubation following esophagectomy was not routinely performed given concerns postoperative complications as well as anastomotic trauma if reintubation was required. Recent data, however, support early extubation as a safe practice that may reduce respiratory complications and decrease the length of intensive care unit stay [41,42]. Most esophagectomy patients can be safely extubated immediately following the procedure provided they are hemodynamically and metabolically stable, pulmonary function is satisfactory, and an adequate postoperative analgesic plan has been instituted. Prior to extubation, the oropharynx and NG tube should be suctioned and the head of the bed elevated to minimize aspiration risk. For patients unable to meet extubation criteria immediately following the procedure, if a DLT was used for lung isolation, it should be exchanged for a single-lumen endotracheal tube in most circumstances prior to operating room departure.

Postoperative Complications

Postoperative pulmonary complications including pneumonia, acute respiratory distress syndrome, and pulmonary embolism are common following esophagectomy. In patients undergoing esophagectomy for cancer, pulmonary complications are the most common cause of postoperative mortality [5]. Swallowing dysfunction and tracheal aspiration can present as an early complication following esophagectomy can increase risk for pneumonia [43].

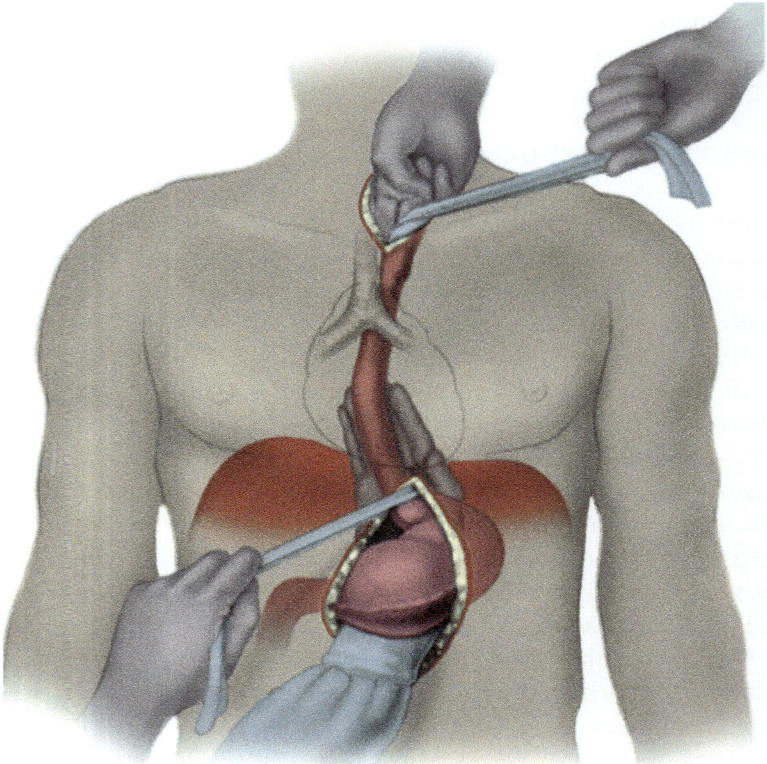

Figure 16.8 Esophageal mobilization during transhiatal esophagectomy.
From Stiles, B. Altorki, N. Traditional techniques of esophagectomy. Surg Clin N Am. 2012;92(5):1249–1263; Orringer MB. Transhiatal esophagectomy without thoracotomy. *Gen Thorac Surg* 2005;10(1):63–83.

Pneumonia is an independent risk factor for postoperative death, and its incidence appears highest in surgical approaches involving thoracotomy [44].

Chyle leaks occur more frequently in patients undergoing esophagectomy than in other thoracic procedures given the close proximity of the thoracic duct to the esophagus. (Figure 16.8) Chyle leaks are estimated to occur in up to 8% of patients undergoing esophagectomy and are associated with mortality rates as high as 18% [45] (Figure 16.9). Management usually involves surgical thoracic duct ligation.

Conduit complications including anastomotic leak and conduit ischemia are among the most feared complications following esophagectomy. The incidence of cervical anastomosis leak has been reported as high as 15% to 37% [5]. Although thoracic anastomosis leak rates are lower, they are associated with a higher morbidity and mortality. Anastomotic leak may present with fever, leukocytosis, pleural effusion, or sepsis although small leaks may be asymptomatic. Conduit ischemia varies in severity, but total conduit ischemia may present as rapidly progressive septic shock [46].

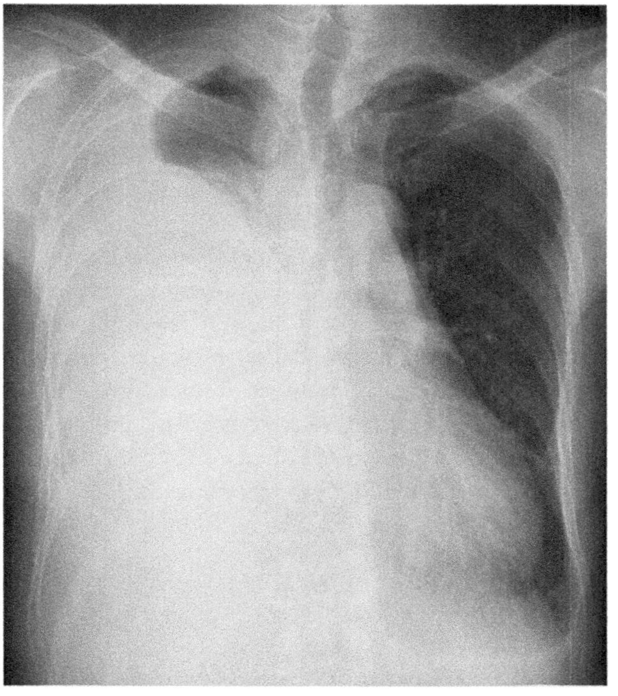

Figure 16.9 Chylothorax following esophagectomy.
Open source image.

Postoperative atrial fibrillation has been reported in up to 25% of esophagectomy patients. Atrial fibrillation has been associated with pulmonary complications and anastomotic leakage and is a marker for poor short-term outcome and increased morbidity and mortality [47].

Recurrent laryngeal nerve injury may occur during esophagectomy as a result of stretching, compression, thermal injury, or vascular compromise during the procedure. Recurrent laryngeal nerve injury most commonly presents as hoarseness. However, severe cases may result in vocal cord paralysis with dyspnea and/or aspiration pneumonia. Reported incidences vary widely but may be as high as 59% [48]. In cases where paralysis persists or is significantly impairing, vocal cord medialization via injection may be necessary.

Later complications following esophagectomy include anastomotic stricture, as well as functional disorders such as dysphagia, delayed gastric emptying, reflux, dumping syndrome, or hiatal hernia. Patients presenting for anesthesia post esophagectomy should be considered at high risk for aspiration and precautions including rapid sequence induction, head of bed elevation, and pretreatment with H_2 receptor antagonists or proton pump inhibitors should be considered [2].

Enhanced Recovery After Surgery

Enhanced recovery after surgery (ERAS) programs provide a multidisciplinary perioperative treatment protocol with the goal of reducing complications, promoting recovery, and improving treatment outcomes [49]. Despite advancements in surgical techniques, esophagectomy remains a high-risk procedure with significant associated morbidity and mortality rates [12]; therefore, it is unsurprising that ERAS protocols for esophagectomy are rapidly gaining traction. Important preprocedure components of esophagectomy ERAS programs include nutritional assessment and optimization, multidisciplinary tumor board planning, and prehabilitation programs. Key intraoperative anesthetic management components include protective lung ventilation, avoidance of volume overload, and adequate pain control via thoracic epidural or paravertebral blocks. Postoperative management recommendations include early extubation when feasible, early mobilization, and early enteral nutrition [50]. Although additional research is needed to standardize protocols and improve adoption, early results for esophagectomy ERAS programs are promising [51].

References

1. Mormando J, Barbetta A, Molena D. Esophagectomy for benign disease. J Thorac Dis. 2018;10(3):2026–2033.
2. Berry MF, Schroeder RA. Esophageal cancer operations. In: Barbeito A, Grichnik K, Shaw AD, eds. *Thoracic Anesthesia*. New York, NY: McGraw-Hill Medical; 2012.
3. Chang AC, Ji H, Birkmeyer NJ, Orringer MB, Birkmeyer JD. Outcomes after transhiatal and transthoracic esophagectomy for cancer. *Ann Thorac Surg*, 2008;85(2):424–429.
4. Connors RC, Reuben BC, Neumayer LA, Bull DA. Comparing outcomes after transthoracic and transhiatal esophagectomy: a 5-year prospective cohort of 17,395 patients. *J Am Coll Surg.* 2007;205(6):735–740.
5. Ng JM. Update on anesthetic management for esophagectomy. *Curr Opin Anaesthesiol.* 2011;24(1):37–43.
6. D'Amico TA. Outcomes after surgery for esophageal cancer. *Gastrointest Can Res.* 2007;1(5):188–196.
7. Slinger P, Campos JH. Anesthesia for thoracic surgery. In Miller RD, Cohen NH, eds. *Miller's Anesthesia.* Philadelphia, PA: Elsevier/Saunders; 2015.
8. Filicori F, Swanström LL. Management of esophageal cancer. In: Cameron JL, Cameron AM, eds. *Current Surgical Therapy.* Philadelphia, PA: Elsevier; 2020.
9. Heitmiller RF. The left thoracoabdominal incision. Anna Thorac Surg. 1988;46(2):250–253.
10. Blank RS, Huffmyer JL, Jaeger M. *Anesthesia for esophageal surgery*. In: Slinger P, ed. *Principles and Practice of Anesthesia for Thoracic Surgery*. Cham, Switzerland: Springer; 2016.
11. Monjazeb AM, Blackstock AW. The impact of multimodality therapy of distal esophageal and gastroesophageal junction adenocarcinomas on treatment-related toxicity and complications. *Semin Radiat Oncol.* 2013;23(1):60–73.
12. Veelo DP, Geerts BF. Anaesthesia during oesophagectomy. J Thorac Dis. 2017;9(Suppl 8):S705–S712.
13. Fleisher LA, Fleischmann KE, Andrew D Auerbach, et al. 2014 ACC/AHA guideline on perioperative cardiovascular evaluation and management of patients undergoing noncardiac surgery: executive summary: a report of the American College of Cardiology/American Heart Association Task Force on Practice Guidelines. *Circulation*. 2014;130(24):2215–2245.
14. Herbella F. Esophagectomy perianesthetic care from a surgeon's point of view. SOJ Anesthesiol Pain Manage. 2014;1(1):1–7.

15. Narayanaswamy M, McRae K, Slinger P, et al., Choosing a lung isolation device for thoracic surgery: a randomized trial of three bronchial blockers versus double-lumen tubes. *Anesth Analg,* 2009;108(4):1097–1101.
16. Visser E, Marsman M, van Rossum PSN, et al. Corrigendum: Postoperative pain management after esophagectomy: a systematic review and meta-analysis. *Dis Esophagus.* 2018;31(4):doy033.
17. Flisberg P, Törnebrandt K, Walther B, Lundberg J. Pain relief after esophagectomy: thoracic epidural analgesia is better than parenteral opioids. *J Cardiothorac Vasc Anesth.* 2001;15:282–287.
18. Rudin A, Flisberg P, Johansson J, Walther B, Johan C, Lundberg F. Thoracic epidural analgesia or intravenous morphine analgesia after thoracoabdominal esophagectomy: a prospective follow-up of 201 patients. *J Cardiothorac Vasc Anesth.* 2005;19(3):350–357.
19. Senturk M, Ozcan PE, Talu GK, et al. The effects of three different analgesia techniques on long-term postthoracotomy pain. *Anesth Analg.* 2002;94(1):11–15.
20. Gu CY, Zhang J, Qian YN, Tang QF. Effects of epidural anesthesia and postoperative epidural analgesia on immune function in esophageal carcinoma patients undergoing thoracic surgery. *Mol Clin Oncol.* 2015;3(1):190–196.
21. Lazar G, Kaszaki J, Abrahám S, et al. Thoracic epidural anesthesia improves the gastric microcirculation during experimental gastric tube formation. *Surgery,* 2003;134(5):799–805.
22. Baidya D, Khanna P, Maitra S. Analgesic efficacy and safety of thoracic paravertebral and epidural analgesia for thoracic surgery: A systematic review and meta-analysis. Interact Cardiovasc Thorac Surg. 2014;18(5):626–635.
23. Davies RG, Myles PS, Graham JM. A comparison of the analgesic efficacy and side-effects of paravertebral vs epidural blockade for thoracotomy: a systematic review and meta-analysis of randomized trials. *Br J Anaesth.* 2006;96(4):418–426.
24. Levy G, Cordes MA, Farivar AS, Aye RW, Louie BE. Transversus abdominis plane block improves perioperative outcome after esophagectomy versus epidural. *Ann Thorac Surg.* 2018;105(2):406–412.
25. Glatz T, Kulemann B, Marjanovic G, Bregenzer S, Makowiec F, Hoeppner J. Postoperative fluid overload is a risk factor for adverse surgical outcome in patients undergoing esophagectomy for esophageal cancer: a retrospective study in 335 patients. *BMC Surg.* 2017;17(1):6.
26. Holte K, Sharrock NE, Kehlet H. Pathophysiology and clinical implications of perioperative fluid excess. *Br J Anaesth.* 2002;89(4):622–632.
27. Chandrashekar MV, Irving M, Wayman J, Raimes SA, Linsley A. Immediate extubation and epidural analgesia allow safe management in a high-dependency unit after two-stage oesophagectomy. Results of eight years of experience in a specialized upper gastrointestinal unit in a district general hospital. *Br J Anaesth.* 2003;90(4):474–479.
28. Brandstrup B, Tønnesen H, Beier-Holgersen R, et al; Danish Study Group on Perioperative Fluid Therapy. Effects of intravenous fluid restriction on postoperative complications: comparison of two perioperative fluid regimens: a randomized assessor-blinded multicenter trial. *Ann Surg.* 2003;238(5):641–648.
29. Buise MP. Proper volume management during anesthesia for esophageal resection. *J Thorac Dis.* 2019;11(Suppl 5):S702–S706.
30. Joshi GP. Intraoperative fluid restriction improves outcome after major elective gastrointestinal surgery. *Anesth Analg.* 2005;101(2):601–605.
31. Nisanevich V, Felsenstein I, Almogy G, Weissman C, Einav S, Matot I. Effect of intraoperative fluid management on outcome after intraabdominal surgery. *Anesthesiology.* 2005;103(1):25–32.
32. Haas S, Eichhorn V, Hasbach T, et al. Goal-directed fluid therapy using stroke volume variation does not result in pulmonary fluid overload in thoracic surgery requiring one-lung ventilation. *Crit Care Res Pract.* 2012;2012:687018–687018.
33. Jeong D, Ahn HJ, Park HW, Yang M, Kim JA, Park J. Stroke volume variation and pulse pressure variation are not useful for predicting fluid responsiveness in thoracic surgery. *Anesth Analg.* 2017;125(4):1158–1165.
34. Theodorou D, Drimousis PG, Larentzakis A, Papalois A, Toutouzas KG, Katsaragakis S. The effects of vasopressors on perfusion of gastric graft after esophagectomy: an experimental study. *J Gastrointest Surg.* 2008;12(9):1497–1501.

35. Zakrison T, Nascimento BA Jr, Tremblay LN, Kiss A, Rizoli SB. Perioperative vasopressors are associated with an increased risk of gastrointestinal anastomotic leakage. *World J Surg.* 2007;31(8):1627–1634.
36. Fumagalli U, Melis A, Balazova J, Lascari V, Morenghi E, Rosati R. Intra-operative hypotensive episodes may be associated with post-operative esophageal anastomotic leak. Updates Surg. 2016;68(2):185–190.
37. Al-Rawi OY, Pennefather SH, Page RD, Dave I, Russell GN. The effect of thoracic epidural bupivacaine and an intravenous adrenaline infusion on gastric tube blood flow during esophagectomy. *Anesth Analg.* 2008;106(3):884–887.
38. Karamanos E, Kane WJ, Mohanty S, Schmoekel N. Is intraoperative use of vasopressors associated with higher leak rate after emergent bowel resection and primary anastomosis? *J Am Coll Surg.* 2016;223:S56–S57.
39. Malhotra SK, Kaur RP, Gupta NM, Grover A, Ramprabu K, Nakra D. Incidence and types of arrhythmias after mediastinal manipulation during transhiatal esophagectomy. *Anna Thorac Surg.* 2006;82(1):298–302.
40. Javed A, Pal S, Chaubal GN, Sahni P, Chattopadhyay TK. Management and outcome of intrathoracic bleeding due to vascular injury during transhiatal esophagectomy. *J Gastroint Surg.* 2011;15(2):262–266.
41. Lanuti M, de Delva PE, Maher A, et al. Feasibility and outcomes of an early extubation policy after esophagectomy. *Ann Thorac Surg.* 2006;82(6):2037–2041.
42. Yap FH, Lau TYW, Joynt GM, Chui PT, Chan ACW, Chung SSC. Early extubation after transthoracic oesophagectomy. *Hong Kong Med J.* 2003;9(2):98–102.
43. Berry MF, Atkins BZ, Tong BC, Harpole DH, D'Amico TA, Onaitis MW. A comprehensive evaluation for aspiration after esophagectomy reduces the incidence of postoperative pneumonia. *J Thorac Cardiovasc Surg.* 2010;140(6):1266–1271.
44. Atkins BZ, Shah AS, Hutcheson KA, et al. Reducing hospital morbidity and mortality following esophagectomy. *Ann Thorac Surg.* 2004;78(4):1170–1176; discussion 1170–1176.
45. Shah RD, Luketich JD, Schuchert MJ, et al. Postesophagectomy chylothorax: incidence, risk factors, and outcomes. *Ann Thorac Surg.* 2012;93(3):897–903; discussion 903–904.
46. Briel JW, Tamhankar AP, Hagen JA, et al. Prevalence and risk factors for ischemia, leak, and stricture of esophageal anastomosis: gastric pull-up versus colon interposition. *J Am Coll Surg.* 2004;198(4):536–541; discussion 541–542.
47. Murthy SC, Law S, Whooley BP, Alexandrou A, Chu K-M, Wong J. Atrial fibrillation after esophagectomy is a marker for postoperative morbidity and mortality. *J Thorac Cardiovasc Surg.* 2003;126(4):1162–1167.
48. Scholtemeijer MG, Seesing MFJ, Brenkman HJF, Janssen LM, van Hillegersberg R, Ruurda JP. Recurrent laryngeal nerve injury after esophagectomy for esophageal cancer: incidence, management, and impact on short- and long-term outcomes. *J Thorac Dis.* 2017;9(Suppl 8):S868–S878.
49. Liu F, Wang W, Wang C, Peng X. Enhanced recovery after surgery (ERAS) programs for esophagectomy protocol for a systematic review and meta-analysis. *Medicine (Baltimore).* 2018;97(8):e0016.
50. Low DE, Allum W, De Manzoni G, et al. Guidelines for perioperative care in esophagectomy: Enhanced Recovery After Surgery (ERAS®) society recommendations. *World J Surg.* 2019;43(2):299–330.
51. Rubinkiewicz M, Witowski J, Su M, Major P, Pędziwiatr M. Enhanced recovery after surgery (ERAS) programs for esophagectomy. *J Thorac Dis.* 2019;11(Suppl 5):S685–S691.

17
Lung Transplantation

Loren Francis and Jared McKinnon

Preoperative Assessment

Introduction

Lung transplant surgery is a high-risk major surgery performed on patients with end-stage lung disease that has the potential to greatly improve quality of life. Thorough evaluation is necessary to identify the causative disease process, qualify the extent of disease, and decide whether the patient would be an acceptable transplant candidate. This evaluation yields data that informs potential patient immune system-donor organ compatibility and helps determine a patient's position on the organ recipient waitlist. In addition to necessary medical evaluation, psychological, financial, and social barriers must be considered.

Medical Evaluation

Patients will arrive on the day of transplant with recent comprehensive workups.
This includes:

- Vital signs, including height, weight, and calculated body mass index
- Complete blood count, complete metabolic panel, and coagulation studies
- ABO type and screen
- Tissue typing for organ compatibility
- Infectious disease tests
- Chest X-ray
- Computed tomography scan of the chest
- Transthoracic echocardiogram
- Electrocardiogram (EKG)
- Heart catheterization
  - Of the left heart to assess coronary artery disease
  - Of the right heart to evaluate right heart function and pulmonary hypertension
- Pulmonary function tests
- 6-minute walk test, to assess functional capacity
- Ventilation-perfusion (V/Q) scan
- Age- and gender-recommended cancer screenings
- Carotid ultrasonography

Cardiac and pulmonary function tests are of particular interest to the anesthesiologist preparing for this case. The results of these may inform surgical approach, use of planned cardiopulmonary bypass (CPB), induction of anesthesia, and intraoperative medication selection.

>> Tip on Technique

The V/Q scan will specify the proportion of blood flow to each lung. Typically, blood flow to each lung is roughly equal, with the right lung receiving 55% and the left lung receiving 45% of cardiac output.[1] The greater the perfusion to the operative lung, the lower the PaO_2 during one lung ventilation.[2] Accordingly, the greater the inequality of lung perfusion demonstrated by V/Q scan, the higher the likelihood that the patient will not tolerate one lung ventilation.

Exclusion Criteria

Absolute and relative exclusion criteria for patients with end-stage lung disease to be listed for a lung transplant have been detailed by the International Society for Heart and Lung Transplantation.[3] Specific criteria are listed in Table 17.1. The preparation, workup, and

Table 17.1 Contraindications to Being Placed on Lung Transplant Waiting List

Absolute Contraindications	Relative Contraindications
Active or recent malignancy	Age > 65
Untreatable significant dysfunction of another major organ system	Body mass index 30–34.9 kg/m^2
Uncorrected or untreatable atherosclerotic disease	Severe malnutrition
Acute medical instability	Severe osteoporosis
Uncorrectable bleeding	Extensive prior chest surgery
Chronic infection that is poorly controlled	Mechanical ventilation or extracorporeal life support
Active *Mycobacterium tuberculosis* infection	Colonization with highly resistant organism
Significant chest wall or spinal deformity	Hepatitis B or C, HIV infection
Body mass index >35 kg/m^2	
History of noncompliance	
Psychiatric/psychological conditions associated with inability to adhere to complex medical therapy	
Absence of reliable social support system	
Severely limited functional status	
Substance abuse or dependence	

follow-up for social support systems posttransplant is extensive. Patients are required to remain within a few hours of the transplant center and be available 24 hours a day before transplant and for several months after transplant.

Transplant Waitlist

Unfortunately, the demand for organs far outstrips the supply of donor organs. An organ waitlist is managed by the United Network for Organ Sharing (UNOS). UNOS bases organ matching on several factors including blood type, height, medical urgency, and time spent on the waitlist. In 2005 a lung allocation score (LAS) was introduced to create a waitlist that accounts for urgency and expected posttransplant survival rate. The LAS has widely been accepted as having improved survival for patients and improved waiting times.

Intraoperative Management

Monitors

Use of standard and invasive monitors is necessary considering the risks of general anesthesia for patients with end-stage lung disease. Rapid fluid shifts, hemodynamic changes, risk of acute heart failure, potential pulmonary hypertension exacerbation, and unique positioning leading to the patient's extremities being inaccessible during the procedure should all be considered.

Standard anesthetic monitors including pulse oximetry, EKG leads, noninvasive blood pressure, temperature, expiratory carbon dioxide analysis, and inspired oxygen analysis should be used. Advanced monitors commonly utilized during lung transplantation include invasive arterial pressure monitoring, pulmonary artery (PA) catheters, and transesophageal echocardiography (TEE).

Besides a temperature monitor, all standard anesthesia monitors should be in place prior to induction of anesthesia. Consider measuring pulse oximetry from multiple locations simultaneously, as patient positioning makes these probes prone to error and redundancy may help achieve consistent oxygen saturation readings. EKG measurement from two leads is standard for rhythm observation. Lead II is used for the clear P-QRS complexes and for identification of arrhythmias. Lead V is used for observation of ST-segment changes of ischemia.

An invasive arterial line should also be placed prior to induction of anesthesia in a radial, brachial, or femoral artery. An arterial line allows for real-time blood pressure measurement and a reliable source for lab draws. During induction of anesthesia and throughout the procedure, large swings in blood pressure can occur rapidly. A radial arterial catheter may be prone to compression or error depending on the patient's arm position, so consider anatomic site choice carefully. Aseptic protocol during invasive line placement procedures is particularly important as this patient population will be immunosuppressed and susceptible to infection.

Pulmonary Artery Catheter

The pulmonary artery catheter (PAC) provides a lot of information to the anesthesiologist. Pulmonary artery pressure and central venous pressure (CVP) are continuously transduced and displayed. Cardiac output is calculated via thermodilution and incorporated with body surface area to calculate cardiac index. Mixed venous oxygen saturation (SvO_2) is measured from pulmonary arterial blood. A simplified Fick equation can assist with the interpretation of SvO_2. The PA occlusion pressure can be used to estimate left atrial and left ventricular end diastolic pressures. Interpretation and clinical application of all this data require practice, repetition, and an in-depth understanding of the physiology and pathology of heart disease.

$$SvO_2 = SpO_2 - \frac{VO_2}{CO \times Hgb \times 1.34}$$

- SvO_2 mixed venous oxygen saturation
- SpO_2 arterial oxygen saturation
- VO_2 systemic oxygen consumption
- *CO* cardiac output
- *Hgb* hemoglobin
- 1.34 is a coefficient for the oxygen-carrying capacity of hemoglobin

A PAC is inserted through a venous introducer sheath into a large central vein using sterile technique. The PAC itself is positioned or "floated" into the PA by inflating a small balloon at the tip of the catheter and incrementally inserting it with consecutive heart beats, allowing blood flow to direct the catheter into place. Confirmation of proper placement is via pressure waveform analysis and/or visualization with TEE. In particularly precarious patients, it might be beneficial to place a PAC prior to induction of general anesthesia to monitor hemodynamics. The right internal jugular (RIJ) vein is the most common anatomic site used for PAC insertion because of its close proximity and relatively straightforward path to the heart. If the RIJ is unsuitable or is likely to be needed for mechanical support cannula access, consider using the left internal jugular (LIJ) vein instead. The LIJ has a more convoluted anatomical path to the heart, and introduction of a large introducer sheath here has a higher risk of vascular injury than placement into the RIJ. The most common complication from PAC placement is arrhythmia, specifically right bundle branch block. Typically line-induced arrhythmias are short lived, but particular caution must be taken in patients with an existing left bundle branch block, as adding a right bundle branch block during insertion can lead to complete heart block. Figure 17.1 shows the expected pressure waveforms when advancing the catheter.

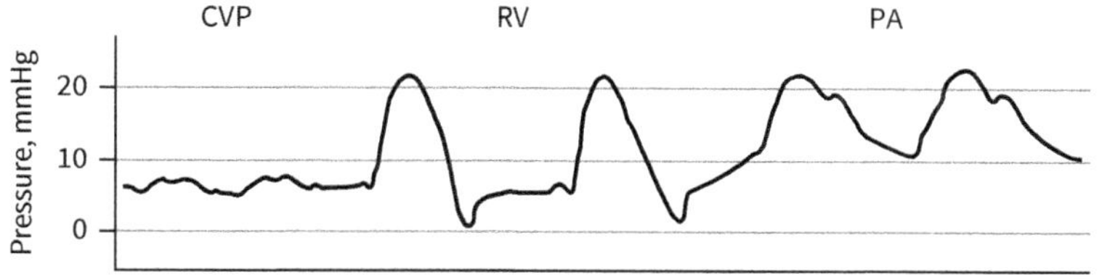

Figure 17.1 Pulmonary Artery Catheter Waveforms. Note low pressure, low amplitude waveform of central venous pressure (CVP) Note the right ventricle (RV) pressure waveform with higher pressure during systole and low diastolic pressure. The pulmonary artery (PA) pressure waveform is similar to RV pressure during systole, but higher diastolic pressure ("step up" in diastolic pressure) and a dicrotic notch indicative of the pulmonic valve closing.
Figure drawn by Jared McKinnon.

Step by Step: Pulmonary Artery Catheter Insertion

- Prepare catheter by connecting the appropriate lumens to pressure transducers, keeping the distal portion of catheter sterile
- Clean the neck with a sterile solution and apply sterile drapes
- Insert venous introducer sheath, using ultrasound guidance
- Place a catheter guard sheath over the PAC
- Flush ports of the catheter and confirm balloon inflation without leaks
- Insert the catheter through the sheath to approximately 25 cm
- Inflate the balloon
- Look for pressure waveform of the PA tracing from the tip of the catheter
- Insert the catheter approximately 1 to 2 cm per heartbeat
- Once a PA pressure waveform is present, advance 1 cm, deflate the balloon, and lock the catheter guard sheath
- Apply sterile dressing

Commonly used cerebral monitors include bispectral index (BiS) and cerebral oximetry. The BiS monitor utilizes scalp electrodes with electroencephalogram monitoring to provide a dimensionless number suggesting depth of anesthesia. Cerebral oximetry applied to each side of the forehead monitors cerebral perfusion. Cerebral oximetry is particularly useful during CPB, when many other monitors of perfusion and oxygenation may be erroneous. A decrease in cerebral oximetry values may indicate decreased delivery of blood, increased oxygen consumption, hypoxia, or anemia.

>> Tip on Technique

The PAC is packaged with a curve in the catheter. Inserting the catheter with this curve directed medially increases chances of success with "floating" the PAC to the appropriate location.

Induction

The main concerns during induction of anesthesia for lung transplantation are airway protection, avoidance of hypoxia and hypercarbia, and maintenance of right ventricular (RV) function. A thorough preoperative evaluation is crucial for planning a safe induction strategy.

Lung transplants are by nature scheduled with little notice and, as such, patients may not be appropriately nil per os (NPO). The risk of aspiration must be balanced with the likelihood of a difficult airway and concern for hemodynamically stable induction. If the patient's airway exam is worrying, an awake fiberoptic intubation may be the best option to avoid the risk of losing the airway. Topicalization and cautiously titrated sedation help minimize sympathetic stimulation that can worsen pulmonary hypertension. If the patient's airway exam is reassuring, a rapid sequence intubation (RSI) may be appropriate. Patients with severe right heart failure or pulmonary hypertension may not tolerate fast medication administration, and a slow induction relying on titrated narcotics with continuous cricoid pressure might be more important than an RSI. All of these factors must be taken into account to appropriately balance the risks and benefits of the chosen induction plan. See Figure 17.2 for a decision tree in planning induction and intubation strategy.

Preoxygenation is critical in patients about to undergo lung transplantation. Supplemental oxygen should be administered via face mask in a closed circuit to denitrogenate the lungs prior to creating apnea. If the patient requires supplemental oxygen at baseline, be prepared for a longer than normal preoxygenation time.

If the patient has significant pulmonary hypertension, having an inhaled pulmonary vasodilator such as inhaled nitric oxide or epoprostenol in the circuit during induction or immediately available may be helpful to limit increases in pulmonary vascular resistance. Hypoventilation during induction can cause hypoxia and hypercapnia, both of which increase pulmonary vascular resistance, and this increased afterload can strain an already abnormal right ventricle. There are many possible pharmacological strategies to induce

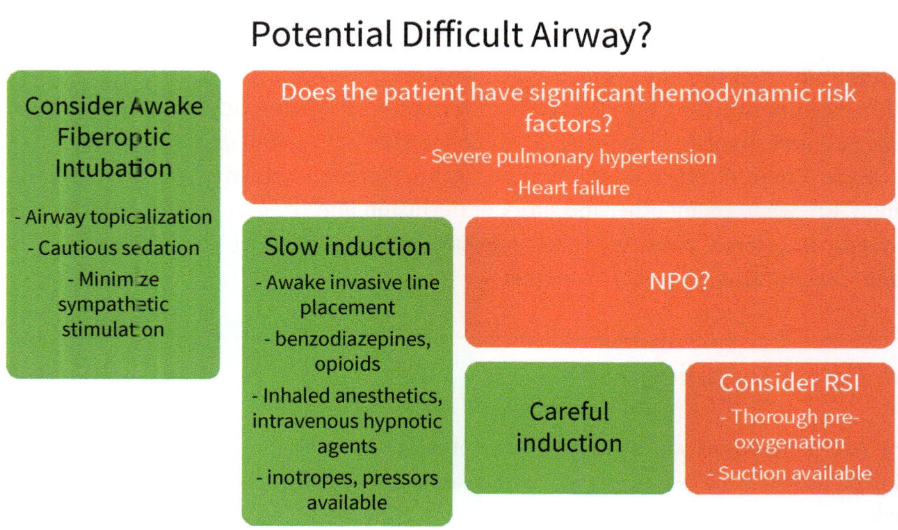

Figure 17.2 Decision tree for planning induction of anesthesia.
Abbreviations: NPO, nil per os; RSI, rapid sequence intubation.

anesthesia for lung transplantation while avoiding hypoxia, hypercapnia, hypotension, and tachycardia. One common strategy is to use a benzodiazepine such as midazolam and an opioid such as fentanyl in combination with inhalational anesthetic like sevoflurane or titrated dose of hypnotic like etomidate or propofol. These medications, when combined with a neuromuscular blocking agent such as rocuronium, provide optimal intubating conditions.

Cardiopulmonary collapse can occur during the transition from negative pressure breathing mechanics to positive pressure ventilation with the concomitant increased intrathoracic pressure and decreased venous return. It is important to be wary of this and to have inotropes and vasopressors immediately available to augment vascular tone and cardiac function as needed.

Intubation can proceed with a single lumen endotracheal tube (SLT) or double lumen endotracheal tube (DLT) based on planned surgical technique and need for lung isolation. If the plan is for a bilateral lung transplant using CPB support, then lung isolation is unnecessary, and a SLT is sufficient. When choosing the size of a SLT endotracheal tube, consider future need for bronchoscopy and the size of available bronchoscopes.

If lung isolation is required, one option is a bronchial blocker placed in conjunction with a SLT, which allows for fewer airway exchanges but also offers less reliable positioning for lung isolation than a DLT. A bronchial blocker will need to be repositioned intraoperatively using a fiberoptic bronchoscope to allow for surgery on the opposite side.

A DLT can alternatively be used for lung isolation. It may be more difficult to place initially because of its large size and stiffness yet results in more reliable positioning. A DLT facilitates switching between lungs and endotracheal suctioning. A left-sided DLT is easier to position than a right-sided DLT and can be used for virtually all lung transplantation surgeries as the left main bronchus anastomosis is well away from the tip of the DLT. A right-sided DLT must have the bronchial lumen precisely in the short distance between the carina and the takeoff of the right upper lobe. If a DLT is used, it may need to be changed for a SLT prior to transfer to the intensive care unit. This airway exchange should be carefully planned to avoid intermittent hypoxia or loss of airway.

Summary of Key Steps

- Preoperative assessment
- NPO status
- Airway exam
- Application of monitors
- Placement of invasive lines
- Preoxygenation
- Induction
- Mask ventilation
- Intubation
- Lung isolation

Position

Patient positioning depends on planned surgical approach. Position choice should account for surgical access, rescue cannulation strategy, venous and arterial line position, and avoidance of nerve injury while the patient is under general anesthesia.

Single lung transplantation is performed via posterolateral thoracotomy, requiring either lateral decubitus position or modified lateral decubitus position with the shoulders tilted sideways but the hips positioned flat. In the modified position, the groin is left exposed and prepped into the field in case CPB or extracorporeal membrane oxygenation (ECMO) support is needed.[4]

Bilateral lung transplantation can be performed via sternotomy, bilateral thoracotomies, or bilateral thoracotomies plus transverse sternotomy that is called a "clamshell" incision, as depicted in Figure 17.3. A sternotomy approach allows for a supine patient with tucked arms. A clamshell incision requires the patient to be supine with arms either out wide or bent at the elbow and positioned over the face.

>> Tip on Technique

Keep in mind the position of line placement in patients positioned for a clamshell incision, as the bent and elevated arm position may hinder peripheral intravenous function or demonstrate inaccurate blood pressures as measured from a radial or brachial artery.

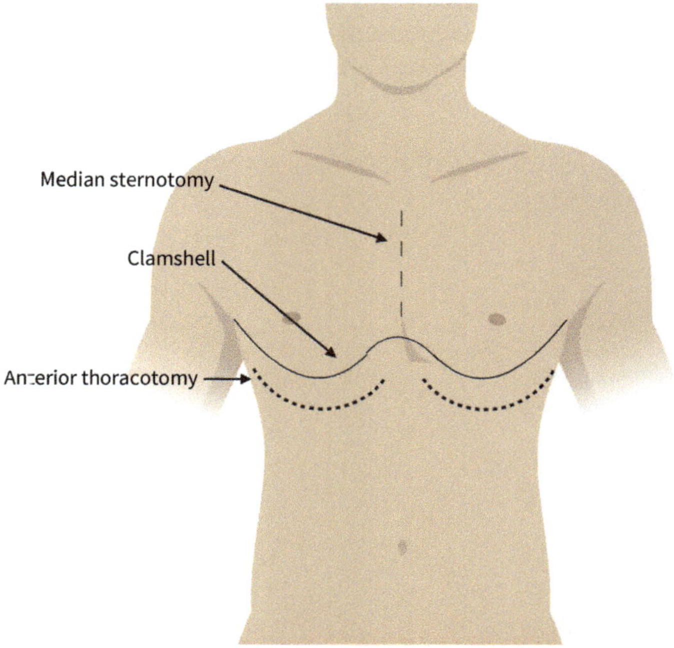

Figure 17.3 Possible surgical incision sites for lung transplantation.

Maintenance of Anesthesia

During surgery, a combination of inhalational and intravenous agents is used to maintain general anesthesia. If ECMO is being utilized, intravenous anesthetics offer the most reliable profile. Common choices for inhalational anesthesia include sevoflurane and isoflurane. Typically, a propofol infusion is selected if using a total intravenous anesthetic technique. A moderate dose of narcotic is a useful adjunct to an anesthetic.

Blood pressure management relies on the use of targeted fluid administration, vasopressors, and inotropes. Vasopressin and norepinephrine are often the vasopressors of choice during lung transplantation. Vasopressin increases systemic vascular resistance without increasing pulmonary vascular resistance, which improves blood pressure without increasing RV afterload. Norepinephrine is a potent vasopressor with action at alpha and beta receptors. Its effect on both types of receptors causes an increase in vasomotor tone along with a small cardiac contractility benefit.

Antibiotics are indicated perioperatively for all patients undergoing lung transplantation. Particular attention should be given to antibiotic choice in patients with cystic fibrosis, as they often have a complex infection and antibiotic history. Consultation with a transplant pharmacist can be helpful to determine the optimal antibiotic choice and intraoperative redosing strategy.

To lessen bleeding risks, it is common to administer antifibrinolytic medications such as tranexamic acid or aminocaproic acid intraoperatively. This is accomplished with an initial bolus dose followed by a continuous infusion for the duration of the case.

The patient should be kept normothermic. Hypothermic patients display more unstable hemodynamics and more coagulopathy. Normothermia can be difficult to maintain in lung transplant surgery because a large surface area of the body is prepped and exposed. In cases that cannot take advantage of the CPB circuit to warm recirculating blood, care must be taken to implement fluid-warming devices and forced air warmers and to optimize operating room temperature to minimize heat loss.

Pretransplant Ventilation Strategy

Ventilation strategy varies based on underlying pathology. If there is predominantly obstructive lung disease, the patient is prone to air trapping and may need longer expiration time to avoid hyperinflation. These patients have highly compliant lungs and may not be able to completely exhale a delivered tidal volume, which may result in an "auto-PEEP" phenomenon with elevated intrapleural pressure and impairment of venous return. Deliberate hypoventilation may ameliorate this effect, at the cost of hypercapnia and possible respiratory acidosis.[4] If restrictive lung disease dominates, high ventilator pressures may be required to adequately oxygenate and ventilate the patient. Be wary of development of pneumothorax either from a ruptured bleb in a patient with emphysematous disease or use of abnormally high airway pressures to achieve adequate oxygenation in fibrotic lungs.

Unsurprisingly, one lung ventilation is often poorly tolerated in patients with end-stage lung disease. Hypoxemia nadirs about 20 minutes after initiation of one lung ventilation.

Maximizing inspired oxygen concentration, pressure control ventilation mode, tolerance of higher airway pressures, intermittent two lung ventilation, and positive end expiratory pressure (PEEP) to the nonventilated lung can help limit hypoxia. Once the PA is clamped, V/Q matching improves, which increases oxygenation at the cost of increased pulmonary vascular resistance and RV afterload. Pulmonary artery clamping can trigger acute RV failure. Patients unable to tolerate one lung ventilation will likely need mechanical support with ECMO or CPB.

Right Heart Failure

RV failure is common during lung transplant surgery. Patients often are already suffering from chronic RV dysfunction and may have reached the limit on adaptation. High intrapleural pressures along with hypoxia and hypercarbia during surgery all further increase pulmonary vascular resistance. Intraoperative hypotension can predispose to RV ischemia, since the right ventricle will have increased oxygen demand with decreased coronary perfusion pressure. Rising CVP and PA pressures, hypoxia, hypotension, and arrhythmias are all signs of potential right heart failure.

RV support strategies include maximizing RV contractility, minimizing RV afterload, optimizing volume status, and controlling conditions as much as possible to avoid hypoxia, hypercarbia, and acidosis. Inotropes such as epinephrine, dobutamine, and milrinone are useful in improving contractility, especially for patients with baseline RV dysfunction. Inhaled pulmonary vasodilators like nitric oxide or epoprostenol decrease pulmonary vascular resistance and improve V/Q matching. Fluids should be administered judiciously. PA pressures, cardiac output monitoring, and real-time TEE can help guide fluid management. See Table 17.2 for a summary of strategies to treat RV failure.

Table 17.2 Strategies to Treat Right Ventricular Failure

Reduce RV Afterload	Augment RV Contractility	Optimize Volume Status
• Avoid increases in PVR • Avoid hypoxia • Avoid hypercarbia • Avoid acidosis • Decrease PVR • Inhaled pulmonary vasodilators • Minimize intrathoracic pressures • Minimize PEEP • Minimize tidal Volumes • Be wary of pneumothorax	• Inotropes • Milrinone • Dobutamine • Epinephrine	• Real-time TEE analysis • Trend filling pressures • Stroke volume variation • Judicious fluid administration

Abbreviations: PEEP, positive end expiratory pressure; PVR, pulmonary vascular resistance; RV, right ventricle; TEE, transesophageal echocardiography.

Transesophageal Echocardiography

TEE is a particularly useful tool during dissection and lung transplantation. Initial echocardiographic evaluation should focus on right and left heart function, taking note of valve function. If an atrial septal defect or patent foramen ovale is present, a right to left shunt can develop if right heart pressures increase during surgery. Real-time TEE is invaluable in the prompt detection of acute RV dysfunction. Indicators on TEE of right heart failure include RV dilation, bowing of interatrial septum and interventricular septum from right to left, increasing tricuspid regurgitation and pulmonic regurgitation, and underfilling of the left ventricle (LV; Figure 17.4).

TEE evaluation after reperfusion initially focuses on ventricular function, presence of intracardiac shunting, and volume status. Once the patient is hemodynamically stable, attention can turn to evaluation of PA anastomoses and flow through bilateral pulmonary veins. Pulmonary artery diameter should be greater than 1 cm.[4] Typically at least the right PA anastomosis can be visualized by TEE. Pulmonary veins should be at least 0.5 cm in diameter and Doppler interrogation should demonstrate flow velocity less than 100 cm/s. If flow velocity is higher, there is suspicion of pulmonary venous stenosis or kinking.[4] The resulting pulmonary venous congestion can cause graft failure, so it is important to note early.[5]

Immunotherapy

After lung transplant, a patient requires immunosuppression for the rest of his or her life. Often there is an induction phase of immunosuppression, followed by lifelong maintenance therapy. These medications are initiated shortly before a recipient arrives to the operating room for the lung transplant procedure. It is important on the day of surgery that the anesthesiologist ensures the lung transplant recipient has received his or her prescribed immunosuppression. The risk of lung rejection is highest in the first 6 to 12 months, and

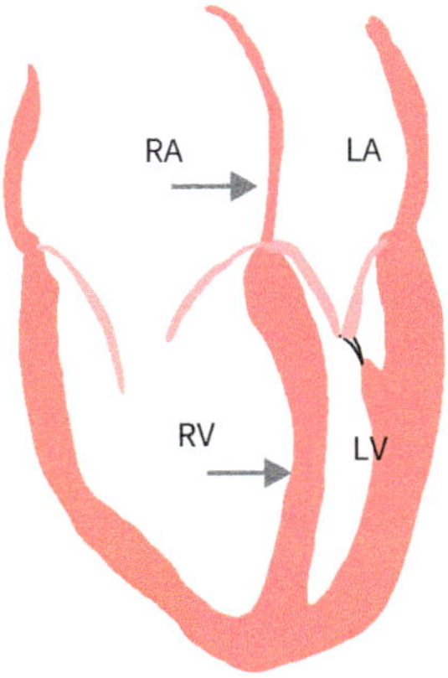

Figure 17.4 Key transesophageal echocardiography findings of right heart failure. Note bowing from right to left of the interatrial septum and interventricular septum. The right atrium and right ventricle are enlarged, and the left side of the heart is underfilled.

immunosuppressive agents are tailored accordingly. A typical posttransplant regimen can be complex. Antibiotics, antiviral, and antifungal medications are prescribed given the patient's increased risk of infection while immunosuppressed. Chronic steroid use can lead to hyperglycemia and the need for glucose-controlling medication. Immunosuppression medications also predispose patients to gastrointestinal ulcer disease.

Glucose Management

Glucose should be measured at least hourly during surgery and managed with an insulin infusion to avoid hyperglycemia. In cardiac surgery, a glucose goal <180 mg/dL is widely accepted standard practice. It is reasonable to adopt the same intraoperative target during lung transplant surgery. The stress of major surgery, need for mechanical cardiopulmonary support using inflammation-inducing cannulae, and inclusion of high-dose steroids intraoperatively for immunosuppression make hyperglycemia and the need for an insulin infusion very likely.

Mechanical Support

Introduction

Mechanical support for lung transplantation can exist in three phases:

1. preoperatively as a bridge to transplant
2. intraoperatively to assist with the procedure
3. postoperatively as a bridge to recovery

Options for mechanical support include ECMO and right ventricular assist device (RVAD).

Preoperative

Patients with end-stage lung disease may require mechanical support while waiting for an organ to become available. In the past, the need for mechanical support was considered a relative contraindication to lung transplantation. As surgical technique has improved and mechanical support complication rates have decreased, there has been a trend toward earlier initiation of mechanical support and survival has improved both pre- and posttransplant. The primary methods of preoperative mechanical support include ECMO and RVAD. When ECMO is used, support can be venoarterial (VA) or venovenous (VV).[6]

VA-ECMO uses a mechanical pump and a membrane oxygenator to provide oxygenation and ventilation as well as cardiac output augmentation. Typically, pretransplant VA-ECMO cannulation is via the femoral vessels. A large bore cannula placed in the femoral vein drains blood from the right atrium to a pump outside the patient, which delivers that blood through an oxygenator and through a cannula in the femoral artery back to the patient (Figure 17.5). These pumps are capable of meeting a patient's entire cardiac output need if necessary, as long as the cannulae are large enough to accommodate the blood flow. Recall that resistance in a

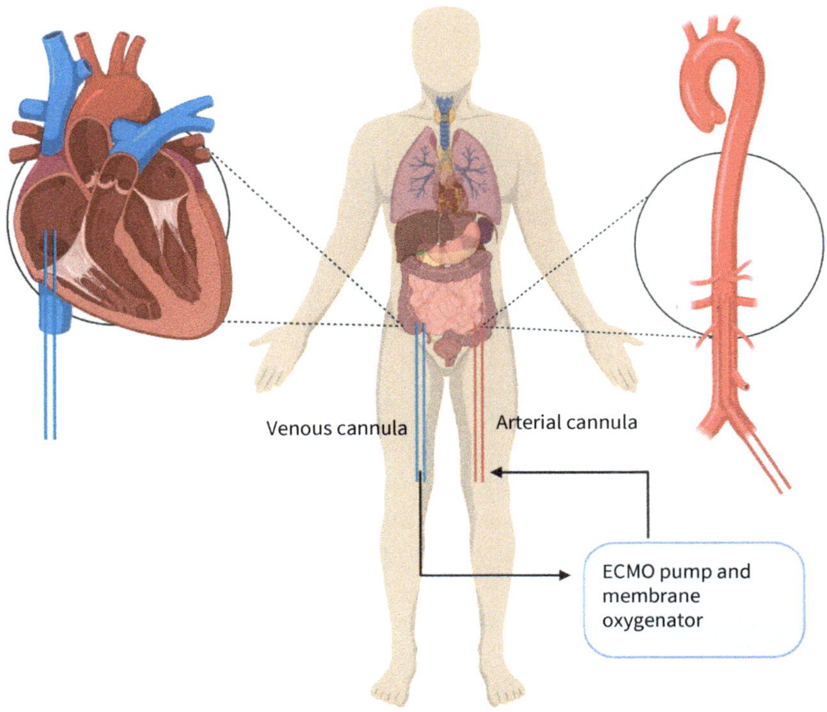

Figure 17.5 Venoarterial extracorporeal membrane oxygenation.
Abbreviation: ECMO, extracorporeal membrane oxygenation.

tube is inversely proportional to the fourth power of the radius, so increasing cannula diameter a small amount makes a large difference in flow capability.

VA-ECMO has the ability to provide cardiac output and to oxygenate and ventilate blood and is thus capable of supporting patients with cardiogenic shock, respiratory failure, or a mixed pathology. Historically ECMO usage was limited as complication rates were high and the concomitant prolonged sedation with mechanical ventilation rapidly deconditioned patients. Newer ECMO cannulation techniques utilizing the upper extremities are being explored in several centers to improve patient mobilization, allowing some degree of "prehab" while waiting on the transplant list.

VV-ECMO also uses a mechanical pump and a membrane oxygenator, but the cannula placement differs from that of VA-ECMO. VV-ECMO can be administered via a single large bore dual-lumen venous catheter. This catheter has a lumen that withdraws blood from the right atrium and vena cava (inferior or superior depending on cannulation site of groin or neck, respectively). Blood then enters a mechanical pump, flows through an oxygenator, then returns through another lumen in the same cannula. The lumen that returns blood to the heart is typically situated in the right atrium to deliver oxygenated blood straight through the tricuspid valve to the RV (Figure 17.6). A key element with this configuration is that cardiac support is not provided—merely pulmonary support. Cardiac output is dependent on the patient's inherent cardiac function. Hypoxia and hypercarbia in these patients is not as much of a concern, but the risk of acute pulmonary hypertension and right heart failure still exists.

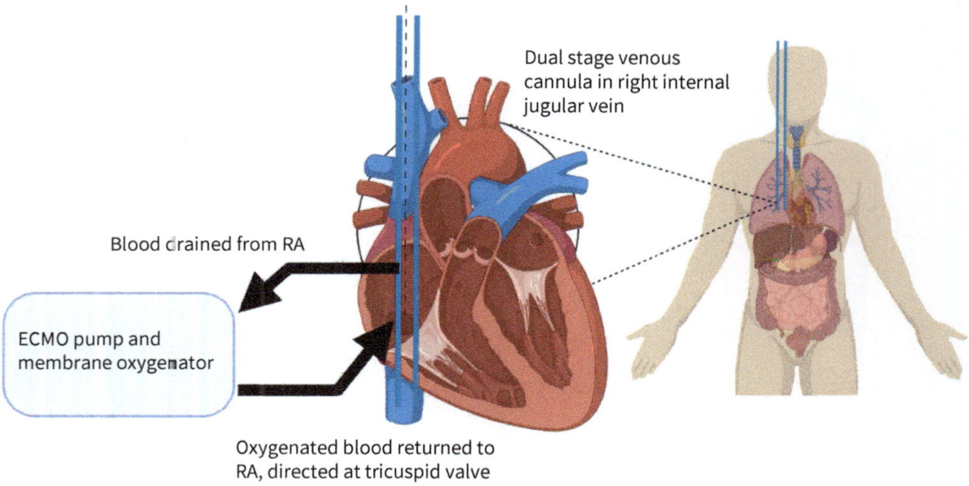

Figure 17.6 Venovenous extracorporeal membrane oxygenation.
Abbreviation: RA, right atrium; ECMO, extracorporeal membrane oxygenation.

RVAD is a device placed for patients with RV failure. In the lung transplant population, this is most commonly due to pulmonary hypertension. The cannula for a preoperative RVAD can be placed centrally or peripherally, typically via the right internal jugular vein. A dual lumen catheter is used, with one lumen draining blood from the right atrium to a pump and the second lumen used to return blood to the main PA (Figure 17.7). This essentially bypasses

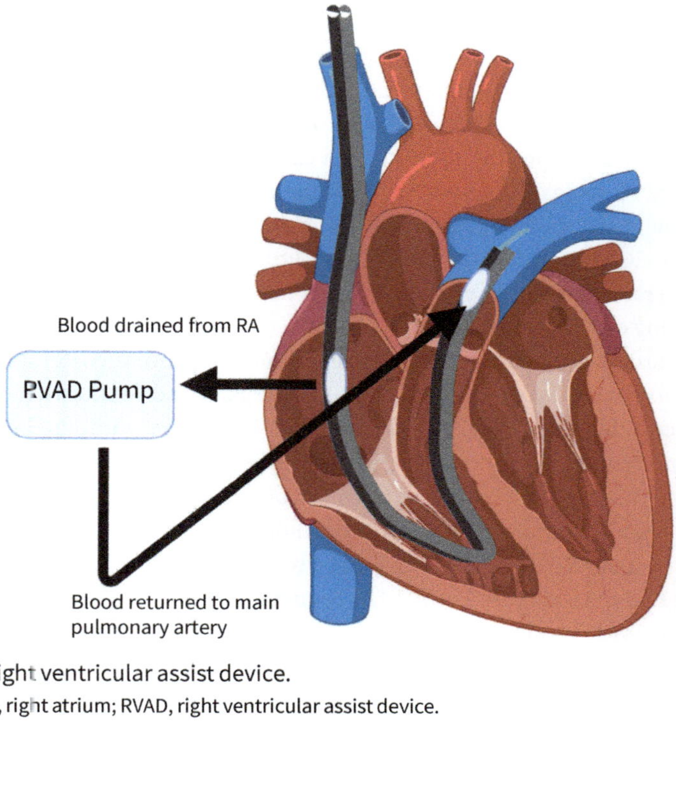

Figure 17.7 Right ventricular assist device.
Abbreviation: RA, right atrium; RVAD, right ventricular assist device.

the RV. In patients with RV failure, this can be lifesaving. An oxygenator can be placed in-line to combine RVAD and VV-ECMO therapies. RVAD flow management requires a delicate balance between providing enough flow to offload the right ventricle and not providing so much flow as to overload the LV or overburden the pulmonary vasculature, which could cause pulmonary edema or pulmonary hemorrhage.

These preoperative mechanical support methods are complex and require multidisciplinary teams for management. Even with mechanical support, these patients are at high risk for complications, and this risk increases with duration of support. Unfortunately, major complications from mechanical support could preclude a patient from remaining on the transplant list.

>> Tip on Technique: Things to Know When Managing a Patient With Mechanical Support

- Reason for placement on support (isolated or combined cardiac or respiratory failure)
- Type of support (VA-ECMO, VV-ECMO, RVAD, RVAD + VV-ECMO)
- Cannulation sites
- Anticoagulation status
- Minor or major complications suffered because of mechanical support

Intraoperative

Lung transplantation is performed with mechanical support in a planned or unplanned fashion or performed with no mechanical support "off pump." Indications for planned support include pulmonary hypertension, decreased heart function, and *en bloc* bilateral lung transplant. Conversion to unplanned mechanical support typically falls into one of several categories: intraoperative hemodynamic instability, impaired gas exchange, acute increases in pulmonary pressures, cor pulmonale, and/or surgical technical difficulties. Traditionally, CPB has been utilized as the mechanical support method of choice intraoperatively for lung transplantation. VA-ECMO has been increasingly adopted as an alternative.

CPB is similar to VA-ECMO in that there is a cannula in the venous system that returns blood to a pump, which pumps blood through an oxygenator and back to the patient via a cannula in the arterial system. These cannulae can be placed peripherally or centrally. The main difference with CPB is the inclusion of a venous reservoir in the circuit, which allows for suction recapturing of blood that has been lost to the surgical field and provides a reserve of blood that can be temporarily called upon in the event of decreased venous drainage to the pump. The downside to CPB is that the air-blood interface in the venous reservoir necessitates a much higher anticoagulation goal than does ECMO. ECMO has less of a systemic inflammatory response and creates less coagulopathy and bleeding than does CPB. A retrospective comparison of outcomes for CPB versus VA-ECMO has suggested that VA-ECMO has better survival and reduced postprocedural complication rates compared to CPB.[7] Another benefit of VA-ECMO, particularly if peripherally cannulated, is that it can be used to support the patient in the postoperative period.

Postoperative

Postoperatively, patients may require mechanical support of the respiratory and/or cardiac systems. RV failure and primary graft dysfunction are common reasons to need such support. If a patient is peripherally cannulated, the surgical team may decannulate at the bedside in the intensive care unit. However, if the patient is centrally cannulated, a return to the operating room for decannulation can be anticipated.

Posttransplant Management

Reperfusion

Lung allograft reperfusion causes hypotension, acidosis, and hyperkalemia as pneumoplegia and inflammatory mediators are released into the systemic circulation. Clear communication between surgical and anesthesia teams allows planning for this event and control of its speed. Preparation by optimizing electrolytes, correcting acidosis, and keeping pressors and inotropes immediately available can help get through reperfusion as smoothly as possible.

Posttransplant Ventilation Strategy

After transplantation and reperfusion of both lungs, ventilation strategy choice is critical. It is important to minimize ventilator pressures to lessen barotrauma. Limiting the inspired fraction of oxygen (FiO_2) as much as possible helps to limit free radical damage and reperfusion injury to fragile lungs. A low tidal volume strategy of 6 mL/kg is commonly employed with a goal of keeping plateau pressures less than 30 cmH_2O.[8] Initial ventilator settings should include moderate PEEP (5–10 cm H_20) and low FiO_2 (0.35–0.4). To keep the $PaO_2 > 65$ mmHg, the FiO_2 and PEEP may be incrementally increased and an inhaled pulmonary vasodilator may be added. Checking frequent arterial blood gas measurements helps correlate measured SpO_2 with PaO_2.

Ventilation strategy gets more complex when the patient receives a single lung transplant, because each lung will have unique compliance. It may be prudent to maintain lung isolation and use two separate ventilators with unique settings tailored to each lung. For example, if the patient's native lung has severe obstructive disease, that lung may require a prolonged expiratory time with less PEEP to minimize the risk of hyperinflation. Vice versa, the pressures high enough to obtain adequate tidal volumes in a native lung with severely restrictive disease may cause significant barotrauma in a newly transplanted lung.

Fluid Management

Ideally, after a lung transplant, a patient will receive minimal intravenous fluids to decrease the development of pulmonary edema. A lung allograft is highly sensitive to low pressure pulmonary edema with reexpansion injury. This can be compounded by microvascular leaks from ischemia-reperfusion and a lack of lymphatic drainage.[1,9] Use of CPB increases inflammation and worsens pulmonary edema. A restrictive fluid management plan helps limit these risks, especially with patients requiring CPB.

On the other hand, often patients require blood products to correct anemia or coagulopathy. Heparin should be reversed with protamine. Point of care elastography tests help give the anesthesiologist almost immediate feedback about the severity of a coagulopathy as well as allow tailoring of blood product therapy to the specific factors that are lacking. Invasive monitors like PACs, CVP, TEE, cardiac output/index, and stroke volume variation help determine the patient's overall fluid status. The balance between appropriate volume resuscitation and minimizing the risk of pulmonary edema can be difficult to strike, so fluid administration should be goal directed.

Analgesia

Large surgical incisions, manipulation of lung and pleura, chest tube placement, prolonged positioning with retraction, underlying pain conditions, and the individual psychologic pain experience of a patient all contribute to postoperative pain. Postoperative pain directly contributes to worse outcomes, as a patient with pain may splint and take shallow breaths. Coughing is necessary but can be painful. After lung transplantation, the cough reflex is lost below the carina. There is some evidence that suggests this reflex returns within 12 months.[10] Mucociliary function also can be depressed for up to a year.[4] Sometimes patients develop bronchial hyperreactivity.[9] Post-thoracotomy pain syndrome can be a debilitating chronic pain syndrome with significantly decreased quality of life for patients, in addition to the possibility of pulmonary complications.

Current standard of care includes placing a thoracic epidural postoperatively and using it in conjunction with a multimodal analgesic medication regimen. This regimen includes acetaminophen, gabapentin, nonsteroidal anti-inflammatory agents, and opioids. Thoracic epidural analgesia has been shown to decrease time to extubation and thus improve overall outcomes in lung transplantation.[11]

Less studied analgesic alternatives include preoperative thoracic epidural catheters and paravertebral catheters. A preoperative thoracic epidural could be used intraoperatively and potentially decrease opioid requirements, but there may be an increased risk of epidural hematoma when combined with systemic heparinization for CPB or ECMO. Paravertebral catheters are more peripheral and have less risk of neurologic sequelae from hematoma formation, but their efficacy is yet to be seen.

References

1. Slinger P, ed. *Principles and Practice of Anesthesia for Thoracic Surgery*. Toronto, ON, Canada: Springer; 2011.
2. Hurford WE, Kolker AC, Strauss HW. The use of ventilation/perfusion lung scans to predict oxygenation during one-lung anesthesia. *Anesthesiology*. 1987;67(5):841–844.
3. Weill D, Benden C, Corris PA, et al. A consensus document for the selection of lung transplant candidates: 2014--an update from the Pulmonary Transplantation Council of the International Society for Heart and Lung Transplantation. *J Heart Lung Transplant*. 2015;34(1):1–15.

4. Quinlan JJ, Murray AW, Casta A. In: Kaplan JA, Reich DL, Savino JS, eds. *Kaplan's Cardiac Anesthesia: The Echo Era*. 6th ed. St. Louis, MO: Elsevier Saunders; 2011: 742–750.
5. Huang YC, Cheng YJ, Lin YH, Wang MJ, Tsai SK. Graft failure caused by pulmonary venous obstruction diagnosed by intraoperative transesophageal echocardiography during lung transplantation. *Anesth Analg*. 2000;91(3):558–560.
6. Javidfar J, Brodie D, Iribarne A, et al. Extracorporeal membrane oxygenation as a bridge to lung transplantation and recovery. *J Thorac Cardiovasc Surg*. 2012;144(3):716–721.
7. Ius F, Kuehn C, Tudorache I, et al. Lung transplantation on cardiopulmonary support: venoarterial extracorporeal membrane oxygenation outperformed cardiopulmonary bypass. *J Thorac Cardiovasc Surg*. 2012;144(6):1510–1516.
8. Brower RG, Matthay MA, Morris A, Schoenfeld D, Thompson BT, Wheeler A. Ventilation with lower tidal volumes as compared with traditional tidal volumes for acute lung injury and the acute respiratory distress syndrome. *N Engl J Med*. 2000;342(18):1301–1308.
9. Anesthesia for thoracic surgery. In: Butterworth JF, Mackey DC, Wasnick JD, eds. *Morgan & Mikhail's Clinical Anesthesiology*. 5th ed. New York, NY: McGraw-Hill; 2013:545–573.
10. Duarte AG, Myers AC. Cough reflex in lung transplant recipients. *Lung*. 2012;190(1):23–27.
11. Pottecher J, Falcoz PE, Massard G, Dupeyron JP. Does thoracic epidural analgesia improve outcome after lung transplantation? *Interact Cardiovasc Thorac Surg*. 2011;12(1):51–53.

18
Postoperative Management and Complications in Thoracic Surgery

Daniel Demos and Edward McGough

Introduction

Thoracic surgery impairs postoperative respiratory function, resulting in a relatively high risk of developing postoperative complications. The incidence of pulmonary and cardiac complications (19%–59%) is much higher than after upper (16%–17%) or lower (0%–5%) abdominal surgery.[1] These complications are most frequently linked to specific risk factors that can be identified before the patient's arrival at the intensive care unit (ICU). These factors include age, results of preoperative pulmonary function tests, cardiovascular comorbidity, smoking status, and chronic obstructive pulmonary disease. Other factors include an American Society of Anesthesiologists score (Table 18.1) of >3 or prolonged mechanical ventilation in the postoperative period.[2]

Patients undergoing thoracic surgery present a unique challenge to the provider in the immediate postoperative setting. Preoperative functional status confounded by lung volume reduction surgeries, specific airway management concerns, pleural devices, mechanical ventilation, and fluid management, as well as pain control, contribute to the complexity of postoperative management. This chapter helps clinicians understand how to mitigate postoperative complications by providing a basic understanding of the management of this patient population.

Immediate Postoperative Concerns

Extubation/Airway Evaluation

Patients frequently arrive in the ICU after being extubated in the operating room. However, various indications support prolonged postoperative mechanical ventilation (Box 18.1). In the event of postoperative mechanical ventilation, we use the same principles to provide gas exchange to the patient. These principles focus on a lung-protective strategy similar to acute respiratory distress syndrome (Figure 18.1). This strategy refers to a tidal volume of 6 to 8 mL/kg with positive end-expiratory pressure to facilitate lung expansion, with an emphasis of limiting peak airway pressures to less than 30 cm of water.[3] It is specifically important in this patient population because barotrauma not only affects the lung parenchyma but also the surgical anastomosis.

Table 18.1 Perioperative Variables in Relation to American Society of Anesthesiologists (ASA) Physical Status Classification

Perioperative Variable	ASA I	ASA II	ASA III	ASA IV
Duration of operation (h)	1.25	1.3	2.1	1.9
Blood loss, intraoperative (L)	0.08	0.1	0.3	1.5
Postoperative ventilation (h)	1	4	8	47
Intensive care unit stay	0.2	1	2	5
Postoperative stay (d)	9	16	21	18
Pulmonary infection (%)	0.5	2	5	12
Pulmonary complication—other (%)	0.6	2	4	10
Cardiac complications (%)	0.1	2	5	18
Urinary infection (%)	2	5	6	5
Wound infection (%)	2	4	6	11
Mortality (%)	0.1	1	4	18

Each variable has a significant difference of $P < 0.05$ according to Fisher's exact test or Student's test between the ASA I and the ASA II, ASA III, or ASA IV classification.

Sources: Data from Sidi A, Lobato EB, Cohen JA. The American Society of Anesthesiologists Physical Status: category V revisited. *J Clin Anesth.* 2000;12:328–334. Reprinted from Sidi A, Yusim Y. Anesthesia in the ICU. In: Gabrielli A, Laydon AJ, Yu M, eds. *Civetta, Taylor, and Kirby's Critical Care.* 4th ed. Philadelphia, PA: Lippincott Williams & Wilkins; 2009:1575, Table 40.1.

Abbreviation: ASA, American Society of Anesthesiologists.

Box 18.1 Indications for Continued Postoperative Ventilation

- Airway compromise due to edema or bleeding
- Inadequate pulmonary reserve post-surgery
- Compromised myocardial function, especially with perioperative infarction
- Expected large fluid shifts with thoracoabdominal procedures
- Severe neurologic impairment
- Continued bleeding with likelihood of return to operating room
- Esophageal surgery patients (risk for reflux and aspiration—delay extubation until airway reflexes have fully recovered as for full stomach intubation)

Reprinted with permission from Higgins T, Mailloux P. Critical care of the thoracic surgery patient. In: Gabrielli A, Laydon AJ, Yu M, eds. *Civetta, Taylor, and Kirby's Critical Care.* 4th ed. Philadelphia, PA: Lippincott Williams & Wilkins; 2009:1[illegible]93, Table 79.4.

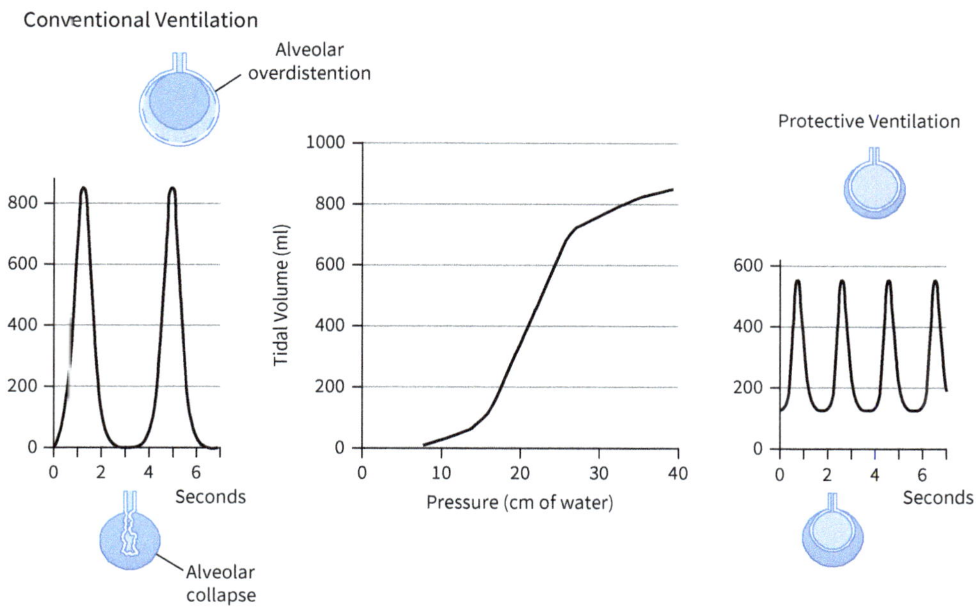

Figure 18.1 Respiratory pressure–volume curve and the effects of traditional as compared with protective ventilation in a 70-kg patient with the acute respiratory distress syndrome. The lower and upper inflection points of the inspiratory pressure–volume curve (center panel) are at 14 and 26 cm of water, respectively. With conventional ventilation at a tidal volume of 12 mL per kilogram of body weight and zero end-expiratory pressure (left-hand panel), alveoli collapse at the end of expiration. The generation of shear forces during the subsequent mechanical inflation may tear the alveolar lining, and attaining an end-inspiratory volume higher than the upper inflection point causes alveolar overdistention. With protective ventilation at a tidal volume of 6 mL per kg (right-hand panel), the end-inspiratory volume remains below the upper inflection point; the addition of positive end-expiratory pressure at 2 cm of water above the lower inflection point may prevent alveolar collapse at the end of expiration and provide protection against the development of shear forces during mechanical inflation.

Reprinted with permission from Tobin MJ. Advances in mechanical ventilation. *N Engl J Med.* 2001;344:1986–1996, Figure 3.

As the patient progresses toward extubation, we recommend performing basic weaning parameters to assess the patient's ability to tolerate removal of mechanical ventilation. These include the negative inspiratory force, which helps determine diaphragmatic strength and can be particularly useful in myasthenia gravis patients after thymectomy. A negative inspiratory force greater than 20 cm of water is generally sufficient. The rapid shallow breathing index, measured as a function of respiratory rate over tidal volume in liters, is a strong indicator of postextubation failure, with numbers greater than 100 being prohibitive to extubation.[4] A significant number of patients in the thoracic population require double-lumen endotracheal tubes in the operating room, which can result in laryngeal and glottic edema postoperatively. To assess this, a cuff leak is tested by deflating the endotracheal tube and observing for auditory signs of air leak as well as loss of tidal volumes on the ventilator. Historically, racemic epinephrine and corticosteroids have been used to reduce airway edema despite a lack of strong data demonstrating their effectiveness.

Postoperative Intrathoracic Hemorrhage

The majority of thoracic surgery patients arrive in the ICU with chest tubes attached to a drainage system. This provides a window into the intrathoracic space and can help guide postoperative decision-making. This is especially true in patients who are bleeding. Hourly chest tube outputs should be monitored and recorded from all chest tubes individually. The surgical team should be made aware of continuous sanguineous output greater than 100 mL/hour over a 4-hour period as well as any hour over 200 mL. In addition to monitoring output, an immediate chest X-ray and coagulation studies should be ordered to identify retained hemothorax and correct coagulopathy. In the event of hemodynamic instability with bleeding, serial hemoglobin and hematocrits should be trended for transfusion. If the pericardium was violated, clinicians should have a high index of suspicion for pericardial tamponade. A point-of-care ultrasound can help diagnose and guide resuscitation. Ongoing bleeding, retained hemothorax, and pericardial tamponade are indications for return to the operating room for exploration and washout.

Early Ambulation/Deep Venous Thromboembolism Prophylaxis

A basic knowledge of postoperative deep venous thromboembolism (DVT) risk is essential to understanding the importance of early ambulation, physical therapy, pneumatic compression devices, and chemical prophylaxis in preventing DVTs. The majority of thoracic surgery patients fall into the high-risk category for DVTs based on age and/or comorbidities. This population has a calf thrombosis rate of 20% to 40%, pulmonary embolism rate of 2% to 4%, and fatality rate of 0.4% to 1%.[5] Because of this risk, patients should be started on prophylactic doses of heparin on postoperative day 1 as well as a pneumatic compression device upon arrival at the ICU. Walking should be encouraged on the morning of postoperative day 1 as pain permits. This is the most important factor in patient recovery and can be significantly aided or hindered by postoperative analgesia. It should be noted that the presence of a DVT is not a contraindication to walking, and physical therapy is still encouraged in the absence of a free-floating thrombus because this carries an increased risk for embolism.[6]

Pain Management

A thoracotomy is one of the most painful operations postoperatively. The pain can be mitigated significantly if a minimally invasive or robotic approach is taken in the operating room. Unfortunately, not all thoracic surgeries can be performed with a minimally invasive approach and, instead, a standard posterolateral thoracotomy is sometimes required. Regardless of the approach, other factors can contribute to significant pain postoperatively. Chest tubes are a source of significant pain and should be evaluated daily for removal. Analgesia is paramount to the progression of patient recovery.

Systemic Analgesia

Intraoperative analgesia is a beneficial adjunct for postoperative pain management and often starts with intravenous (IV) acetaminophen. After arrival at the ICU, a stepwise approach to pain management is recommended with the addition of oral acetaminophen as a first-line agent. Opioid analgesia remains the mainstay of acute pain control in the ICU setting. However, using multimodal pain management is far more beneficial to the patient and far more effective for the provider. By using multiple pathways for pain control, we can minimize negative side effects associated with analgesic medications (Table 18.2). Tramadol, a partial mu receptor agonist with an unclear mechanism, and gabapentin provide quality nonopioid analgesia with relatively benign side effects and are often given alongside a patient-controlled analgesia device. The device provides the added benefit of delivering IV pain medication in smaller doses on demand. Additionally, because it is patient triggered, it can bypass the time-consuming ritual of as-needed administration and keep pain control at a more consistent steady state.[7]

Nonsteroidal anti-inflammatory drugs work by inhibiting the cyclooxygenase enzyme responsible for the release of inflammatory mediators leading to pain. They are commonly given alongside opiates and are generally an effective adjunct to pain control. However, their propensity to exacerbate renal dysfunction as well as their inhibitory properties to platelet function limit their use in certain patients. Adverse effects are more commonly seen after

Table 18.2 Adverse Effects of Analgesic Drugs

Drugs	Adverse Events
Opioids	Respiratory depression Nausea and vomiting Urinary retention Pruritus
Local anesthetics	Seizures Hypotension Cardiac dysrhythmias
Ketorolac	Renal impairment Platelet dysfunction Gastrointestinal bleeding
COX-2 inhibitors	Side effects minimal
Ketamine	Hallucinations Emergence delirium Catecholamine release with resulting hypertension and tachycardia Increased intracranial pressure Increased secretions

Reprinted with permission from Soto RG, Fu ES. Acute pain management for patients undergoing thoracotomy. *Ann Thorac Surg*. 2003;75:1349–1357, Table 1.

prolonged use (greater than 5 days), and they are associated with higher rates of gastrointestinal bleeding.[8]

Other modes of systemic therapy include ketamine, a direct N-methyl-D-aspartate receptor antagonist, and lidocaine infusions. These agents are reserved for patients with refractory pain despite a multimodal approach with systemic and local analgesic strategies. A thorough understanding of the dosing and side effects are critical to their safe administration in the ICU, but that falls outside the scope of this chapter.

In summary, there are several systemic options to manage postoperative pain. We suggest a multimodal approach as well as a graded escalation of treatment. Initial management begins pre- and intraoperatively with oral and IV acetaminophen and transitions back to oral, pending enteral access postoperatively. The addition of nonsteroidal anti-inflammatory drugs when appropriate and gabapentin are reasonable second-line agents, but most patients will require some level of opioid analgesia. If pain persists, adding IV lidocaine and/or ketamine infusions is the next appropriate option for systemic therapy.

Epidural and Paravertebral Anesthesia

Regional anesthesia has become an integral part of postoperative pain management, with a significant focus in thoracic surgery. Regional blocks can be loosely categorized as peripheral or central. The most notable peripheral block performed currently is the paravertebral block. This form of anesthesia is different than epidural anesthesia, the mainstay of centrally acting regional analgesia. The On-Q pain pump, a type of peripherally acting regional block, is a novel technique used more recently that allows for the continuous administration of a local anesthetic at the operative site. A catheter is placed intraoperatively by the surgeon and connected to a pump that provides local anesthesia until it is removed in the ICU or in an outpatient facility (Figure 18.2).

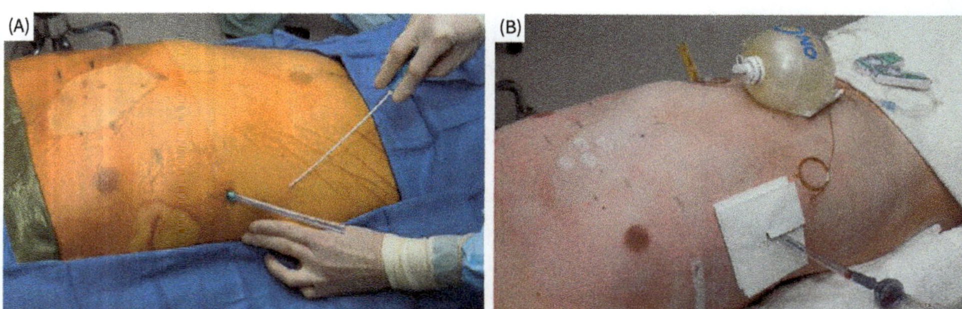

Figure 18.2 On-Q catheters are placed at the end of the procedure to provide local anesthesia and postoperative pain control. (A) 7.5-inch catheters are tunneled in the subcutaneous tissue, posterior axilla bilateral. (B) A 750-mL reservoir is utilized to infuse local anesthetic.

Reprinted with permission from Jaroszewski D, Ewais M, Lackey J. et al. Revision of failed, recurrent or complicated pectus excavatum after Nuss, Ravitch or cardiac surgery. *J Vis Surg*. 2016;2:74, Figure 10.

Paravertebral blocks can be provided as a single injection or as a continuous infusion of local anesthetic. Ideally, the point of injection is within the intercostal space at the level of the incision and is 3 cm lateral to the corresponding posterior spinous process. Advancing the needle too far medial risks epidural penetration. Pleural and/or lung puncture are encountered if the needle is advanced too deep (Figure 18.3). When performed correctly, this regional block should cover multiple dermatome levels on the ipsilateral side of the injection as it travels up and down the paravertebral space as well as through the intercostal space.

Epidural administration of a local anesthetic achieves analgesia through blocking conduction at the nerve root or spinal cord level and at the level of the dorsal horn if spinal opioids are being administered.[7] Ideally, this catheter is placed preoperatively. This will allow for patient-driven feedback to ensure proper catheter positioning, which increases pain control postoperatively. Using a continuous infusion epidural catheter (ropivacaine or bupivacaine) is associated with hypotension postoperatively. This is most likely secondary to blunting of the sympathetic response leading to decreased heart rate (in the case of an upper thoracic block) and loss of sympathetic tone. Providers need to be diligent in recognizing epidural-related hypotension because excessive resuscitation in patients who have undergone thoracic surgery can be detrimental to their recovery. The preferred management is to decrease the epidural dosing followed by a low dose of peripheral vasoconstrictors if the patient is adequately resuscitated.

Studies have shown peripheral and central regional anesthesia to be equally effective. However, one randomized, double-blinded controlled study examined the effects of thoracic epidural bupivacaine with and without opioid analgesia and compared it to continuous infusion paravertebral bupivacaine. This study suggested equal efficacy of both modalities when using bupivacaine alone. However, the addition of the opioid showed a reduction in postoperative hypotension. This was likely due to decreased basal infusion rates required to achieve analgesia, thus reducing sympathectomy.[9] Pain control scores appeared to be improved in the latter group as well.

Other Techniques for Postoperative Analgesia

Other forms of postoperative analgesia are available to the anesthesia and surgical team. These include intercostal as well as cryoablation therapy. The former is performed by the anesthesiologist while the latter is achieved during the operation by the surgeon.

Intercostal blocks provide the benefit of local anesthesia without the risk for systemic effects associated with centrally acting regional anesthesia. However, these blocks have risks because they are usually performed as a single injection. Therefore, repeated treatments are required, which increases the risk of pneumothorax. This has led to the use of liposomal bupivacaine as a slow-release agent for long-acting analgesia from a single injection. Liposomal bupivacaine has a duration of action of 72 to 96 hours after a single dose. This is due to the encapsulation of the local anesthetic into multivesicular liposomes, which allows for a slow release of the drug at the injection site.[10] However, more studies are needed to prove its true benefit because of its high costs. A single vial of liposomal bupivacaine costs $285 compared to bupivacaine hydrochloride, which is $5 per vial.[11] The potential to eliminate

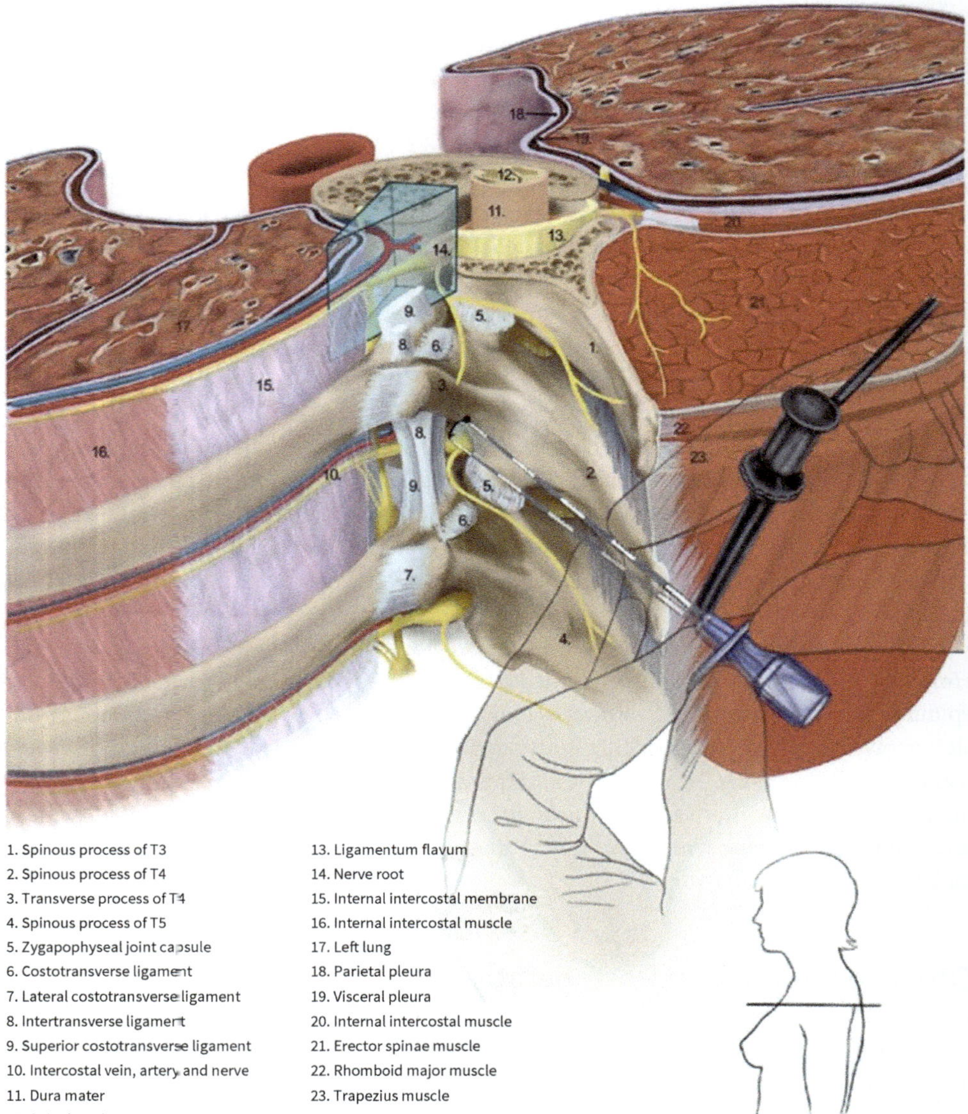

Figure 18.3 The Tuohy needle enters from posterior, contacts the transverse process of the appropriate vertebra, penetrates the costotransverse or intertransverse ligament, and enters the thoracic paravertebral space.
Illustration ©brysonbiomed.com. Reprinted with permission.

continuous infusion catheters and their complications has not yet been shown to overcome the cost of implementing such an expensive drug to formulary use.

Cryoablation therapy is a form of peripheral regional anesthesia in which a cryoprobe is applied to the intercostal nerve fibers at the level of incision as well as two intercostal spaces above and two intercostal spaces below the surgical site. The probe is cooled to −70°C to cause freezing damage to the nerve and its surrounding vasa vasorum. This type of block has proved effective and has been shown to decrease opioid requirements in the postoperative setting.[12] In some cases, it has eliminated the need for other forms of regional anesthesia.

Chest Tube Management

The vast majority of postoperative thoracic surgery patients arrive at the ICU with a chest tube drainage system in place. In general, two tubes will be placed intraoperatively, and their placement location should be noted upon admission. This helps to identify sources of bleeding and/or the location of an air leak. Generally, one curved chest tube rests over the diaphragm to drain any accumulation of fluid and an apical chest tube aids in reexpansion of the lung. The provider should avoid clamping in transport due to the risk of tension pneumothorax.

Upon arrival at the ICU, the chest tube should be placed under −20 cm of water continuous suction. This will help to evacuate any pneumothorax that developed in transport as well as aid in lung reexpansion. The main exception to this rule is in post-pneumonectomy patients in whom the chest tube is always left to water seal to avoid mediastinal shift and loss of venous return. The function of the pleural evacuation system (pleurevac) is to remove air and fluid from the thoracic cavity under a controlled negative pressure system (Figure 18.4). It should be noted that applying continuous negative pressure to the pleurevac system can increase broncho-pleural air leaks due to a higher transpulmonary pressure. This is the pressure difference between the alveoli and pleural space.[13] In the case of a continuous air leak, it may be beneficial to remove suction to seal the leak. This can be identified by looking for air bubbles within the water seal chamber of the pleurevac system. When placing a patient on water seal, check a chest X-ray to ensure air has not rapidly accumulated within the pleural space.

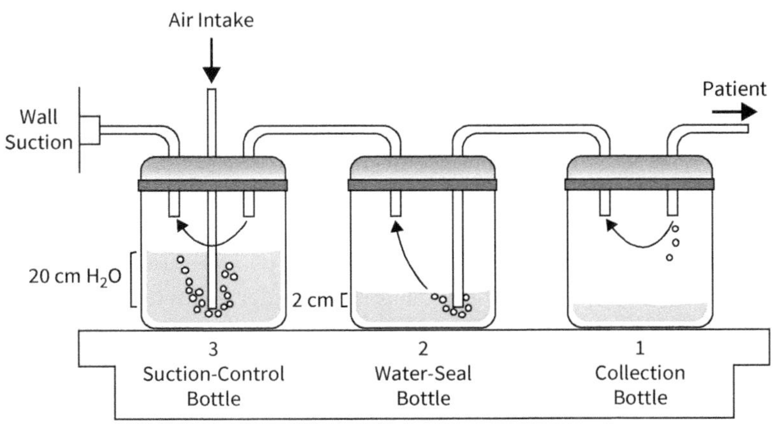

Figure 18.4 A standard pleural drainage system for evacuating air and fluid from the pleural space. Air that is evacuated from the pleural space passes through the water in the second bottle and creates bubbles. Thus, the presence of bubbles in the water-seal chamber (called bubbling) is used as evidence for a continuing broncho-pleural air leak.

Reprinted with permission from Marino P. *The ICU Book*. 3rd ed. Philadelphia, PA: Lippincott Williams & Wilkins; 2007: Figure 26.7.

Chest tube removal criteria vary from physician to physician, but a general guide is to assess for air leak and identify chest tube output. When there is no air leak and chest tube output has decreased to 100 to 200 mL per day, it is safe to remove the chest tube. To do so, pull the chest tube during the expiratory phase of ventilation or while the patient performs a Valsalva maneuver to avoid air entrapment within the pleural space.

Postoperative Fluid Management

Fluid management in postthoracic surgery patients can be challenging in the immediate postoperative setting due to multiple intraoperative factors that affect the lung parenchyma. While in the operating room, the surgical lung is exposed to a significant amount of manipulation while the ventilated lung undergoes an extended period of single-lung ventilation. These factors, combined with intraoperative resuscitation, can lead to significant pulmonary edema postoperatively despite achieving an euvolemic state.

We recommend using standard forms of volume assessment for resuscitation. These include monitoring urine output, blood pressure, heart rate, central venous pressure, and blood lactate levels. Goal-directed fluid management is strongly encouraged for postoperative fluid resuscitation. If a pulmonary arterial catheter is in place, more invasive measurements can be obtained, including central venous oxygen saturations, left ventricular end-diastolic pressures, and cardiac output.[14]

An arterial pressure-based monitoring device can be implemented in the absence of a pulmonary artery catheter to obtain similar parameters. The Flotrac/Vigileo system is an example. This device can provide useful measurements, including systemic vascular resistance, cardiac output, and stroke volume variation with varying reliability. The latter is specifically useful in volume resuscitation. Stroke volume variation reflects variation in left ventricular output secondary to intrathoracic pressure changes induced by ventilation and has been shown to be an accurate predictor of fluid responsiveness. It is calculated as the percentage of change between the maximal and minimal stroke volumes during a defined period of time divided by their mean value.[15]

Point-of-care ultrasound to assess fluid status has become increasingly useful and should be used serially to assess volume status changes. Evaluation of left ventricular filling, overall cardiac function, the presence or absence of pericardial/pulmonary effusions, and right-sided heart pressures/inferior vena cava collapsibility can be used to aid resuscitation.

It is important to note that the preference is for the patient to be euvolemic or slightly hypovolemic in the first 24 hours postoperatively to avoid postresection pulmonary edema. If resuscitation is required, crystalloid or colloid are appropriate options; both were equally effective in a randomized trial.

Complications

Given the complexity of these operations, postoperative complications should be expected and are most often directly related to the procedure performed. The relationship between procedure and complication is depicted in Table 18.3. In this section, we discuss the most common issues that arise in the thoracic ICU and their management.

Table 18.3 Complications of Specific Thoracic Procedures

Procedure	Complications
Anterior mediastinotomy (Chamberlain)	Damage to recurrent laryngeal nerve (particularly left)
Bronchoscopy/mediastinoscopy	Bleeding from major vessels if torn, air leak with biopsy of bronchus
Bronchopleural fistula repair	Persistent leak, dehiscence
Bronchopulmonary lavage	Respiratory distress/contralateral spillage
Bullectomy	Tension pneumothorax, air leak
Chest wall reconstruction	Blood loss, altered chest wall compliance, unstable chest, infection prosthetic material
Clagett window	Air leak
Collis–Belsey	Gastric leak, splenic injury
Decortication	Blood loss, air leak(s)
Esophageal dilatation	Esophageal perforation, pleural effusion, airway obstruction
Esophagoscopy	Esophageal perforation
Esophagogastrectomy	Third-spacing of fluids, anastomotic leak, gastric devascularization, splenic injury, gastric torsion
Heller myotomy	Esophageal tear
Lobectomy	Bronchial leak, lobar collapse, lobar torsion
Mediastinal tumor excision	Airway obstruction with sedation/anesthesia, damage to recurrent laryngeal nerve
Nissen fundoplication	Esophageal obstruction (with tight wrap), splenic injury
Pectus repair	Costochondritis, unstable sternum
Pleuroscopy	Pharyngeal laceration, air leak
Pneumonectomy	Atrial arrhythmias (atrial fibrillation, MAT), mediastinal shift, cardiac torsion, air embolism, disrupted bronchus
Thoracic aortic aneurysm	Paraplegia, bleeding, aortobronchial fistula, esophageal injury
Thymectomy	In myasthenics, possible weakness and respiratory failure
Lung transplant	Rejection (day 5), reperfusion injury, infection, overdistention of native lung, dehiscence
Tracheal resection	Fixed neck flexion postoperatively, dehiscence, air leak

Reprinted with permission from Higgins TL. Selected issues in postoperative management. In: American College of Chest Physicians: The ACCP Critical Care Board Review. Northbrook, IL; 1998:323–334.

Airway

As discussed previously, laryngeal edema related to airway manipulation and double-lumen endotracheal tubes can lead to a critically swollen airway upon extubation. Corticosteroids and racemic epinephrine remain first-line treatment options. However, in refractory cases of upper airway edema or tracheal stenosis after resection, heliox remains an appropriate adjunct to therapy. Heliox is a mixture of helium and oxygen that is significantly less dense than nitrogen. This allows for laminar flow through a narrow opening and may convert a critical airway to a stable airway.[16]

Recurrent laryngeal nerve injury, usually from excessive traction or dissection of the surrounding tissue, can lead to hoarseness with the inability to clear secretions and increases aspiration risks. These patients should recover function over time if the nerve was not sacrificed intraoperatively. If hoarseness persists, this should prompt an evaluation for vocal cord injection to medialize the cord on the affected side.

Cardiac

Atrial tachyarrhythmias and cardiac ischemia are common in this patient population and worth noting, but their management is beyond the scope of this chapter.

Right-to-left shunting arises postoperatively but sometimes not until after discharge. It is estimated that upward of 20% of the general population has a patent foramen ovale. After lung resection surgery, specifically pneumonectomy, patients can develop shunting due to increased right-sided pressures.[17] Patients will present with dyspnea and hypoxia, which improves when lying flat. A diagnosis can be made with arterial blood gas analysis as well as echocardiography after ruling out more common causes of these symptoms. Treatment options include surgical closure versus intravascular occlusion.

A rare but dreaded complication is cardiac herniation. Herniation generally occurs early in the postoperative course and presents as hemodynamic instability, superior vena cava syndrome, and abnormally located heart sounds on the right side of the chest. This is due to evisceration of the heart from its pericardial sac, usually following pneumonectomy with intrapericardial dissection. Management is immediate surgical exploration with closure of the pericardial defect.

Lung resection or lung reduction surgery carries the added risk of right ventricular dysfunction/failure. This is thought to be in relation to an alteration in pulmonary vascular resistance due to a reduction in the cross-sectional area of the pulmonary capillary bed. Elevated central venous pressures with hemodynamic instability should alert the provider to this potential diagnosis. A transthoracic echocardiogram with/without pulmonary artery catheter placement can lead to a diagnosis. Management with ionotropic support, diuresis, and afterload reduction with pulmonary vasodilators is the mainstay of treatment but is beyond the scope of this chapter.

Pulmonary

Atelectasis and pulmonary edema remain the most common complications in thoracic surgery patients. However, more complex issues may arise in the ICU.

Postpneumonectomy syndrome is a counterclockwise rotation of the mediastinum typically following right pneumonectomy. Patients present with dyspnea on exertion, stridor, and recurrent pulmonary infections usually due to left main stem bronchus compression.[18] Treatment is surgery, and it should be noted that this condition most often presents following discharge.

Of more immediate concern is bronchial stump leak after pneumonectomy. These patients present with worsening fevers and leukocytosis in conjunction with opacification of the hemithorax due to endobronchial secretions leaking into the chest cavity. This is managed with antibiotics and surgical exploration that usually requires flap closure of the stump with repeated washouts.

Following lobectomy, lobar torsion may occur as a segment of lung twists about its hilar structures. These may initially present as atelectasis on chest X-ray but will progress to opacification with evidence of tissue necrosis. This can be diagnosed by bronchoscopy and requires detorsion intraoperatively if diagnosed. A lobectomy may be required if necrotic tissue is encountered.

In the event of worsening oxygenation and ventilation despite maximal ventilatory and ancillary support, more invasive techniques are sometimes required. Veno-venous extracorporeal membrane oxygenation is the final treatment modality for refractory respiratory failure and should be considered when the patient fails other modalities to improve oxygenation and ventilation. These modalities include inverse ratio ventilation/airway pressure release ventilation, paralytics with sedation, pulmonary vasodilators, and prone positioning in severe acute respiratory distress syndrome.

Pleural

Pneumothorax is second only to atelectasis in the frequency of postoperative complications.[19] Patient presentation can vary widely and can include a subclinical presentation, dyspnea on exertion, hypoxia, decreased breath sounds on the affected side, and, if ventilated, rising airway pressures as positive pressure forces air into the pleural space. If the patient has developed a tension pneumothorax, hemodynamic instability arises. In a stable patient, a chest X-ray should be ordered to rule out pneumothorax. Point-of-care ultrasound can also be used to identify the presence or absence of pleural sliding and may be more efficient than waiting for radiology. In an unstable patient, it is prudent to decompress the thoracic cavity based on clinical findings. This may be done with a needle decompression at the second intercostal space in the midclavicular line or with a traditional chest tube. If the former is performed, providers must place a chest tube for long-term drainage.

If the pneumothorax is identified on the surgical side with chest tubes in place, it is prudent to check the circuit for any obstruction. Commonly, the drainage tube may be kinked or inadvertently clamped, leading to an accumulation of air behind the level of obstruction.

It should be noted that multiple meta-analyses have suggested that point-of-care ultrasound is a more sensitive study to rule out pneumothorax (Table 18.4) with similar specificity.[20] This is most likely due to the presence of an anterior pneumothorax that chest X-rays will not always identify (Figure 18.5) but can be diagnosed when lack of sliding with the characteristic "barcode" sign is seen on M mode. A bedside ultrasound is also very effective at identifying "b lines" in pulmonary edema, large effusions, and lung consolidation/atelectasis (Figure 18.6).

Thoracic duct injury is a complication of thoracic surgery requiring dissection within the posterior mediastinum and is commonly encountered in esophageal resection. A high index of suspicion is warranted when chest tube output turns from serous/serosanguinous to milky white with increasing output after the initiation of fatty foods. A diagnosis should be made by sending pleural fluid for triglycerides and chylomicrons, which will be elevated. Conservative management includes a medium chain fatty acid diet versus elemental tube feed formulas to decrease fatty acid content within the lymphatic system. If that treatment is unsuccessful, transitioning to parenteral nutrition may be necessary while the surgeon decides if operative intervention is necessary. It is prudent to rule out other sources of purulent

Table 18.4 Diagnostic Accuracy of Ultrasound in Pleural Chest Syndromes: Evidence From Systematic Reviews

Pneumothorax	Number of Studies	Population, Unit of Analysis	US Features, Comparator	Reference Standard	Prevalence and Number	Sensitivity	Specificity
Wilkerson RG, Stone MB. Sensitivity of bedside ultrasound and supine anteroposterior chest radiographs for the identification of pneumothorax after blunt trauma. *Acad Emerg Med.* 2010;17:11–17.	4 studies; no meta-analysis	Blunt trauma, by patient (3 studies), by hemithorax (1 study)	Not stated; CXR	Chest CT or release of air	21.5%–30.1% of 497 patients, 11.5% of 218 hemithoraces	US: 86%–98% CXR: 28%–75%	US: 97%–100% CXR: 100%
Ding W, Shen Y, Yang J, et al. Diagnosis of pneumothorax by radiography and ultrasonography: a meta-analysis. *Chest.* 2011;140:859–866.	20 studies	Trauma, post-lung biopsy, critically ill, by hemithorax[a]	Absent lung sliding, absent comets, lung point; CXR	Chest CT or clinical findings and release of air	13.2% of 7569 hemithoraces	US: 88% CXR: 52%	US: 99% CXR: 100%
Alrajhi K, Woo MY, Vaillancourt C. Test characteristics of ultrasonography for the detection of pneumothorax: a systematic review and meta-analysis. *Chest.* 2012;141:703–708.	8 studies	Trauma, iatrogenic, by patient[a]	Absent lung sliding, absent comets; CXR	Chest CT or release of air	Not stated (unable to calculate), 1048 patients	US: 90.9% CXR: 50.2%	US: 98.2% CXR: 99.4%
Alrajab S, Youssef AM, Akkus NI, et al. Pleural ultrasonography versus chest radiography for the diagnosis of pneumothorax: review of the literature and meta-analysis. *Crit Care.* 2013;17:R208.	13 studies	Trauma, post-lung biopsy, critically ill, by hemithorax	Not defined; CXR	Chest CT	22.5% of 3028 hemithoraces	US: 78.6% CXR: 39.8%	US: 98.4% CXR: 99.3%
Ebrahimi A, Yousefifard M, Mohammad Kazemi H, et al. Diagnostic accuracy of chest ultrasonography versus chest radiography for identification of pneumothorax: a systematic review and meta-analysis. *Tanaffos.* 2014;13:29–40.	28 studies	Trauma, iatrogenic, critically ill, by patient[a]	Not stated; CXR	Chest CT	20% of 5314 patients	US: 87% CXR: 46%	US: 99% CXR: 100%

Pleural effusion							
Grimberg A, Shigueoka DC, Atallah AN, et al. Diagnostic accuracy of sonography for pleural effusion: systematic review. *Sao Paulo Med J.* 2010;128:90–95.	4 studies	Trauma, heart failure, ICU patients with ARDS By patient	Not stated; CXR	CT or drainage	27.6% of 924 patients	US: 92%–96% CXR: 24%–100%	US: 88%–100% CXR:85%–100%
Yousefifard M, Baikpour M, Ghelichkhani P, et al. Screening performance characteristic of ultrasonography and radiography in detection of pleural effusion; a meta-analysis. *Emerg (Tehran)*. 2016;4:1–10.	12 studies	Trauma, heart failure, critically ill, surgical patients By patient	Not stated; CXR	CT, US, CXR	41.5% of 1554 patients	US: 94% CXR: 51%	US: 98% CXR: 91%

Abbreviations: CXR, chest radiography; CT, computed tomography; ICU, intensive care unit; ARDS, acute respiratory distress syndrome.
[a]Included and pooled studies reporting the alternative unit of analysis, by doubling the number of patients or halving the number of hemithoraces in those studies. Reproduced with permission of the ©ERS 2019: *European Respiratory Review* 2016;25(141):230–246; DOI: 10.1183/16000617.0047-2016 Published 31 August 2016.

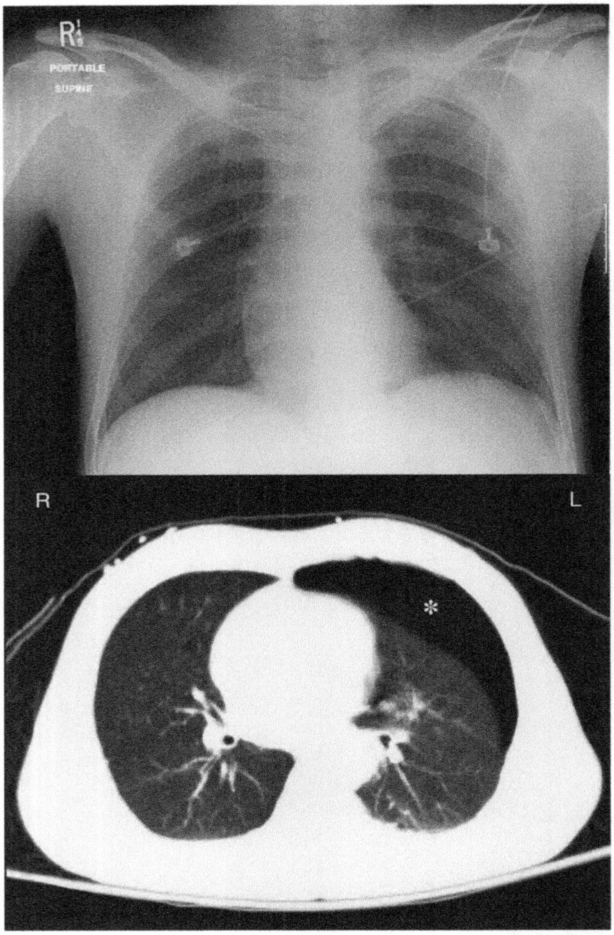

Figure 18.5 A portable chest X-ray and computer tomography image of the thorax in a young male with blunt trauma to the chest. An anterior pneumothorax is evident on the CT image (indicated by the asterisk) but is not apparent on the chest X-ray.

Reprinted with permission from Marino P. *The ICU Book*. 3rd ed. Philadelphia, PA: Lippincott Williams & Wilkins; 2007: Figure 26.5.

chest tube drainage, especially after esophageal surgery. Amylase levels will aid in the diagnosis of esophageal leak/anastomotic breakdown and should be checked alongside protein, lactate dehydrogenase levels, and cell counts to assess for a transudative versus exudative effusion.

The mainstay of treatment for esophageal injury has evolved in recent years. After evaluation/diagnosis of esophageal leak with computed tomography esophagram, the immediate focus of the provider should be to ensure adequate source control with chest tube drainage and the addition of broad-spectrum antibiotics/antifungals. This may be accomplished at the bedside, in the interventional radiology suite, or in the operating room depending on the degree of contamination and location of spillage. After source control, gastroenterology should be consulted to assess for esophageal stenting versus operative repair, depending on injury.

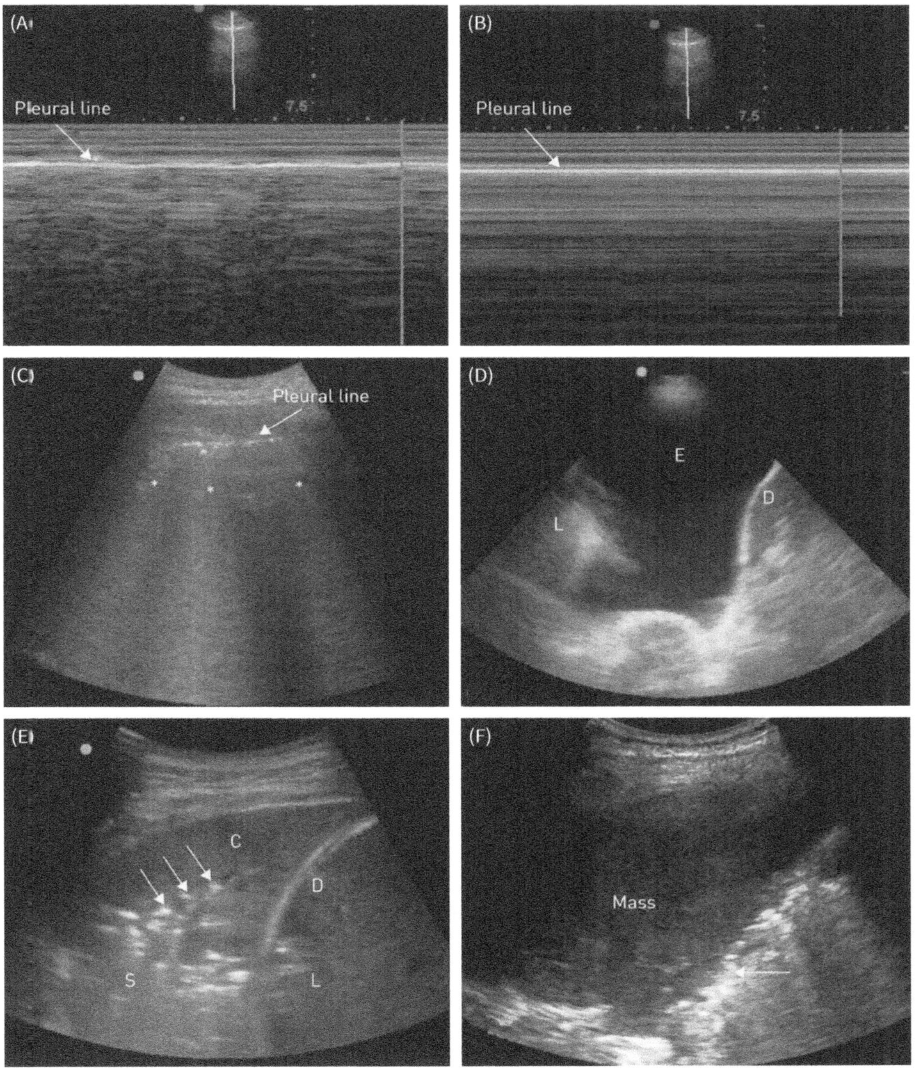

Figure 18.6 Selected chest ultrasound images. (A) Seashore sign. Granular "seashore" appearance of normal lung sliding on M mode. (B) Barcode sign. Horizontal "barcode" appearance with loss of lung sliding on M mode. (C) B-lines. Asterisks indicate comet tail artefacts arising from the pleural line (B-lines). (D) Simple pleural effusion. "E" indicates anechoic free-flowing effusion. "L" indicates compressed atelectatic lung. "D" indicates diaphragm. (E) Consolidation. "C" indicates consolidation. "D" indicates diaphragm. "L" indicates liver. "S" indicates serrated distal margins of the consolidation. Arrows indicate air bronchograms. (F) Lung tumor. The arrow indicates the smooth distal margin of the mass.

Reproduced with permission of the ©ERS 2019: *European Respiratory Review* 2016;25(141):230–246; DOI: 10.1183/16000617.0047-2016 Published 31 August 2016.

Infections

Infection after thoracic surgery is centered around nosocomial pneumonia, empyema, and surgical site infections. With the use of perioperative antibiotics, surgical site infections have become exceedingly rare. However, providers must maintain a high index of suspicion in the setting of emergency department thoracotomies and surgeries for empyema, lung abscesses, and perforated esophagus because these increase the risk of postoperative infection. It is also important to encourage early ambulation and have an aggressive physical therapy strategy to prevent atelectasis and its conversion to pneumonia.

If there is a clinical suspicion for pneumonia and the patient is ventilated, we recommend a bronchoscopy with bronchial alveolar lavage sent for cultures. This is followed by empiric broad-spectrum antibiotic coverage with methicillin-resistant staphylococcus aureus coverage as well as antipseudomonal coverage. Our institution favors vancomycin and cefepime while awaiting speciation and sensitivities. If the patient is extubated, a deep tracheal aspirate may suffice in guiding the antibiotic course.

The frequency of empyema is decreasing, but it remains a risk in prolonged air leaks and may be confounded by prolonged mechanical ventilation. Cultures may be sent from the chest tube, and broad-spectrum antibiotics should be started. In some cases, these may necessitate operative intervention.

References

1. Iyer A, Yadav S. Postoperative care and complications after thoracic surgery. In: Firstenberg S, ed. *Principles and Practice of Cardiothoracic Surgery.* London: IntechOpen; 2013.
2. Stéphan F, Boucheseiche S, Hollande J, et al. Pulmonary complications following lung resection: a comprehensive analysis of incidence and possible risk factors. *Chest.* 2000;118:1263–1270.
3. Brower RG, Matthay M, et al; Acute Respiratory Distress Syndrome Network. Ventilation with lower tidal volumes as compared with traditional tidal volumes for acute lung injury and the acute respiratory distress syndrome. *N Engl J Med.* 2000;342:1301–1308.
4. Vallverdu I, Calaf N, Subirana M, Net A, Benito S, Mancebo J. Clinical characteristics, respiratory functional parameters, and outcome of a two-hour t-piece trial in patients weaning from mechanical ventilation. *Am J Respir Crit Care Med.* 1998;158:1855–1862.
5. Shaw J, LoCicero J. General principles of postoperative care. In: Shields TW, LoCicero J, Reed CE, Feins RH, eds. *General Thoracic Surgery.* 7th ed. Philadelphia, PA: Lippincott Williams & Wilkins; 2009:571–579.
6. Pacouret G, Alison D, Pottier JM, Bertrand P, Charbonnier B. Free-floating thrombus and embolic risk in patients with angiographically confirmed proximal deep venous thrombosis: a prospective study. *Arch Intern Med.* 1997;157:305–308.
7. Stevens D, Edwards T. Management of pain after thoracic surgery. In: Pearson FG, Cooper JD, Deslauriers J, et al., eds. *Thoracic Anesthesia*, 2nd ed. New York, NY: Churchill Livingstone; 1991: 563–591.
8. Strom BL, Berlin JA, Kinman JL, et al. Parenteral ketorolac and risk of gastrointestinal and operative site bleeding. A postmarketing surveillance study. *JAMA.* 1996;275:376–382.
9. Grinder JS, Mullet TW, Saha SP, Harned ME, Sloan PA. A randomized, double-blind trial comparing continuous thoracic epidural bupivacaine with and without opioid in contrast to continuous paravertebral infusion of bupivacaine for post-thoracotomy pain. *J Cardiothorac Vasc Anesth.* 2012;26:83–89.
10. Bulbake U, Doppalapudi S, Kommineni N, Khan W. Liposomal formulations in clinical use: an updated review. *Pharmaceutics.* 2017;9(2):12.

11. Pedoto A, Amar D. Liposomal bupivacaine for intercostal nerve block: pricey or priceless? *Semin Thorac Cardiovasc Surg.* 2017;29:538–539.
12. Ju H, Feng Y, Yang BX, Wang J. Comparison of epidural analgesia and intercostal nerve cryoanalgesia for post thoracotomy pain control. *Eur J Pain.* 2008;12:378–384.
13. Marino P. *The ICU Book.* 3rd ed. Philadelphia, PA: Lippincott Williams & Wilkins; 2007.
14. Kendrick JB, Kaye AD, Tong Y, et al. Goal-directed fluid therapy in the perioperative setting. *J Anaesthesiol Clin Pharmacol.* 2019;35(Suppl 1):S29–S34.
15. Berkenstadt H, Margalit N, Hadani M, et al. Stroke volume variation as a predictor of fluid responsiveness in patients undergoing brain surgery. *Anesth Analg.* 2001;92:984–989.
16. Skrinkas GJ, Hyland RH, Hutcheon MA. Using helium-oxygen mixtures in the management of acute upper airway obstruction. *Can Med Assoc J.* 1983:128:555–558.
17. Bakris NC, Siddiqi AJ, Fraser CD Jr, Mehta AC. Right-to-left interatrial shunt after pneumonectomy. *Ann Thorac Surg.* 1997;63:198–201.
18. Jansen JP, Brutel de la Rivière A, Alting MP, Westermann CJ, Bergstein PG, Duurkens VA. Postpneumonectomy syndrome in adulthood. Surgical correction using an expandable prosthesis. *Chest.* 1992;101:1167–1170.
19. Amini S, Gabrielli A, Caruso L, Layon AJ. The thoracic surgical patients: initial postoperative care. *Semin Cardiothorac Vasc Anesth.* 2002;6:169–188.
20. Ding W, Shen Y, Yang J, He X, Zhang M. Diagnosis of pneumothorax by radiography and ultrasonography: a meta-analysis. *Chest.* 2011;140:859–866.

19
Pulmonary Pathophysiology in Anesthesia Practice

Gary R. Haynes and Brian P. McClure

Introduction

Maintaining and controlling respiratory function is fundamental to anesthesia practice. General anesthesia and mechanical ventilation interfere with pulmonary function, and their effect on pulmonary physiology can be exaggerated in patients with pulmonary disease. Restoring pulmonary function to normal, or as near to normal as possible after surgery, is a primary responsibility of the anesthesiologists.

Restoring arterial carbon dioxide ($PaCO_2$) and oxygen (PaO_2) levels prevents injury to critical organ systems and delayed emergence from general anesthesia. Control ventilation is necessary because patients breathing spontaneously during anesthesia risk airway obstruction and tend to hypoventilation, leading to hypercarbia. Airway obstruction and depressed ventilation occurring from sedation, general anesthesia, nerve blocks, neuraxial anesthesia, or positioning must be immediately addressed. Managing respiratory function under anesthesia requires knowledge of neurological controlling mechanisms, what airway and lung volumes changes occur, and how ventilation-perfusion (V/Q) relationships are altered during anesthesia and surgery. Basic pulmonary physiology, emphasizing the relationship to clinical practice, is reviewed here.

Pulmonary pathology can be grouped into four main categories: obstructive disease, restrictive disease, infectious disease, and neoplastic disease. While pulmonary diseases and their effects on pulmonary function are categorized for educational and research purposes, there often is considerable overlapping of these classes. On a clinical level, pulmonary pathophysiology becomes essentially a problem of either inadequate lung ventilation or perfusion. However, the clinical problem is often one of both inadequate ventilation and inadequate perfusion of pulmonary blood flow. While some disease processes elicit a specific pathophysiological response, patients often present with multiple comorbid conditions, resulting in a complex pathophysiological picture.

Signs and Symptoms of Pulmonary Disease

Anesthesiologists' initial encounter with patients occurs in a variety circumstances and conditions. With elective surgery there is an opportunity for scheduled patient interviews and examination, but emergent patients or critically ill intensive care unit (ICU) patients may be unconscious, intubated, or on ventilator support at the first opportunity for evaluation.

Recognizing physical manifestations of lung disease and making a quick assessment is necessary to anticipating problems with ventilation and oxygenation.

Recognizing the physical signs of pulmonary disease is necessary as sedation and general anesthesia mask some pulmonary symptoms. Common signs include dyspnea and tachypnea, or difficulty with breathing and rapid breathing, indicating shortness of breath. These are often accompanied with increased breathing effort, a sign of narrowed airways and greater respiratory effort. Forceful movement of air through constricted airways can cause audible wheezing or heard when auscultating the chest. In severe instances, conscious patients have retractions of accessory muscles of breathing on inspiration. Flaring of the nostrils with inspiration and expiration often accompanies difficult, labored breathing.

Coughing is the mechanism to expel fluid or mucous from the airways. Expectorant coughing is a productive cough. Irritation of the airway triggering coughing without production of sputum is a nonproductive cough. Causes include acute upper respiratory tract infections, sinus drainage into the trachea, asthma, and gastroesophageal disease. A chronic productive cough is a characteristic of chronic bronchitis from tobacco smoking or other irritants. Chronic exposure to smoke or other irritants is another cause of chronic bronchitis.

An important physical sign is cyanosis, a bluish and mottled appearance that develops with increases in in deoxygenated hemoglobin. Peripheral cyanosis occurs when vasoconstriction in the extremities decreases blood flow to allow more time for extraction of oxygen. Cyanosis from cold exposure is an example. Central cyanosis occurs when the pulmonary system cannot oxygenate blood adequately. Failure to oxygenate blood can result from multiple causes: when the number of respiratory units falls below a critical level, when the movement of oxygen across the alveolar walls and into the blood is obstructed, when the blood flow distributed in the lungs is not matched to ventilation (a ventilation-perfusion mismatch), or with an interruption in the pulmonary blood flow. Clubbing of the nail beds and tips of fingers and toes is a common physical finding with chronic hypoxemia.

Chest pain is a common symptom but one not specific for pulmonary disease. Pain that is respiratory in origin originates from the pleural lining of the inner chest wall and surface covering the lungs, the bronchial airways, or from the muscles or skeletal structures in the chest wall. Splinting, or limiting breathing movements, is frequently associated with a disease process involving the chest wall or pleural lining of the thorax.

Patients in respiratory failure often present with dyspnea and tachypnea. Drowsiness and visual and mental status changes may be present. Patients may experience headaches that are secondary to cerebral vasodilation. In advancing cases sedation, obtundation, and loss of consciousness occurs.

Respiratory Function in the Conscious Patient

Respiratory function consists of (i) neural control mechanisms, (ii) chest wall and diaphragm action, (iii) air movement in the upper airways, and then into (iv) the lung parenchyma. Anesthetic drugs effect the pulmonary system on every level. Sedatives, hypnotics, opioids, and inhalational agents depress the neural control; sedatives and paralytic drugs relax oropharyngeal muscles promoting airway obstruction; sedative and hypnotic drugs, as well as inhalational anesthetics, can relax bronchial smooth muscle resulting in bronchodilation; and anesthetics can depress cardiac function, altering pulmonary perfusion.

Normal Control of Breathing

In normal conditions there is autonomic nervous system and conscious control over ventilation. Changes in minute ventilation (V_E) are primarily controlled by the levels of carbon dioxide and oxygen in the blood using a closed-loop negative feedback system (see Figure 19.1). The partial pressure of $PaCO_2$ and the change in hydrogen ion concentration (H^+) it causes is sensed by chemoreceptors in the medulla of the brainstem. Peripheral chemoreceptors in the carotid and aortic vessels are sensitive to PaO_2 as well as $PaCO_2$, pH, and aortic blood pressure. Those chemoreceptors are most sensitive to PaO_2, and they stimulate ventilation when the PaO_2 falls to 50 to 60 mmHg. The carotid body chemoreceptors have a more important role in controlling PaO_2 than the aortic arch chemoreceptors. It has been shown in animal models with denervated carotid bodies that they fail to increase ventilation when breathing hypoxic gas mixtures. Instead, uncorrected hypoxia only further depresses the central respiratory center in the brain. When patients become hypoxic, it is the action of the carotid bodies that overrides the central respiratory depression and stimulates ventilation.[1]

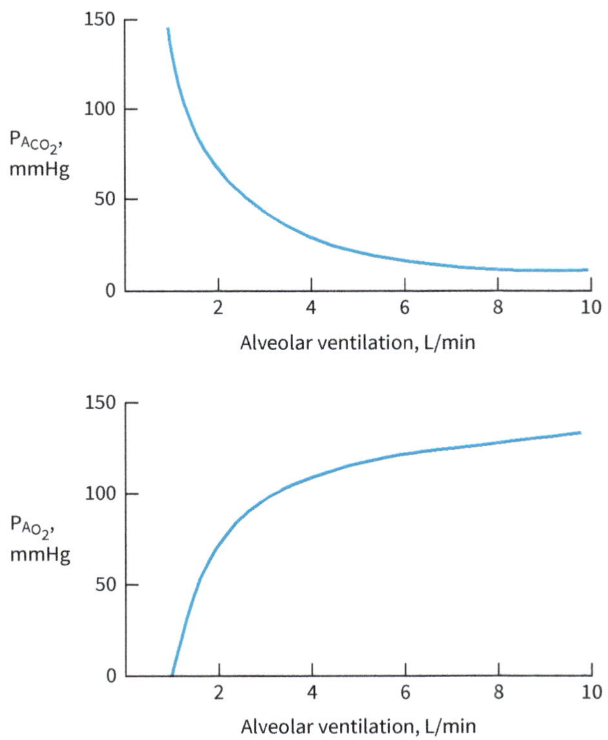

Figure 19.1 Alveolar ventilation is controlled by central chemoreceptors responding to changes in $PaCO_2$ in cerebrospinal fluid. The normal set point is to keep the $PaCO_2$ 40 mm Hg and the PaO_2 at about 104 mm Hg.

From Levitzky MG. Pulmonary Physiology. 9th ed. New York, NY: McGraw-Hill Education; 2012. Copyright McGraw-Hill Education © All rights reserved.

The $PaCO_2$ transiently increases with exercise, and in response slight hyperventilation acts to return it to the normal resting level. The hyperventilation response is quick, but with exercise the response is even faster, suggesting greater sensitivity of the chemoreceptors to carbon dioxide. When at rest the central chemoreceptors in the brainstem appear dominant when controlling $PaCO_2$ but, with exercise, the carotid body chemoreceptors are probably recruited to heighten the response.[2]

Since the carbon dioxide level primarily drives ventilation, apnea is an important consequence of lowering $PaCO_2$. The apneic threshold is the $PaCO_2$ level that fails to stimulate spontaneous breathing. When the $PaCO_2$ level falls below this level, there is no stimulus to breathe. The patient will not breathe spontaneously until the $PaCO_2$ rises above the apneic threshold point. Lowering the $PaCO_2$ by 5 to 10 mmHg is usually enough to reach the apneic threshold.

Neural control centers in the brainstem direct the rate and degree of thoracic expansion by acting on the muscles of the chest wall and diaphragm. Regulatory feedback is provided by peripheral and medullary chemoreceptors that sense the hydrogen ion (H^+) concentration and $PaCO_2$ in the blood and cerebrospinal fluid. Stretch receptors in skeletal muscles of the chest wall and mechanoreceptors in the lung provide feedback to the central nervous system about the degree of chest expansion. Through coordination of these influences, the supply of oxygen and elimination of carbon dioxide are maintained over a wide range of conditions.

Basic Principles of Pulmonary Physiology

Lung Volumes and Capacities

Pulmonary ventilation is quantified by four lung volumes and capacities. The lung volumes are the *tidal volume*, the volume of air inspired and expired with a breath, the *inspiratory reserve volume*, or that amount of air that can be inhaled over and above a normal tidal volume breath; the *expiratory reserve volume*, the amount of air that can be forcefully exhaled after a normal breath and the *residual volume*, or that volume of air remaining after the most forceful exhalation possible[3] (see Figure 19.2).

The lung capacities are the *inspiratory capacity*, the maximum amount of air that can be inhaled from the end of a normal exhalation, and the *functional residual capacity*, or the amount of air remaining in the lungs after a normal exhalation. The *vital capacity* is the combination of the inspiratory reserve volume, tidal volume, and expiratory reserve volume. It represents the maximum amount of air that can move in and out of the lungs when expending maximal effort. The *total lung capacity* is the combination of all lung volumes and is the maximum volume of the lungs.

The position of the patient effects pulmonary function and requires consideration because lung volumes can change significantly with repositioning. In normal subjects the total lung capacity, vital capacity, and residual volumes do not change significantly when moving from standing to supine. However, the functional reserve capacity (FRC) decreases due to an increase in the inspiratory reserve volume and a decrease in the expiratory reserve volume (see Figure 19.3). The change has implications for patients, especially the morbidly obese. Gas exchange occurs continuously with air contained in the FRC. A decrease in the FRC means less air, and thus less oxygen, is available. An increased body mass index is associated with rapid

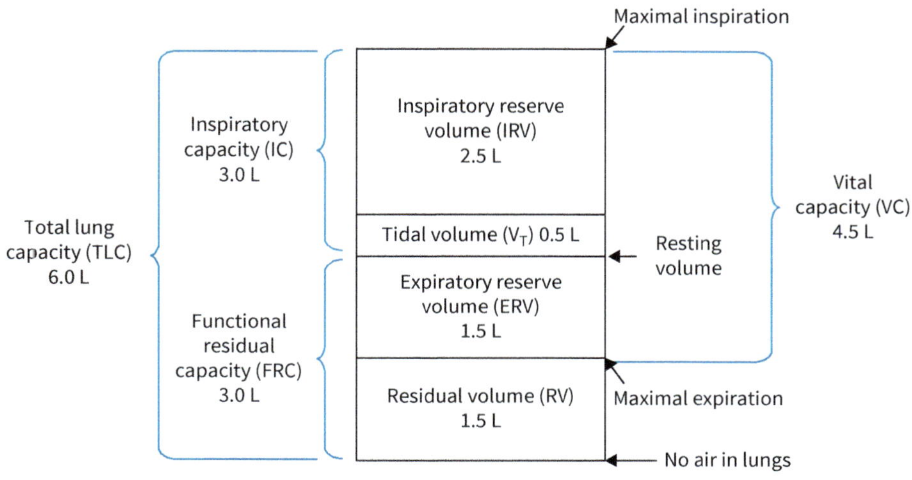

Figure 19.2 Lung volumes and capacities for a 70 kg subject.

From Levitzky MG. Pulmonary Physiology. 9th ed. New York, NY: McGraw-Hill Education; 2012. Copyright McGraw-Hill Education © All rights reserved.

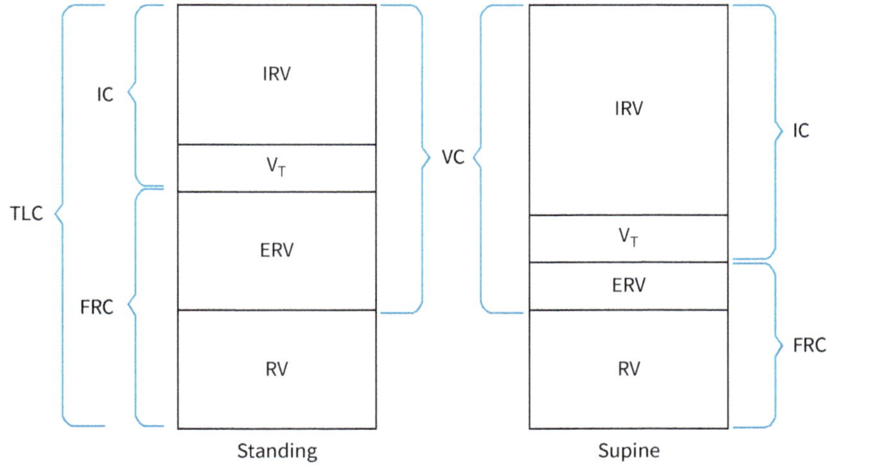

Figure 19.3 Changes in the lung volumes and capacities when moving from standing to the supine position.

From Levitzky MG. Pulmonary Physiology. 9th ed. New York, NY: McGraw-Hill Education; 2012. Copyright McGraw-Hill Education © All rights reserved.

Abbreviations: ERV, expiratory reserve volume; FRC, functional residual capacity; IC, inspiratory capacity; IRV, inspiratory reserve volume; RV, residual volume; TLC, total lung capacity; VC, vital capacity; VT, tidal volume.

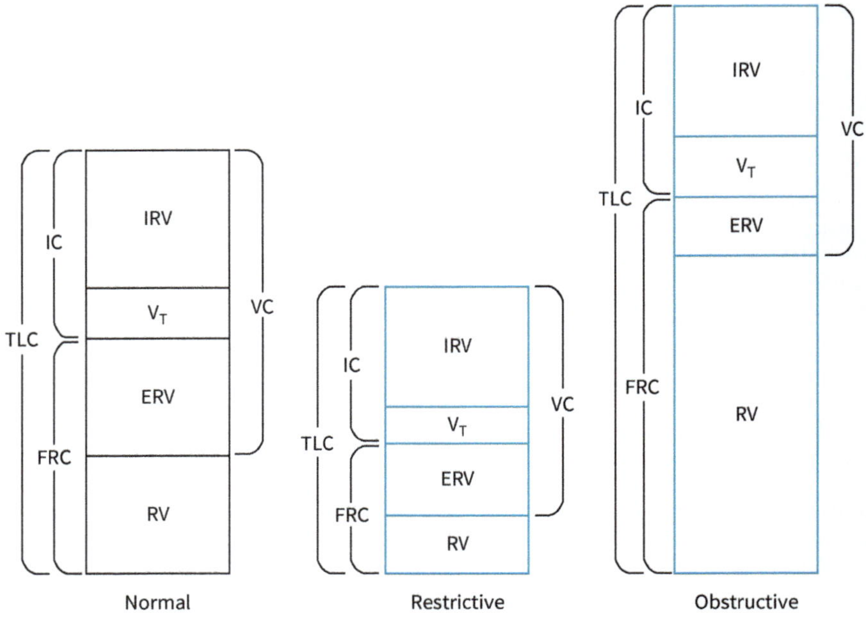

Figure 19.4 Altered lung volumes and capacities in obstructive and restrictive lung disease. Typical examples for obstructive disease include emphysema and asthma.
Abbreviations: ERV, expiratory reserve volume; FRC, functional residual capacity; IC, inspiratory capacity; IRV, inspiratory reserve volume; RV, residual volume; TLC, total lung capacity; VC, vital capacity; VT, tidal volume.

oxygen desaturation during induction of general anesthesia due to a markedly decreased FRC. This is a form of restrictive lung disease caused by the added weight on the chest wall and abdominal compression on the diaphragm (see Figure 19.4). These patients can be difficult to manage with positive pressure mask ventilation because of a less compliant thorax and airway obstruction is likely. Shifting a morbidly obese patient to a 25° head-up position before and after preoxygenation improves the PaO_2.[4]

Gas exchange occurs only at the level of the terminal respiratory bronchioles and alveoli, so it is the movement of *alveolar air* that is most important to oxygenation and CO_2 removal. Air in the tracheobronchial tree not participating in gas exchange is termed the *anatomic dead space* ($V_{D\ anat}$). The *minute ventilation* ($V_{E\ min}$), that volume of gas that is moving in and out of the lungs each minute, is the *tidal volume* (V_T) multiplied by the *respiratory frequency* (f). Under normal circumstances the anatomic dead space is not subject to any significant change.

Assessment of Gas Exchange

Determining how well the lungs function in gas exchange during anesthesia care is an important assessment. Gas exchange depends on pulmonary blood flow reaching the alveolar air sacs. Oxygen and carbon dioxide move across alveolar walls by diffusion, and their movement is determined by the concentration gradient, or partial pressure of the gas in the alveoli, the thickness of the alveolar wall, and the solubility of these gases in blood.[5]

Carbon dioxide diffuses easily and rapidly in biological systems. The effectiveness of the lungs in eliminating it is largely a function of the dead space volume at any time. To a lesser extent it also depends on how rapidly it is produced. Establishing what part of the tidal volume participates in gas exchange requires measuring the dead space volume. However, measuring V_D directly is technically difficult and is rarely, if ever, done in routine clinical settings. A suitable estimate can be made by determining the dead space to tidal volume ratio (V_D/V_{TV}). Using monitoring and blood gas data, the equation to estimate the ratio is:

$$V_D/V_{TV} = \frac{paCO_2 - P_{ET}CO_2}{paCO_2}$$

Blood flow in the lungs is not uniform (see Figure 19.5). When a person is standing, blood tends to perfuse the lower portion of the lungs rather than the apical regions. Air drawn into the lungs moves to the most compliant alveoli. As a result, in the standing position alveoli at the lung's apex will overexpand while alveolar compression in the lower part of the lung limits their expansion. Oxygen transfer depends on reasonable matching of perfusion and ventilation (see Figure 19.6). The efficiency for pulmonary transfer of oxygen is assessed by evaluating the alveolar to arterial oxygen gradient. The formula for estimation is:

$$P_AO_2 = FiO_2\left(P_{baro} - P_{H2O}\right) - \frac{PaCO_2}{RQ}$$

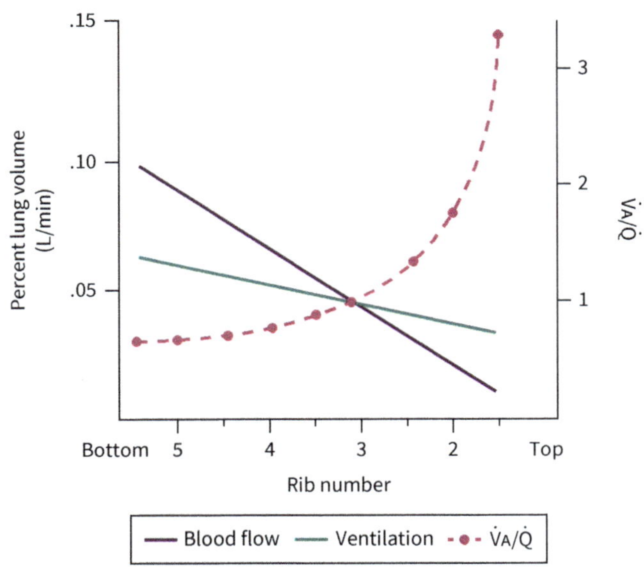

Figure 19.5 Distribution of ventilation and perfusion (left axis) and the V̇/Q̇ ratio (right axis) in healthy young individuals. Blood flow and ventilation are in liters per minute per percentage of alveolar volume. The dashed line with closed circles is the V̇/Q̇ ratio ate different anatomic levels based on a cardiac output of 6.0 L/min and an alveolar ventilation of 5.1 L/min.

Redrawn with modification from West JB. *Ventilation/Blood Flow and Gas Exchange*. 4th ed. Oxford, UK: Blackwell Scientific, 1970.

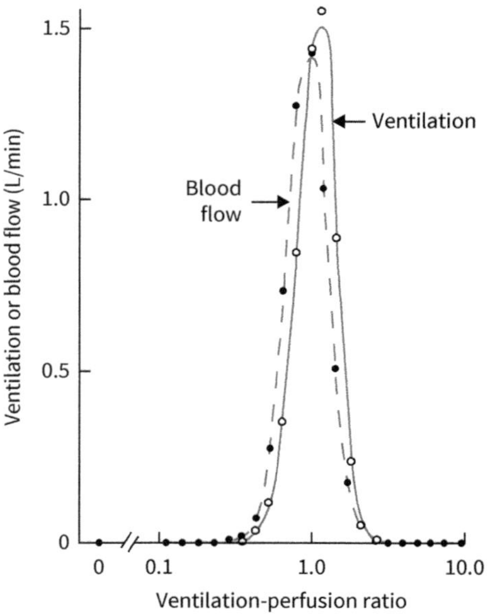

Figure 19.6 Experimental measurement of ventilation–perfusion ratio in young subjects demonstrating areas that are over ventilated and under perfused ($\dot{V}/\dot{Q} > 1$) and areas with greater perfusion than ventilation ($\dot{V}/\dot{Q}$), but normally most areas show well-matched ($\dot{V}/\dot{Q} = 1.0$).

From Wagner PD, Laravuso RB, Uhl RR, West JB. Continuous distributions of ventilation–perfusion ratios in normal subjects breathing air and 100% O_2. *J Clin Invest.* 1974;54:54–68.

where alveolar partial pressure of oxygen (P_AO_2), fraction inspired oxygen (FiO_2), barometric pressure (P_{baro}), vapor pressure of water (P_{H2OH}), and respiratory quotient (RQ) is assumed to be 0.8 under normal dietary conditions.[6] The gradient between oxygen contained in the alveolar space and that in the blood is the "A-a gradient":

$$A - a\ gradient = P_AO_2 - PaO_2$$

Pulmonary Pathophysiology and Anesthesia Effects

Respiratory Failure

Respiratory failure is when there is inadequate oxygenation of blood and removal of carbon dioxide occurs. It can present as an acute or a chronic problem, and it is often encountered as an acute exacerbation superimposed on chronic disease process. Acute failure can occur with pulmonary parenchymal, airway or chest wall pathology. Respiratory failure also occurs secondarily from the loss of neural control mechanisms with brain or spinal cord injury. Chronic failure occurs with persistent obstruction to air flow or restriction of lung expansion due to structural changes in the pulmonary parenchyma, bronchi, or adjacent structures.

There are two patterns of respiratory failure: hypoxic failure and combined hypoxic and hypercapnic failure. Hypoxic failure occurs when the partial pressure of arterial oxygen (PaO_2) falls below 60 mmHg. Usual causes of hypoxic pulmonary failure include chronic bronchitis, lung consolidation in pneumonia, and acute respiratory distress syndrome (ARDS).

Progressive hypoxia initially causes weakness and tiredness but may eventually lead to progressive sedation if unchecked. Hypoxia poses considerable risk to the brain, heart, kidneys, and liver because of their high metabolic requirement for oxygen. Total system failure and death can occur when brain stem hypoxia causes loss of cardiovascular control and circulatory shock. Respiratory failure can involve hypercapnia, $PaCO_2$ exceeding 45 mmHg. Retention of CO_2 will result in a respiratory acidosis.

Compensatory mechanisms for respiratory failure include tachycardia and peripheral vasodilation to increase cardiac output and deliver more oxygen to the body. The clinical signs of these changes are warm and moist skin, and tremors may be present from autonomic nervous system activation. As the disease advances, drowsiness occurs, and coma is a symptom of end-stage disease. This can lead to a low cardiac output state with depressed neurologic function, fluid and electrolyte imbalances, and a lessened ability to eliminate metabolic wastes.

Respiratory Function in the Anesthetized Patient

General anesthesia causes atelectasis in normal subjects.[7,8] A high fraction of inspired oxygen (FiO_2) also contributes to atelectasis. However, the margin of safety provided by breathing a high concentration of O_2 to displace nitrogen in the air contained in the FRC prior to general anesthesia outweighs this effect. Morbidly obese patients are at risk of hypoxia because anesthesia-induced atelectasis occurs to a greater extent in obese patients[9] (see Figure 19.7).

Blood flow is shunted away from areas of the lung that are not ventilated by the hypoxic pulmonary vasoconstriction (HPV) mechanism (see Figure 19.8). HPV improves matching

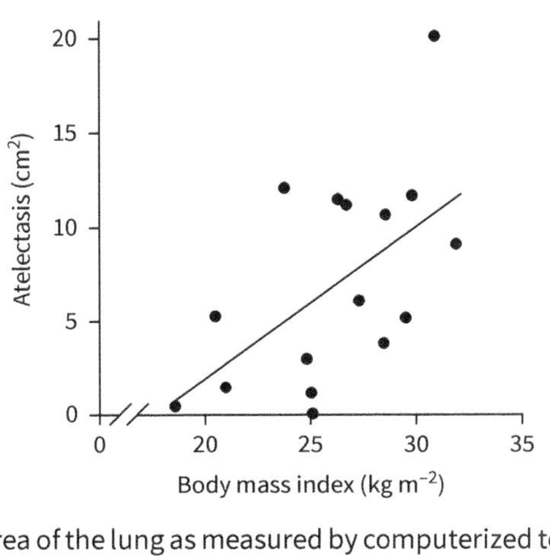

Figure 19.7 Atelectatic area of the lung as measured by computerized tomography versus body mass index (BMI); correlation, r = 0.66 and $P = 0.010$.

From Rothen HU, Sporre B, Engberg G, Wegenius G, Hedenstierna G. Re-expansion of atelectasis during general anaesthesia: a computed tomography study. *Brit J Anaesth.* 1993;71(6):788–795.

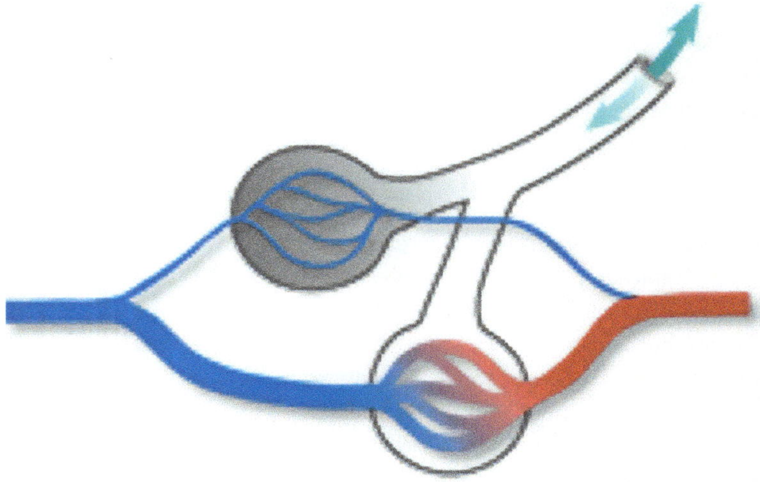

Figure 19.8 Illustration of hypoxic pulmonary vasoconstriction mechanism to maintain PaO_2 by shunting pulmonary blood flow away from areas of atelectasis. The hypoxic pulmonary vasoconstriction mechanism is unique to the lungs.

Modified from Lumb AB and Slinger P. Hypoxic pulmonary vasoconstriction. Physiology and anesthetic implications. *Anesthesiology*, 2015; 122(4):932–946.

of ventilation with pulmonary perfusion by reducing blood flow to areas that are not ventilated. This happens when small pulmonary arterioles constrict and shunt blood to alveoli in areas that are ventilated. The effect increases systemic PaO_2 and occurs within minutes when parts of the lung are not ventilated.[10]

Atelectasis can result in clinically significant hypoxia as blood flow is directed away from areas of collapsed lung parenchyma. It was once common practice to ventilate anesthetized patients using large tidal volumes, 12 to 14 ml/kg body weight, to minimize atelectasis and avoid high inspired concentrations of oxygen (FiO_2).[11,12] Ventilation with large tidal volumes was initially found to increase pulmonary injury and mortality in patients with ARDS (see Figure 19.9). Ventilation with smaller tidal volumes minimized ventilator-associated lung injury. Large tidal volume ventilation was discovered to also cause lung injury in the absence of ARDS.[13,14,15,16] The practice of ventilating with large tidal volumes yielded to using lower tidal volumes, generally 7 to 9 ml/kg body weight, although this decreases P_{max} in ICU patients, and not in operating room patients, nor did positive end-expiratory pressure, plateau pressures, or FiO_2 requirements change in either ICU or surgical patients.[17]

Effects of Anesthesia on Pulmonary Function

Control of Ventilation

Patients hypoventilate when breathing spontaneously under general anesthesia, resulting in hypercarbia although patients can maintain an adequate PaO_2. Many drugs used for sedation

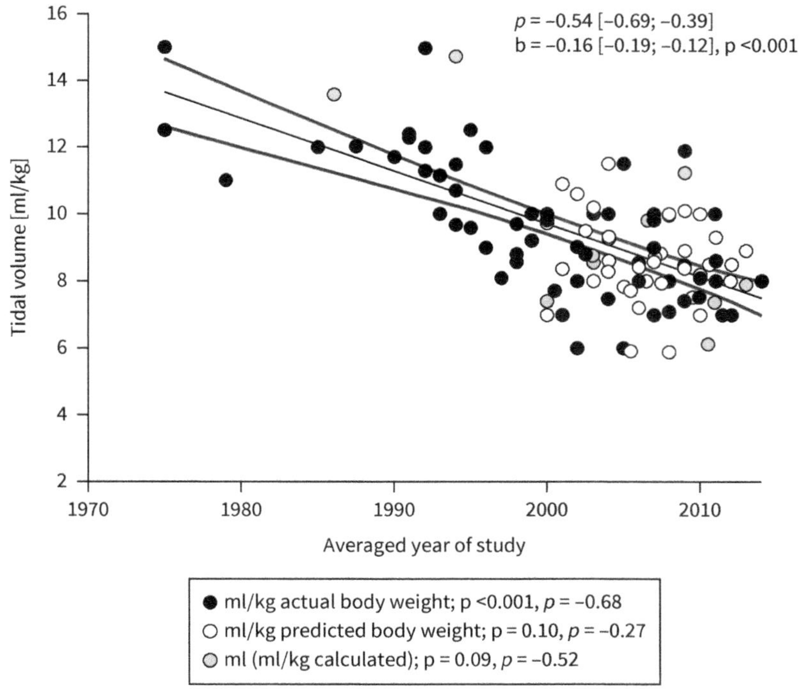

Figure 19.9 Progressive decrease in tidal volume over time in intensive care unit patients. Black line is the linear regression of tidal volume over time with the 95% confidence interval (blue lines). Each dot represents a single clinical study.

From Schaefer MS, Serpa Neto A, Pelosi P, et al. Temporal changes in ventilator settings in patients with uninjured lungs: a systematic review. *Anesth Analg*. 2019;129(1):129–135.

and general anesthesia depress ventilation by inhibiting the central and peripheral chemoreceptor responses to CO_2 and O_2. The effect of combining these drugs is additive.

Propofol

Propofol (2,6-diisopropylphenol) is used extensively for sedation, induction, and maintenance of general anesthesia. Propofol depresses ventilation[18,19,20] and depresses the sensitivity of the carotid body in a dose-dependent fashion[21] (see Figure 19.10).

Endotracheal intubation following induction of general anesthesia often causes bronchoconstriction and increased airway resistance.[22] This response is thought to result from light anesthesia or failure to suppress reflexes triggered in response to manipulation of the larynx and the presence of a foreign body in the airway. In comparison to thiopental or etomidate, induction of general anesthesia with propofol is associated with less airway resistance and no detectable wheezing on auscultation. The effect in patients with a smoking history is even more pronounced[23] (see Figure 19.11).

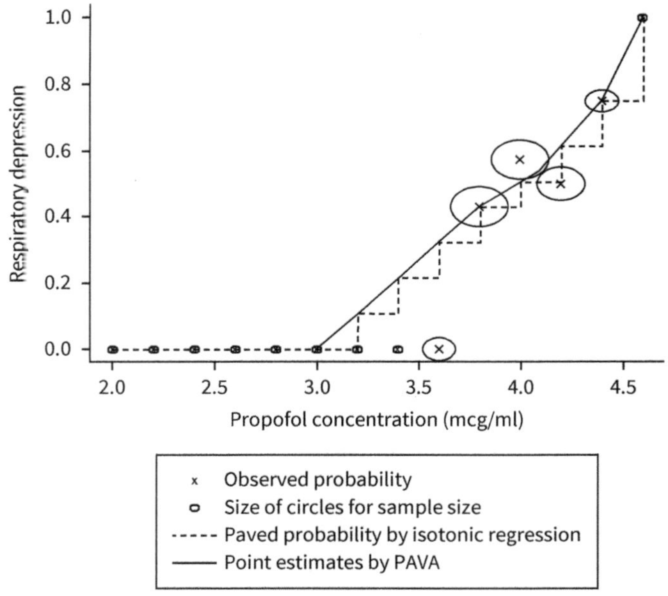

Figure 19.10 The plasma propofol concentration at which 5% (EC_5) and 50% (EC_{50}) of subjects experience respiratory depression. Respiratory depression is first seen with plasma concentrations just over 3 mcg/mL and increases in a dose-dependent manner.

From Lee MH, Yang K-H, Lee CS, Lee HS, Moon SY, Hwang S-I, Song J-H. The effect-site concentration of propofol producing respiratory depression during spinal anesthesia. *Korean J Anesthesiol.* 2011;61(2):122–126.

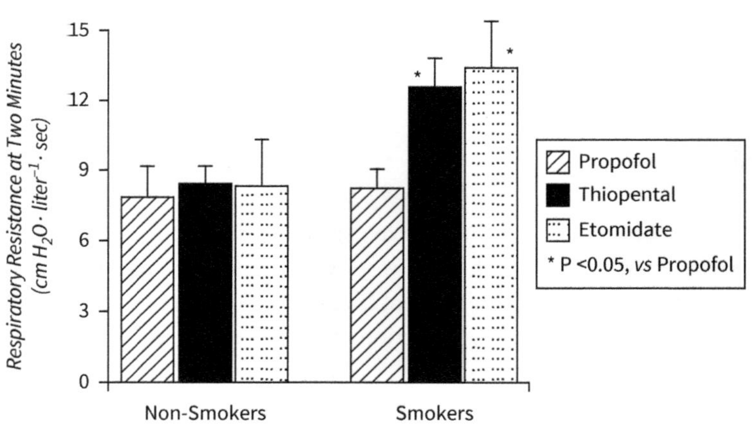

Figure 19.11 Airway resistance following induction of general anesthesia and endotracheal intubation in tobacco smokers and nonsmokers demonstrates smokers who received propofol was less than for those who received thiopental or etomidate.

From Eames WO, Rooke GA, Wu RS-C, Bishop MJ. Comparison of the effects of etomidate, propofol, and thiopental on respiratory resistance after tracheal intubation. *Anesthesiology*, 1996; 84:1307–1311.

Volatile Anesthetics

Inhalation of volatile anesthetics causes rapid, shallow breathing and blunts the responses to hypoxemia and hypercarbia. When a patient is breathing spontaneously and without clinical interventions, volatile anesthetics will increase the $PaCO_2$ about 5 to 15 mmHg. As the tidal volume decreases, dead space ventilation becomes a more significant part of each breath. With less fresh gas reaching the alveoli, hypoxia and hypercarbia ensue.

When comparing older agents, we find isoflurane causes more significant depression of ventilation than halothane. The response to hypoxia under isoflurane anesthesia (1 MAC) was depressed by 50% when tested in healthy volunteers.[24] When a patient is transitioning from an awake to a sedated state, low doses of isoflurane reduce the minute ventilation by about 34% whereas it does not change significantly with halothane. At higher doses, the minute ventilation is still reduced to a greater extent by isoflurane than by halothane. Respiratory rate changes are no different between these two agents.[25] In contrast to these older volatile agents, low-dose sevoflurane (0.1 MAC) of sevoflurane has little effect on the ventilatory response to hypoxia.[26] In experimental settings where subjects breathe a mildly hypoxic gas while the $PaCO_2$ is held constant, there is no increase in ventilation, and ventilation does not increase even in the presence of hypercarbia when the hypoxic drive is inhibited by volatile anesthetics.[27] All of the volatile anesthetics produce this result, as does propofol[28,29] (see Figure 19.12).

Results of past studies to determine the effect volatile anesthetics have on the acute ventilatory response to hypoxia have been controversial. This came about because different results were obtained when human subjects were studied under different conditions. The state of alertness of study subjects and whether changes creating hypoxia were introduced gradually or abruptly influenced the results. The same conditions may also matter in everyday clinical settings. However, earlier studies revealed that at low doses (less than 0.2 MAC) halothane

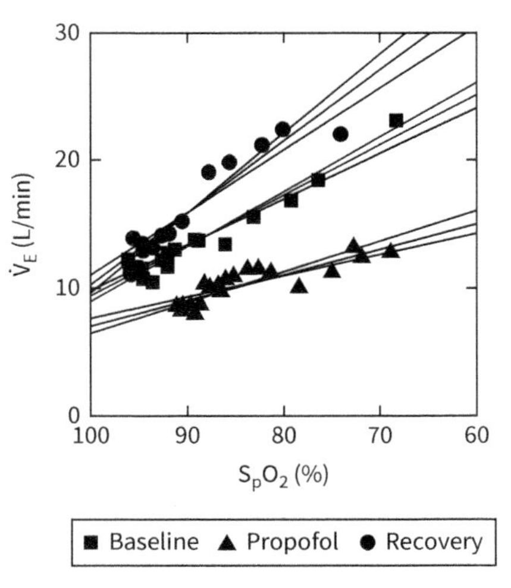

Figure 19.12 Hypoxic ventilatory response curves before, during, and 30 minutes after propofol infusion. Propofol infused for sedation decrease the slope and causes a downward shift of the hypoxic ventilatory response curve and is associated with decreased in minute ventilation and tidal volume decrease.

From Blouin RT, Seifert HA, Babenco HD, Conard PF, Gross JB. Propofol depresses the hypoxic ventilatory response during conscious sedation and isohypercapnia. *Anesthesiology*. 1993;79:1177–1182.

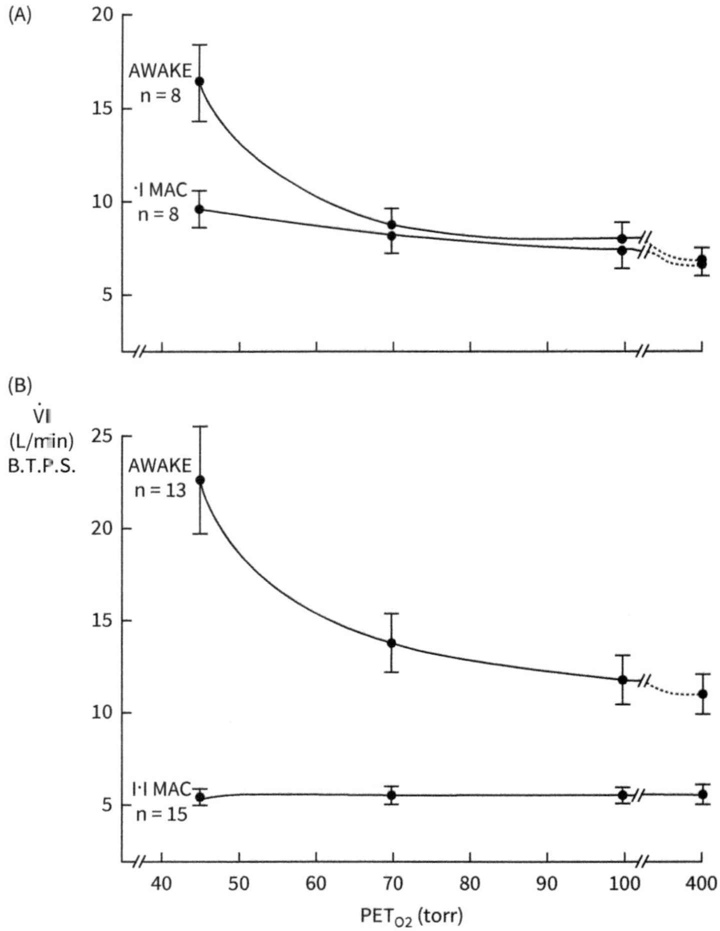

Figure 19.13 The effect of volatile anesthetic (in this case halothane) on the ventilatory response to hypoxia. At isocapnic states halothane sedation (A) and anesthesia (B) depresses or abolishes the ventilatory response to hypoxia.
From Knill RL and Gelb AW. *Anesthesiology.* 1978; 49:244–251.

profoundly depresses the acute ventilatory response to hypoxia.[30,31] (see Figure 19.13). Newer results support this conclusion, showing halothane, at about two-thirds MAC, significantly depressed carotid body response by 24%. There were no differences between individual halothane, enflurane, isoflurane.[32]

Opioids

The opioids are a group of drugs with potent analgesic and sedative effects. They are used extensively in hospitals for treatment of acute pain and sedation and in outpatient settings for chronic pain. Opioids include morphine, a naturally occurring compound extracted from the sap of poppies, and the semi-synthetic derivatives known as fenylpiperidines. This subgroup includes fentanyl, sufentanil, alfentanil, remifentanil, and the related compounds buprenorphine, oxycodone, and methadone.[33]

Opioids express their pharmacologic effect through binding with multiple μ-, δ-, and κ- opioid receptors.[34] The μ-opioid receptor is expressed on neurons in the brainstem, and there is convincing evidence it is this receptor that mediates opioid-induced respiratory depression.

Opioids induce slow, irregular respiration and will cause hypercarbia and hypoxia. However, the pharmacologic action of opioids on ventilation depends to great extent on the drug, the route, and the rate of administration. A slow infusion of opioid will result in the gradual onset of hypercapnia, while a bolus injection will cause apnea. Opioids profoundly depress the ventilatory responses to hypoxia and hypercarbia by depressing chemoreceptor activity.[35] This is characteristic of all opioids, and none are free of respiratory depression.

Excessive sedation, respiratory depression, pulmonary aspiration, chest wall rigidity, noncardiogenic pulmonary edema, bronchospasm, and depressed immunity are some of the pulmonary complications reported with opioid use. Deaths from respiratory depression and pulmonary complications have been reported with the abuse of opioid including illness from the route of drug administration.[36]

Noncardiogenic pulmonary edema (NCPE) is an unusual problem associated with opioids, although most cases involve diacetyl morphine, or heroin. The mechanism for this is unclear, but association with hypoxia, a neurogenic effect, an action increasing capillary permeability, or some direct effect of heroin have been proposed. Another mechanism may be attempting to inspire against an obstructed airway, thereby generating significant negative intrathoracic pressure.[37] In most instances NCPE usually resolves within 48 hours with supportive treatment.[38]

Chest wall rigidity can occur with opioid administration. Thoracic compliance changes rapidly and the chest simply becomes stiff. This is a well-known side effect with high-dose sufentanil anesthesia but is less frequent with fentanyl and other opioids. Chest wall rigidity is related to the dose and speed of administration. When it occurs during the induction of general anesthesia, it can make positive pressure mask ventilation difficult. This can be managed by administering a neuromuscular blocking drug or by administering an opioid antagonist such as naloxone.

Special Pathophysiological Situations

Pulmonary Hypertension

Pulmonary arterial hypertension (PAH) is the common result of a group of pulmonary diseases that is debilitating and associated with poor survival.[39] PAH can be caused by inheritable conditions and a variety of pulmonary diseases, secondary to systemic and cardiac disease, but, in many cases, it is idiopathic; it is also referred to as primary pulmonary hypertension. Historically PAH has been uncommon in the general population; increased awareness and more frequent testing with Doppler echocardiography may explain why it is now recognized more often. Management of patients with PAH requires regular evaluation and treatment assessment. Because it is relatively rare in the general population, patients with PAH are optimally managed at medical centers with experience with this disorder.

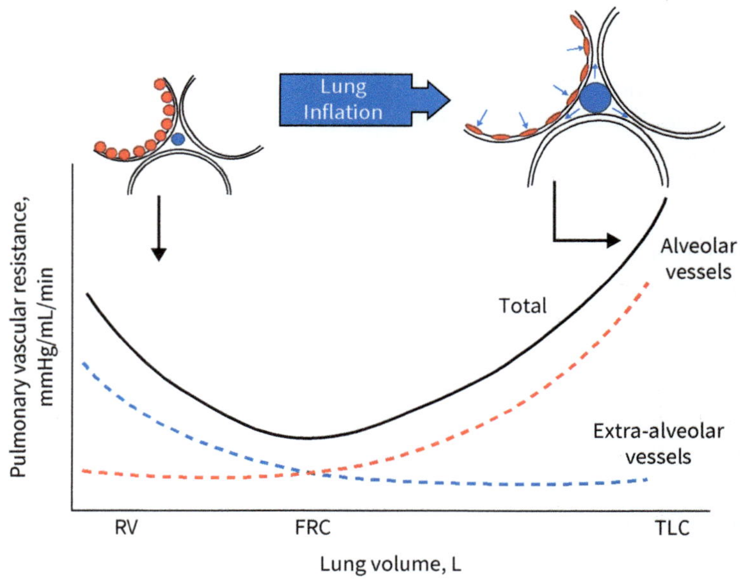

Figure 19.14 The minimum pulmonary vascular resistance occurs at the function reserve capacity volume and increases with over- or underexpansion of alveoli.

From Cortes-Puentes GA, Oeckler RA, Marini JJ. Physiology-guided management of hemodynamics in acute respiratory distress syndrome. *Ann Transl Med*. 2018;6(18):353. doi: 10.21037/atm.2018.04.40.

The normal mean PA pressure is 8 to 20 mmHg. PAH is the sustained elevation of a resting mean pulmonary arterial pressure 25 mmHg at rest or 30 mmHg with exercise and pulmonary capillary wedge pressure and left ventricular end-diastolic pressure <15 mmHg.[40,41] Progressive remodeling of the resistance pulmonary arteries and increasing pulmonary blood pressure occur during the course of this disease.

The pulmonary vasculature is normally a low-pressure system. Pulmonary arteries have thin walls and are easily distensible. This structure allows them to accommodate increases in blood flow from the right ventricle (RV) with little increase in pressure or resistance. The lowest pulmonary vascular resistance occurs at the FRC, that point where the outward pull from chest wall expansion is in equilibrium with the intrinsic elastic recoil of the pulmonary parenchyma. Pulmonary vascular resistance increases at extremes of under- or overexpansion of the lungs (see Figure 19.14). Pulmonary vascular resistance (PVR) is calculated by the difference between the measured pulmonary artery (PA) and pulmonary capillary wedge pressure and divided by the cardiac output. The normal range is 20 to 130 dynes•sec^{1}•cm^{-5}, about one-fifth the normal systemic vascular resistance.[42]

As PAH progresses, the pulmonary vessels become less distensible and reach a point where they cannot accommodate increased blood flow without increasing pulmonary pressure (see Figure 19.15). Patients with PAH have limited exercise tolerance and experience fatigue when activity requires increases in cardiac output.[43] Serious complications from PAH include hypoxia and right ventricular failure. Both can rapidly worsen during general anesthesia and surgery.

Patients with PAH often have systemic hypertension and obstructive sleep apnea, and both conditions contribute to the severity of PAH. Initial medical management of PAH requires demonstrating the pulmonary vasculature will respond to calcium channel blockers without

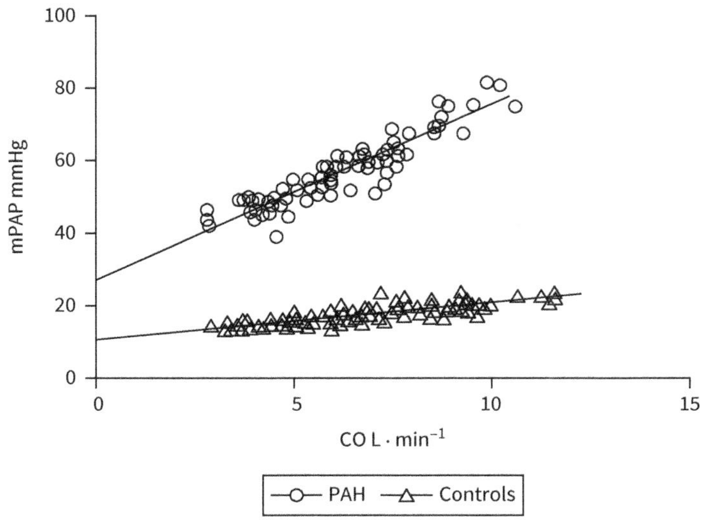

Figure 19.15 Arterial remodeling in pulmonary hypertension makes vessels less compliance and subject to greater pressures with increases in cardiac output.

From Simonneau G, Montani D, Cetermajer SD, Denton CP, Gatzoulis MA, Krowka M, Williams PG, Souza R. Haemodynamic definitions and updated clinical classification of pulmonary hypertension. *European Respiratory Journal* Jan 2019, 53 (1) 1801913; DOI: 10.1183/13993003.01913-2018.

significant side effects. First-line treatments include the calcium channel blockers nifedipine, diltiazem, or amlodipine. With increasing disease severity, the addition of ambrisentan (an endothelial receptor antagonist) or tadalafil or sildenafil (phosphodiesterase-type 5 inhibitors) are recommended in PAH. Other endothelial receptor antagonists, bosentan, macitentan, and riociguat (a cGMP stimulator) are recommended to slow the progression of PAH. In severe cases, continuous administration of prostacyclin derivatives epoprostenol by the intravenous route or treprostinil subcutaneously are recommended. These drugs are often used in combination to attain treatment goals.[44]

PAH is exacerbated by chronic obstructive pulmonary disease (COPD), pulmonary thromboembolism, hypoxia, hypercarbia, acidosis, cardiopulmonary bypass, reperfusion injury, micro-emboli, or systemic inflammatory mediators. Optimization of COPD in the preoperative surgical patient with bronchodilators, antibiotics, and steroids is essential. Anticoagulation prior to surgery in those patients prone to thromboembolism is also important.

Pulmonary blood pressure increases during general anesthesia when surgical triggers stimulate PVR. Increases in PVR can stress the RV, and for patients with coronary artery disease this may cause myocardial ischemia and a decrease in right ventricular contractility. Close attention must be given to any electrocardiographic changes, hypoxemia, and systemic low blood pressure because they may reflect right heart strain and ischemia. Treatments approaches include optimizing the RV preload and reducing afterload.[45]

Several actions can be taken during anesthesia to minimize sympathetic stimulation that may worsen pulmonary blood pressures (see Box 19.1). Correcting hypoxemia and acidosis are useful, and optimizing right-sided cardiac preload requires carefully titrating intravenous fluids and observing for an increased mean arterial pressure response. Intravascular fluid volume in excess of what the RV can handle will likely cause complications. Intravenous anesthetics have a significant role in managing these patients. Propofol, fentanyl, sufentanil,

Box 19.1 Anesthetic Interventions to Minimize Increases in Pulmonary Arterial Pressure

1. Avoid hypoxia—insure adequate oxygenation with > 60% F_iO_2
2. Avoid hypercarbia and respiratory acidosis with moderate hyperventilation (P_aCO_2 30-35 mm Hg)
3. Avoid metabolic acidosis
4. Avoid high airway pressure—ventilate with 6-8 mL/kg ideal body weight
5. Utilize recruitment maneuvers to avoid atelectasis and $\dot{V}/\dot{Q}$ mismatch
6. Maintain normothermia (36–37°C)
7. Employ goal-directed fluid management to avoid excess fluid administration

Source: Adopted from Gille J, Seyfarth H-J, Gerlach S, Malcharek M, Czeslick E, Sablotzki A. Perioperative anesthesiological management of patients with pulmonary hypertension. *Anesthesiology Research and Practice*. 2012, Article ID 356982, 16 pages. doi:10.1155/2012/356982.

and ketamine have all been used with success as they have minimal effects on hypoxic ventilation, vascular reactivity, and oxygenation during one lung ventilation. Pharmacologic treatment of right ventricular failure in the face of increased PVR requires vasodilating drugs rather than vasopressors. There are several options available for long-term treatment of PAH. However, immediate options for improving RV function during anesthesia include adenosine and phosphodiesterase inhibitors.[46]

Pulmonary Embolism

Pulmonary embolism is a very serious problem that carries a high risk of mortality. In a composite study of 14 publications that totaled 11,218 Asian patients, the incidence of PE averaged 0.18%, ranging from 0% to 0.58%.[47] A cohort study from the UK analyzed 18,151 trauma and elective orthopedic patients with symptoms suggesting a PE, which were then examined by computer tomography (CT) scan for confirmation, found the overall incidence was only 0.47%. Among those patients who developed a PE, however, the mortality was 15.29%.[48] Like similar studies, these reports do not separate intraoperative from postoperative PE occurrence. The intraoperative incidence of embolization has been estimated to range from 0.6% to 10%.[49]

PE is often encountered in patients with deep vein thrombosis presenting for vascular procedures to prevent a thrombus from embolizing to the lungs. Depending on the extent of pulmonary vascular obstruction, pulmonary symptoms can range from mild dyspnea to hypotension or shock, and often the pulmonary embolism (PE) presents as acute cardiovascular collapse and death.

Principle physical signs of acute PE are worsening dyspnea, chest pain, or sustained hypotension without other identifiable cause. In stable patients the optimal evaluation includes CT scan to detect emboli in the pulmonary arteries. Patients experiencing a PE can be hemodynamically unstable with severe hypotension or cardiac arrest with pulseless electrical activity. As an alternative in emergency situations, transthoracic echocardiography or transesophageal echocardiography (TEE) can be used to assist in the diagnosis of pulmonary thromboembolism. Some signs suggesting PE include right heart strain with dissension of the RV, hypokinesis of the RV apex, and thrombi in the RV or pulmonary arteries.[50] Echocardiography does not always provide a definitive diagnosis, however; only with TEE is it possible to visualize thrombi in the main and right pulmonary arteries, as the left is obscured from view by the left main stem bronchus.[51]

Pulmonary embolism increases dead space ventilation as the lungs continue receiving ventilation but with reduced blood flow. This creates a right to left shunt where oxygenation of pulmonary arterial blood is compromised. When thrombi lodge in distal pulmonary arteries, the blood flow redirects and increases flow in areas of the lung with continuing perfusion. This can cause pulmonary edema and alveolar hemorrhage. Thrombi lodging in the main, right, or left pulmonary arteries can result in hypotension, often severe, and severe elevation of RV and right atrial pressures, leading to low cardiac output. The effect on the RV is dilation with increased RV afterload. This increases RV wall stress and, when combined with systemic hypotension, can decrease RV myocardial perfusion and cause myocardial ischemia or infarction.

Single-Lung Ventilation Scenarios

Laparoscopic procedures offer challenges in anesthesia management because of abdominal insufflation and the steep head-down positioning required. Insufflation of the abdomen with carbon dioxide gas and the patient's position push the diaphragm cephalad. With insufflation the inspiratory ventilatory pressures, arterial CO_2, and end-tidal carbon dioxide ($EtCO_2$) increase, and there are corresponding decreases in lung compliance and tidal volume.[52] These changes are usually not difficult to manage.

When repositioning patients for surgery, endotracheal tubes may be dislodged. During laparoscopic surgery with reverse Trendelenburg positioning, effective movement of the endotracheal tube can be easily missed because the tube is anchored to the head while cephalad movement of the lungs can cause the tube to slide into a main stem bronchus. In this setting, movement of the endotracheal tube during laparoscopy is common, with the tube moving toward the carina in 50% of cases and with right main bronchus intubation in over 15% of patients. Despite this, no significant changes in SpO_2, $EtCO_2$, or inspiratory peak pressure were observed.[53] Laparoscopic procedures present risks for other events with potential for pulmonary implications including hypotension, subcutaneous emphysema, pneumothorax, and carbon dioxide embolism.[54]

Maintaining HPV to shunt blood away from nonventilated area of the lung is important, particularly in thoracic procedures. Separation of lung ventilation with double lumen endotracheal tubes allows for ventilation of one lung while the operative lung is deflated. Usually the blood flow to the deflated lung is not interrupted during these surgical procedures. When single-lung ventilation begins, the complete mismatch of ventilation and perfusion in the deflated lung would cause significant hypoxemia if the reflex is suppressed by anesthetics.[55]

References

1. Levitzky MG, ed. *Pulmonary Physiology*. 9th ed. New York, NY: McGraw-Hill.
2. Jacobi MS, Patil CP, Saunders KB. The transient ventilatory response to carbon dioxide at rest and in exercise in man. *Resp Physiol*. 1989;(77):225–238.
3. West JB Luks AM. West's Respiratory Physiology (11th ed). Wolter Kluwer; 2021.

4. Dixon FJ, Dixon JB, Carden JR, Burn AJ, Schachter LM. Pre-oxygenation is more effective in the 25° head-up position than in the supine position in severely obese patients: a randomized controlled study. *Anesthesiology.* 2005;102(6):1110–1115.
5. Forster RE. Exchange of gas between alveolar air and pulmonary capillary blood: pulmonary diffusing capacity. *Physiological Reviews*, 1957; 37(4):391–452.
6. Raymond LW The alveolar air equation abbreviated. *Chest.* 1978;74(6):675–676.
7. Brismar B, Hedenstierna G, Lundquist H, et al. Pulmonary densities during anesthesia with muscular relaxation: a proposal of atelectasis. *Anesthesiology.* 1985;62:422–428.
8. Lundquist H, Hedenstierna G, Strandberg A, et al. CT-assessment of dependent lung densities in man during general anaesthesia. *Acta Radiol.* 1995;36:626–632.
9. Rothen HU, Sporre B, Engberg G, Wegenius G, Hedenstierna G. Re-expansion of atelectasis during general anaesthesia: a computed tomography study. *Brit J Anaesth.* 1993;71(6):788–795.
10. Moudgil R, Michelakis ED, Archer SL. Hypoxic pulmonary vasoconstriction. *J Appl Physiology.* 2005;98:390–403.
11. Bendixen HH, Henley-Whyte J, Laver MB. Impaired oxygenation in surgical patients during general anesthesia with controlled ventilation. a concept of atelectasis. *N Engl J Med.* 1963;269:991–996.
12. Visick WD, Farley HB, Hickey RF. The effects of tidal volume and end-expiratory pressure on pulmonary gas exchange during anesthesia. *Anesthesiology.* 1973;39:285–290.
13. Sherpa Neto A, Cardozo SO, Manetta JA, et al. Association between use of lung-protective ventilation with lower tidal volumes and clinical outcomes among patients without acute respiratory distress syndrome: a meta-analysis. *JAMA.* 2012;308:1651–1659.
14. Sherpa Neto A, Simonis FD, Barbas CS, et al. Association between tidal volume size, duration of ventilation, and sedation needs in patients without acute respiratory distress syndrome: an individual patient data meta-analysis. *Intensive Care Med.* 2014;40:950–957.
15. Putensen CK, Theurkauf N, Zinserling J, Wrigge H, Pelosi P. Meta-analysis: ventilation strategies and outcomes of the acute respiratory distress syndrome and acute lung injury. *Ann Intern Med.* 2009;151:566–576.
16. Brower RG, Matthau MA, Morris A, Schoenfeld D, Thompson BT, Wheeler A; Acute Respiratory Distress Syndrome Network. Ventilation with lower tidal volumes as compared with traditional tidal volumes for acute lung injury and a the actuate respiratory distress syndrome. *N Engl J Med.* 2000;342:1301–1308.
17. Schaefer MS, Serpa Neto A, Pelosi P, et al. Temporal changes in ventilator settings in patients with uninjured lungs: a systematic review. *Anesth Analg.* 2019;129(1):129–135.
18. Goodman NW, Black AM, Carter JA: Some ventilatory effects of propofol as sole anaesthetic agent. *Br J Anaesth.* 1987;59:1497–503.
19. Goodman, NW Black, AM Carter, JA, Lee YS: Effects of propofol target-controlled infusion on haemodynamic and respiratory changes with regard to safety. *J Int Med Res.* 2004;32:19–24.
20. Lee M-H, Yang K-H, Lee C-S, et al. The effect-site concentration of propofol producing respiratory depression during spinal anesthesia. *Korean J Anesthesiol.* 2011;61(2):122–126.
21. Malin M. Jonsson, Sten G. E. Lindahl, Lars I. Eriksson. Effect of propofol on carotid body chemosensitivity and cholinergic chemotransduction. *Anesthesiology.* 2005;102(1):110–116.
22. Dohi S, Gold MI. Pulmonary mechanics during general anaesthesia: the influence of mechanical irritation on the airway. *Br J Anaesth.* 1979;51:205–213; Gal TJ. Pulmonary mechanics in normal subjects following endotracheal intubation. *Anesthesiology.* 1980;52:27–35.
23. Wendell OE, Rooke AG, Sai-Chuen Wu R, Bishop MJ; Comparison of the effects of etomidate, propofol, and thiopental on respiratory resistance after tracheal intubation. *Anesthesiology.* 1996;84(6):1307–1311.
24. D. Sjogren, S.G. Lindahl, A. Sollevi. Ventilatory responses to acute and sustained hypoxia during isoflurane anesthesia. *Anesth Analg.* 1986;86:403–409.

25. Canet J, Sanchis J, Zegrí A, Llorente C, Navajas D, Casan P. Effects of halothane and isoflurane on ventilation and occlusion pressure. *Anesthesiology.* 1994;81(3):563–571.
26. Pandit JJ, Manning-Fox J, Dorrington KL, Robbins PA. Effects of subanaesthetic sevoflurane on ventilation. 2: Response to acute and sustained hypoxia in humans. *Br J Anaesth.* 1999;83(2):210–216.
27. Pandit, J.J. Effect of low dose inhaled anaesthetic agents on the ventilatory response to carbon dioxide in humans: a quantitative review. *Anaesthesia.* 2005;60:461–469.
28. Pandit JJ. Volatile anaesthetic depression of the carotid body chemoreflex-mediated ventilatory response to hypoxia: directions for future research. Scientifica 2014;2014:394270
29. Blouin RT, Seifert HA, Babenco HD, Conard PF, Gross, JB. Propofol depresses the hypoxic ventilatory response during conscious sedation and isohypercapnia. *Anesthesiology.* 1993;79:1177–1182.
30. Knill RL, Gelb AW. Ventilatory responses to hypoxia and hypercapnia during halothane sedation and anesthesia in man. *Anesthesiology.* 1978;49:244–251.
31. Knill RL, Clement JL. Site of selective action of halothane on the peripheral chemoreflex pathway in humans. *Anesthesiology.* 1984;61:121–126.
32. Pandit JJ, O'Gallagher K. Effects of volatile anesthetics on carotid body response to hypoxia in animals. In: Poulin MJ, Wilson RJA, eds. *Integration in Respiratory Control. Advances in Experimental Medicine and Biology.* Vol 605. New York, NY: Springer; 2008.
33. Dahan A, Niesters M, Olofsen E, Smith T, Overdyk F. Opioids. In Barash PG, Cullen BF, Stoelting RK, Cahalan MK, Stock MC, Ortega R, eds. *Clinical Anesthesia.* 7th ed. Philadelphia: Lippincott, Williams & Wilkins; 2013: 501–522.
34. Martin WR. Opioid antagonists. *Pharmacol Rev.* 1967;19:463–521.
35. Weil JV, McCullough RE, Kline JS, Sodal IE. Diminished ventilatory response to hypoxia and hypercapnia after morphine in normal man. *N Engl J Med.* 1975;292:1103–1106.
36. Radke JB, Owen KP, Sutter ME, Ford JB, Albertson TE. The effect of opioids on the lung. *Clinic Rev Allerg Immunol.* 2014;46:54–64.
37. Sterrett C. Patterns of presentation in heroin overdose resulting in pulmonary edema. *Am J Emerg Med.* 2003;21:32–34.
38. Horng HC, Ho MT, Huang CH, Yeh CC, Cherng CH. Negative pressure pulmonary edema following naloxone administration in a patient with fentanyl-induced respiratory depression. *Acta Anaesthesiol Taiwan.* 2010;48:155–157.
39. Prins KW, Thenappan T. WHO Group I pulmonary hypertension: epidemiology and pathophysiology. *Cardiol Clin.* 2016;34(3):363374.
40. Badesch DB, Champion HC, Gomez Sanchez MA, et al. Diagnosis and assessment of pulmonary arterial hypertension. *J Am Coll Cardiol.* 2009;54(1 Suppl):S55–S66.
41. Farber HW, Loscalzo J. Pulmonary arterial hypertension. *N Engl J Med.* 2004;351(16):1655–1665.
42. Kelly CR, Rabbani LE. Pulmonary-artery catheterization. *N Engl J Med.* 2013;369(25):e35.
43. Lau EMT, Vanderpool RR, Choudhary P, et al. Dobutamine stress echocardiography for the assessment of pressure-flow relationships of the pulmonary circulation. *Chest.* 2014;146:959–966.
44. Therapy for pulmonary arterial hypertension in adults: update of the CHEST Guideline and Expert Panel Report. *Chest.* 2019;155(3):565–586.
45. Fisher L, Van Aiken H, Bürkle H. Management of pulmonary hypertension: physiological and pharmacological considerations for anesthesiologists. *Anesth Analgesic.* 2003;96:1603–1616.
46. Fisher L, Van Aiken H, Bürkle H. Management of pulmonary hypertension: physiological and pharmacological considerations for anesthesiologists. *Anesth Analgesic.* 2003;96:1603–1616.
47. Yeo DXW, Junnarkar S, Balasubramaniam S, et al. Incidence of venous thromboembolism and its pharmacological prophylaxis in Asian general surgery patients: a systematic review. *World J Surg.* 2015;39:150–157.
48. Gudipati S, Fragkakis EM, Ciriella V, et al. A cohort study on the incidence and outcome of pulmonary embolism in trauma and orthopedic patients. *BMC Med.* 2014;12:39.

49. Koesssler MJ. Fabianai R, Hamer H, Pitto RP. The clinical relevance of embolic events detected by TEE during cemented total hip arthroplasty: a multicenter clinical trial. *Anesth Analg.* 2001;92:49–55.
50. Rosenberger P, Shernan SK, Body S, Eltzschig HK. Utility of intraoperative transesophageal echocardiography for diagnosis of pulmonary embolism. *Anesth Analg.* 2004; 99(1):12–16.
51. Rosenberger P, Shernan SK, Body SC, Eltzschig HK. Utility of intraoperative transesophageal echocardiography for diagnosis of pulmonary embolism. *Anesth Analg.* 2004; 99:12–16.
52. Iwasaka H, Miyakawa H, Yamamoto H, Kitano T, Taniguchi K, Honda N. Respiratory mechanics and arterial blood gases during and after laparoscopic cholecystectomy. *Can J Anaesth.* 1996;43(2):129–133.
53. Ezri T, Hazin V, Warters D, Szmuk P, Weinbroum AA. The endotracheal tube moves more often in obese patients undergoing laparoscopy compared with open abdominal surgery. *Anesth Analg.* 2003;96:278–282.
54. Wahba Ma RWM, Tessler MJ. Tessler, Kleiman SJ. Acute ventilatory complications during laparoscopic upper abdominal surgery. *Can J Anaesth.* 1996;43(1):77–83.
55. Nagendran J, Stewart K, Hoskinson M, Archer SL. An anesthesiologist's guide to hypoxic pulmonary vasoconstriction: implications for managing single-lung anesthesia and atelectasis. *Curr Opin Anaesthesiol.* 2006;19(1):34–43A.

20 Anesthetic Management Techniques (Regional Anesthesia)

Tyler Kabes, Rene Przkora, and Juan C. Mora

Thoracic Epidural

Introduction

The thoracic epidural is one of the earliest developed regional techniques. It was first described by Fidel Pagés in 1921, and in the 1930s it became a more widely accepted form of anesthesia.[1] Today, the epidural is an essential component of perioperative pain management with broad clinical applications, including abdominal, thoracic, gynecologic, and urologic surgeries.[2] A growing body of research has suggested that local anesthetics in the epidural space can provide a multitude of benefits such as improved postoperative pain control and reduced postoperative pulmonary dysfunction, duration of mechanical ventilation, and ileus.[3]

Thoracic epidural procedures are generally regarded as safe but must be performed with caution and precision due to their inherent anatomic environment: deep to the epidural space is the spinal cord and subarachnoid space, laterally are the thoracic nerve roots, and throughout the epidural space is a significant vascular burden, both arterial and venous. Epidural hematoma, although rare, is a serious complication that can be mitigated through appropriate assessment of coagulation status and platelet abnormalities (see Table 20.1). The hemodynamic effects of epidural anesthetics, secondary to sympathetic blockade, may also limit their use in selected patients.

Indications

Indications include breast, cardiac, chest wall, esophageal, and thoracic wall surgery, as well as multiple rib fractures (see Table 20.2).

Anatomy

Thoracic epidural anesthesia is thought to be achieved through local anesthetic distribution to the spinal nerves within the paravertebral space, as well as from penetration through the dura mater to the spinal cord and thoracic nerve roots.[4] Needle entry within the epidural space requires traversing several tissue planes when performed in a midline approach: skin, subcutaneous fat, supraspinous ligament, interspinous ligament, and ligamentum flavum.

Table 20.1 Clinical Characteristics and Complications of Techniques

Block Type	Allows Use of Catheter	Ultrasound Required	Requires Holding Anticoagulation	Complications
Thoracic epidural	Yes	No (could be used to identify landmarks)	Yes	• Accidental intrathecal injection • Epidural abscess • Epidural hematoma • Intravascular injection • Local anesthetic systemic toxicity • Nerve root or spinal cord injury • Pneumothorax
Thoracic paravertebral	Yes	No (could be used to identify landmarks and perform block)	Yes	• Accidental epidural or intrathecal injection • Hematoma • Horner syndrome (transient) • Intravascular injection via intercostal artery or vein • Local anesthetic toxicity • Pneumothorax • Spinal or intercostal nerve injury
Intercostal nerve block	Yes	No (could be used to identify landmarks and perform block)	No	• Intercostal nerve injury • Intravascular injection via intercostal artery or vein • Local anesthetic toxicity • Pneumothorax
Pecs I and II blocks	No	Required	No	• Intravascular injection via pectoral branch of the thoracoacromial artery • Local anesthetic toxicity • Neuraxial spread • Pneumothorax
Serratus anterior plane block	No	Required	No	• Intercostal nerve injury • Intravascular injection via intercostal artery or vein • Local anesthetic toxicity • Pneumothorax
Erector spinae plane block	Yes	Required	No	• Local anesthetic toxicity • Pneumothorax
Transversus thoracis muscle plane block	No	Required	No	• Intravascular injection via internal thoracic artery or vein • Local anesthetic toxicity • Pericardial puncture • Pneumothorax

Table 20.2 Regional Coverage, Indications, and Technical Degree of Techniques

Block Type	Regional Coverage	Indications	Technical Degree
Thoracic epidural	Anterior, lateral, and posterior thoracic wall	Breast, cardiac, chest wall, esophageal, and thoracic wall surgery; multiple rib fractures	High
Thoracic paravertebral	Anterior, lateral, and posterior thoracic wall Internal organs of thorax (e.g., esophagus, heart, lungs)	Breast, cardiac, chest wall, esophageal, thoracic wall surgery, multiple rib fractures	High
Intercostal nerve block	Anterolateral, lateral, posterolateral thoracic wall	Breast, chest wall, and thoracic wall surgery; chest tube placement; rib fracture(s)	Intermediate
Pecs I and II blocks	Anterolateral and lateral thoracic wall	Breast surgery including axillary dissection; chest wall and thoracic wall surgery	Intermediate
Serratus anterior plane block	Anterolateral and lateral thoracic wall	Breast surgery including axillary dissection; chest wall and thoracic wall surgery	Low
Erector spinae plane block	Anterolateral, lateral, posterolateral thoracic wall	Breast, chest wall, and thoracic wall surgery	Low
Transversus thoracis muscle plane block	Anterior thoracic wall	Anterior thoracic wall and breast surgery, ICD placement	Intermediate

Abbreviation: ICD, implantable cardioverter-defibrillator.

The paramedian approach, commonly used in thoracic epidurals due to the inferiorly angled spinous processes, bypasses the supraspinous and interspinous ligaments to enter the epidural space (Figure 20.1B and 20.1C).

The posterior epidural space contains several important structures: vessels, adipose tissue, spinal nerve roots, and the dural sac. Arterial supply to the epidural space is derived from the posterior arterial arcade, which runs up and down the spinal canal. The venous drainage includes two posterior longitudinal veins that are part of a broad vertebral venous plexus connecting to the anterior epidural space.[5] The rich vascularity of the posterior epidural space contributes to a risk of vessel puncture, intravascular catheter or injection, and epidural hematoma, as well as increased local anesthetic absorption when performing neuraxial techniques. Adipose tissue is abundant throughout the posterior epidural space and is thought to play an important role in the variability of local anesthetic duration, onset, sensitivity, and spread.[6] The spinal nerve roots, each comprising a dorsal and ventral root, arise as direct branches of the spinal cord. Within the thoracic segments, the dorsal nerve roots carry afferent sensory fibers, while the ventral nerve roots carry efferent motor and sympathetic fibers. These nerve roots travel laterally to the intervertebral foramen and fuse to become a single spinal nerve.[7] The dural sac is a protective membrane surrounding the spinal cord; it comprises the ventral limit of the posterior epidural space.

Local Anesthetic

Commonly used local anesthetics include 2-chloroprocaine, lidocaine, bupivacaine, and ropivacaine. Surgical anesthesia may be achieved with 3% 2-chloroprocaine and 2% lidocaine formulations, as well as higher concentrations of bupivacaine and ropivacaine (e.g., 0.5%). Lower concentrations of bupivacaine and ropivacaine (0.1%–0.25%) are preferred for perioperative analgesia to decrease motor fiber blockade. Local anesthetic dosing encompasses a variety of surgical- and patient-related factors and must be determined within the immediate, or anticipated, clinical context.

Equipment

- 17- or 18-gauge epidural Tuohy needle
- 3 mL of 1.5% lidocaine with epinephrine (1:200,000)
- Loss of resistance syringe
- Sterile draping
- Syringe and needle for cutaneous local infiltration
- Syringe with extension tubing for block injection or epidural catheter for continuous infusion

Procedural Technique

Position the patient seated with the neck and upper back flexed. Identify the target interspace by palpation and surface anatomic landmarks or by using ultrasound.

>> Tip on Technique

The C7 vertebra has a distinctly prominent spinous process. The scapular spine and inferior border correlate to T3 and T7 levels, respectively.

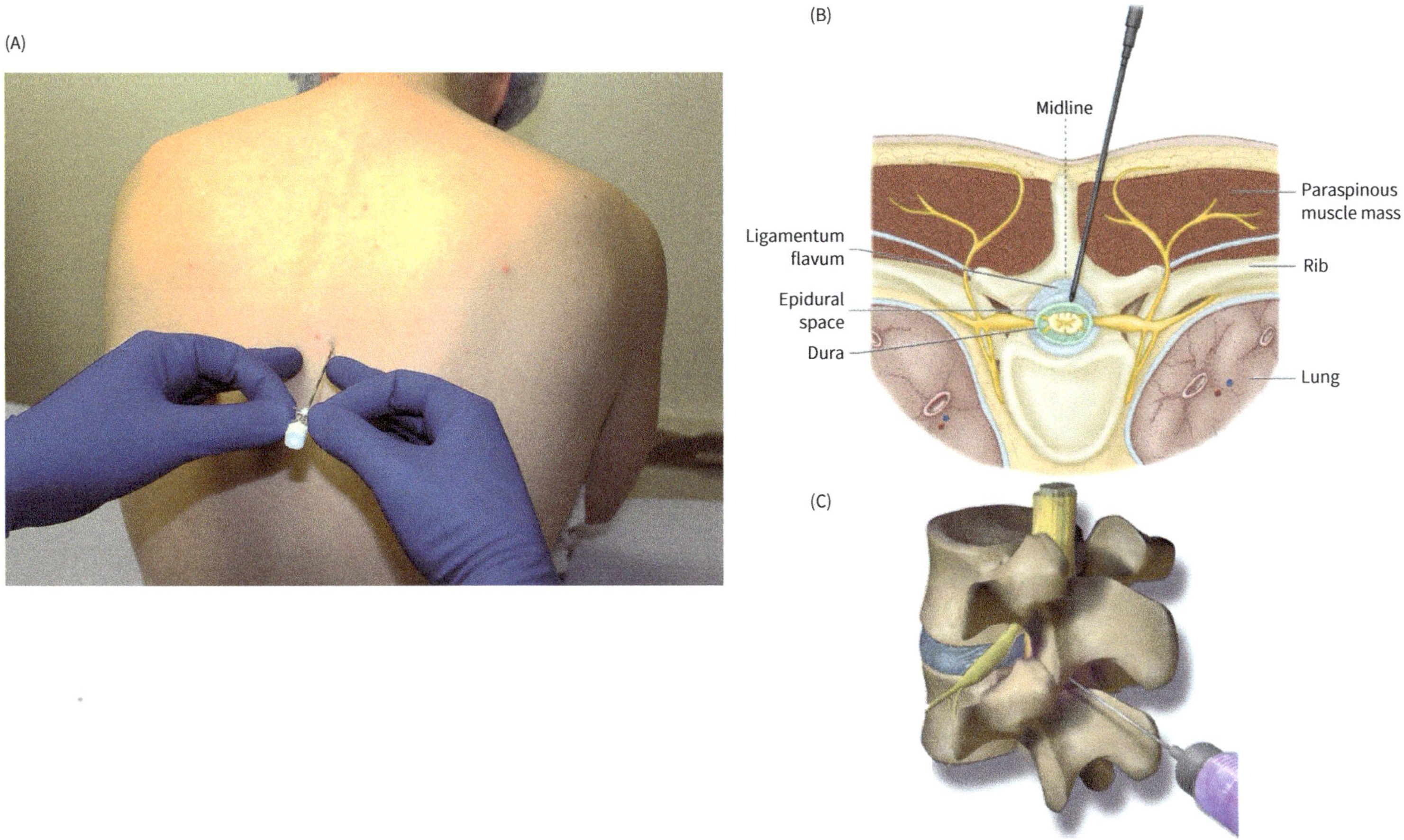

Figure 20.1 (A) Needle positioning for the thoracic epidural with a paramedian approach. (B) Anatomy of the thoracic epidural performed with a paramedian approach. (C) Paramedian approach to epidural placement.

(B) Reprinted with permission from Butterworth JF, Mackey DC, Wasnick JD. *Morgan and Mikhail's Clinical Anesthesiology*. McGraw-Hill Education. Figure 45-15.

(C) Modified from Blausen.com staff (2014) "Medical gallery of Blausen Medical 2014." WikiJournal of Medicine 1(2)/CC BY3.0.

> **>> Tip on Technique**
>
> This can be performed by anchoring the middle fingertips on the patient's back with the thumbs and index fingers holding the needle wings.
>
> Prepare and drape the targeted interspace(s) in a sterile fashion. Infiltrate a local anesthetic (most commonly, 1% lidocaine) 1 cm lateral to the inferior margin of the target spinous process. The local anesthetic needle should be used to create a large skin wheal and then advanced to the lamina or transverse process to anesthetize periosteum. Advance a styletted epidural Tuohy needle, bevel facing cephalad, within the previous local anesthetic trajectory until the lamina or transverse process is contacted (Figure 20.1A).

> **>> Tip on Technique**
>
> Administering a test dose of 3 mL of 1.5% lidocaine with epinephrine (1:200,000) 3 to 5 minutes prior to initiating a bolus or infusion regimen can help identify intrathecal or intravascular placement.

The epidural needle should be retracted and readvanced medially until the lamina is contacted more superficially, indicating a near midline needle trajectory. Again, retract the epidural needle and advance cephalad with a similar medial angle. When the epidural needle depth exceeds that of the medial lamina and bone has not been contacted, the epidural needle stylet should be removed and a loss of resistance syringe applied. Advance the needle until loss of resistance is achieved, remove the loss of resistance syringe, and, after negative aspiration, inject a local anesthetic or advance the catheter 3 to 6 cm within the epidural space.

Complications

- Accidental intrathecal injection
- Epidural abscess
- Epidural hematoma
- Intravascular injection
- Local anesthetic systemic toxicity
- Nerve root or spinal cord injury
- Pneumothorax

Thoracic Paravertebral

Introduction

The thoracic paravertebral block (TPVB) was first performed in 1905 by Hugo Sellheim of Leipzig in an effort to replace spinal anesthetics while still providing analgesia and abdominal muscle relaxation. It provides analgesia in a unilateral and segmental fashion through local anesthetic infiltration within a wedge-shaped region near the vertebral body called the paravertebral space.[8]

Imaging and cadaveric studies have demonstrated variable distributions of injectate spread when performing a TPVB: remaining localized, craniocaudal spread to adjacent paravertebral spaces, lateral movement to the intercostal space, and medial movement to the epidural space. Single injections have demonstrated craniocaudal coverage of three to four dermatomes, although this distribution is inconsistent. Multiple site injection techniques, where local anesthetic injections are performed in small volumes at consecutive or alternating levels (e.g., T3, 5, 7), may be preferred when the TPVB is the sole anesthetic.[8,9]

The TPVB has demonstrated similar analgesic efficacy compared to the thoracic epidural for thoracotomy.[10] Patients undergoing breast, inguinal hernia, and nephrectomy surgeries have also shown significant improvement in perioperative pain scores.[8,11] This regional technique offers the advantage of a more targeted unilateral coverage, reduced perioperative hypotension and urinary retention, reduced postoperative nausea and vomiting, and a lower rate of block failure compared to thoracic epidurals.[8,10,11]

Indications

Indications are breast, cardiac, chest wall, esophageal, and thoracic wall surgery and multiple rib fractures.

Anatomy

The TPVB provides unilateral and segmental analgesic coverage through local anesthetic infiltration within the paravertebral space. This wedge-shaped region found on either side of the vertebral column extends from the cervical spine to the sacrum. At the thoracic level, it is bounded anteriorly by the parietal pleura, posteriorly by the superior costotransverse ligament, and medially by the vertebral body and disc. Laterally, it is in continuity with the intercostal space (Figure 20.2C). The thoracic paravertebral space is filled with adipose tissue and contains several important vascular and nervous structures: the intercostal artery and vein, sympathetic trunk, and dorsal and ventral rami of the thoracic spinal nerve.[8] The intercostal artery and vein begin in an anteromedial position and move posterolaterally within the intercostal space. Prior to their distal entry in the subcostal groove, these vessels remain unprotected and can be a source of intravascular injection or hematoma.[12] The sympathetic trunk is found at the anteromedial limit of the paravertebral space and contributes to a segmental sympathectomy.[8] Local anesthetic distributions reaching the cervical paravertebral space and stellate ganglion may also induce transient ipsilateral Horner syndrome.[8,11] The thoracic spinal nerve enters from the medial aspect via the intervertebral foramen and quickly branches into the dorsal and ventral rami. The dorsal rami move posteriorly to provide motor and sensory innervation to the posterior thorax. The ventral rami continue laterally to become the intercostal nerves, which travel within the subcostal groove to provide motor and sensory innervation from the posterolateral to the anterior thorax.

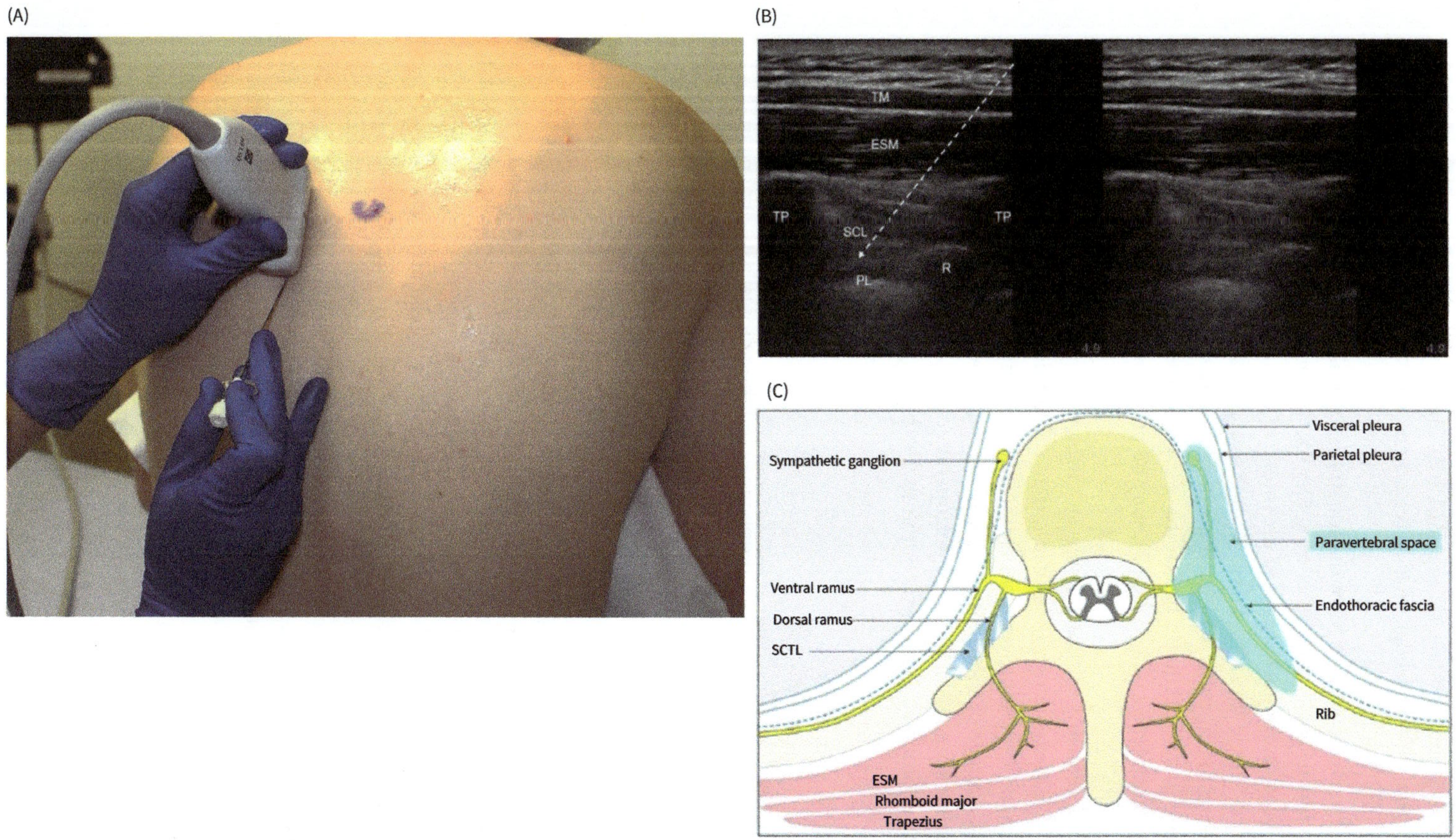

Figure 20.2 (A) Ultrasound transducer and needle positioning for the thoracic paravertebral block. (B) Ultrasound anatomy and needle trajectory of the thoracic paravertebral block. (C) Anatomy of the thoracic paravertebral space.

Reprinted from Pawa A, Wojcikiewicz T, Barron A, El-Boghdadly K. Paravertebral blocks: anatomical, practical, and future concepts. *Curr Anesthesiol Rep*. 2019;9:263–270/CC BY4.0.

Abbreviations: ESM, erector spinae muscles; PL, pleura; R, rib; SCL, superior costotransverse ligament; SCTL, superior costotransverse ligament; TM, trapezius muscle; TP, transverse process.

Local Anesthetic

Long-acting local anesthetics, such as bupivacaine or ropivacaine, are most commonly used: 0.5% bupivacaine or 0.5% ropivacaine can be given as a single injection of 20 mL or as multiple injections of 4 to 5 mL at consecutive or alternating levels (e.g., T3, 5, 7). For continuous infusions, 0.25% bupivacaine or 0.2% ropivacaine can be used at 0.1 mL/kg/h.

Equipment

- 17- or 18-gauge epidural Tuohy needle
- Linear, high-frequency ultrasound transducer (ultrasound-guided technique)
- Loss of resistance syringe (landmark-based technique)
- Marking pen
- Sterile draping
- Syringe and needle for cutaneous local infiltration
- Syringe with extension tubing for block injection or epidural catheter for continuous infusion

Procedural Technique

Landmark-Based Technique

Position the patient seated with the head resting in the forward position. Identify the target thoracic vertebral levels and their corresponding spinous processes. Mark the skin 2.5 cm lateral to the cephalad portion of each targeted spinous process. Each skin mark represents a needle entry point that overlies the transverse process of one lower thoracic vertebrae. Prepare and drape the targeted interspace(s) in a sterile fashion. Infiltrate a local anesthetic (most commonly, 1% lidocaine) within the marked area to create a skin wheal, then advance the needle until contact with the transverse process is made and anesthetize the periosteum. If the transverse process is not contacted by 4 cm, the proceduralist should withdraw the needle and readvance in a cephalad or caudad direction before advancing further. Advance a styletted Tuohy needle, bevel facing cephalad, until the transverse process is contacted (Figure 20.3). Walk the needle off the inferior border of the transverse process, then remove the Tuohy needle stylet and apply a loss of resistance syringe. Advance until loss of resistance is achieved, approximately 1 cm beyond the transverse process. This will indicate that the needle has penetrated the superior costotransverse ligament and passed into the thoracic paravertebral space. Remove the loss of resistance syringe and, after negative aspiration, inject a local anesthetic or advance the catheter 1 to 3 cm within the paravertebral space.

Ultrasound-Guided Technique

Position the patient seated with the head resting in the forward position. Identify the target thoracic vertebral levels and their corresponding spinous processes. Prepare and drape the

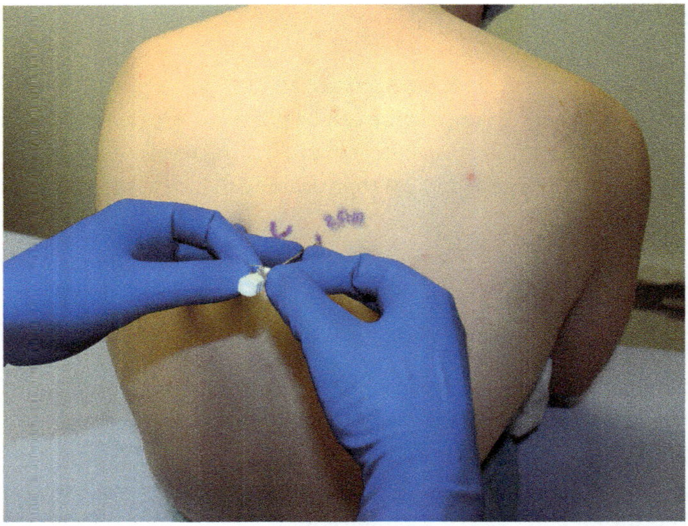

Figure 20.3 Needle positioning for the landmark-based technique of the thoracic paravertebral block.

target thoracic paraspinal region. Place a linear, high-frequency ultrasound transducer in the parasagittal plane 2.5 cm lateral to the tip of the spinous process. Move the ultrasound probe laterally and medially to identify the transverse processes, superior costotransverse ligament, and pleura (Figure 20.2B). The pleura appears as a bright, shimmering structure running below the transverse processes. The superior costotransverse ligament is identified as a white line extending between adjacent transverse processes, just above the pleura.

Move the transducer along the sagittal plane until the midpoint between two adjacent transverse processes is reached. Infiltrate a local anesthetic (most commonly, 1% lidocaine) at the caudal end of the ultrasound probe to create a skin wheal. With an in-plane approach, advance a styletted Tuohy needle in a cephalad direction to the paravertebral space, just beyond the superior costotransverse ligament (Figure 20.2A). Avoid bony contact with a needle trajectory midway between adjacent transverse processes. Saline may be injected in small volumes (e.g., 3 mL) to confirm position. Remove the epidural stylet and inject a local anesthetic or advance the catheter 1 to 3 cm within the paravertebral space.

Complications

- Accidental epidural or intrathecal injection
- Hematoma
- Horner syndrome (transient)
- Intravascular injection via intercostal artery or vein
- Local anesthetic systemic toxicity
- Pneumothorax
- Spinal or intercostal nerve injury

Intercostal Nerve Block

Introduction

The intercostal nerve block (ICNB) was first described in 1907 and is one of the earliest peripheral nerve blocks performed.[13] It provides analgesia to the upper abdomen and thoracic wall in a band-like pattern through local anesthetic infiltration at the neurovascular bundle just below the rib. The ICNB is unique in that each intercostal nerve is blocked individually to achieve broad analgesic coverage. It is also important to note that the intercostal spaces are highly vascular and permit high levels of systemic absorption, which may increase the risk of local anesthetic toxicity.[14]

The ICNB is a well-established regional technique with clear benefit in reducing perioperative pain scores, opioid use, and postoperative respiratory complications.[15,16] It may be preferred over neuraxial techniques where coagulopathy or hemodynamic instability precludes their use.

Indications

Indications are breast, chest wall, and thoracic wall surgery, chest tube placement, and rib fracture(s).

Anatomy

The ICNB provides a band-like pattern of analgesia across the thorax and upper abdomen through local anesthetic infiltration of the intercostal nerve along its course from the angle of the rib to the midaxillary line. The intercostal nerves are mixed motor and sensory nerves that originate from the ventral rami of the thoracic spinal nerves (Figure 20.4B). They provide motor innervation to intercostal muscles, serratus posterior superior and inferior, and transversus thoracis, in addition to sensory innervation to the parietal pleura and skin of the anterior, lateral, and posterolateral thorax.[14,17]

Beginning in the posterior thorax, the intercostal nerves move laterally between the parietal pleura and posterior intercostal membrane. As they continue, the intercostal nerves move between the innermost intercostal muscle and internal intercostal muscle within the costal groove of the rib above. The costal groove also provides a surface for the intercostal artery and vein to travel; they are collectively termed the neurovascular bundle.[14,17]

As the intercostal nerves approach the midaxillary line, the lateral cutaneous branches are formed. These sensory branches penetrate through the intercostal muscles and serratus anterior and bifurcate into the anterior and posterior branches to provide cutaneous innervation from the anterolateral to the posterolateral thorax. The lateral cutaneous branch of T2 is unique in that it does not divide into anterior and posterior branches but provides sensory innervation to the arm as the intercostobrachial nerve.[14,17]

Beyond the midaxillary line, the intercostal nerves terminate as the anterior cutaneous branches. These penetrate the overlying external intercostal muscles and pectoralis major to provide cutaneous innervation of the anterior thoracic wall.[14,17]

Local Anesthetic

Long-acting local anesthetics such as bupivacaine or ropivacaine are most commonly used: 0.25% to 0.5% bupivacaine or 0.25% to 0.5% ropivacaine can be given in volumes of 3 to 5 mL per injection. Lower concentrations are frequently chosen for blocks performed at multiple levels.

Equipment

- 22-gauge regional block needle
- Marking pen
- Sterile draping
- Syringe and needle for cutaneous local infiltration
- Syringe with extension tubing for block injection

Procedural Technique

Position the patient seated with arms forward holding a pillow. Allow the patient to lean forward slightly with support. Identify the spinous processes of each target block level, then locate the angle of the rib and mark the skin at its inferior border for each level. The angle of the rib can be identified as a superficial bony prominence approximately 7 cm from the midline.

>> Tip on Technique

Intercostal nerve blocks can be blocked anywhere between the angle of the rib and midaxillary line.

Prepare and drape the targeted ribs in a sterile fashion. Infiltrate a local anesthetic (most commonly, 1% lidocaine) within the marked area to create a skin wheal. Position the nondominant hand onto the patient's back and apply upward traction on the skin with the index finger, moving the skin mark over the mid to lower rib. With the dominant hand, advance a 22-gauge needle 10° cephalad until the rib is contacted (Figure 20.4A). Slowly release skin traction and grasp the needle and syringe with the nondominant hand. Maintain a cephalad angle as the needle is walked off the lower rib border (Figure 20.4C). Advance the needle 4 mm beneath the rib, aspirate, and inject 3 to 5 mL.

(A)

(B)

(C)

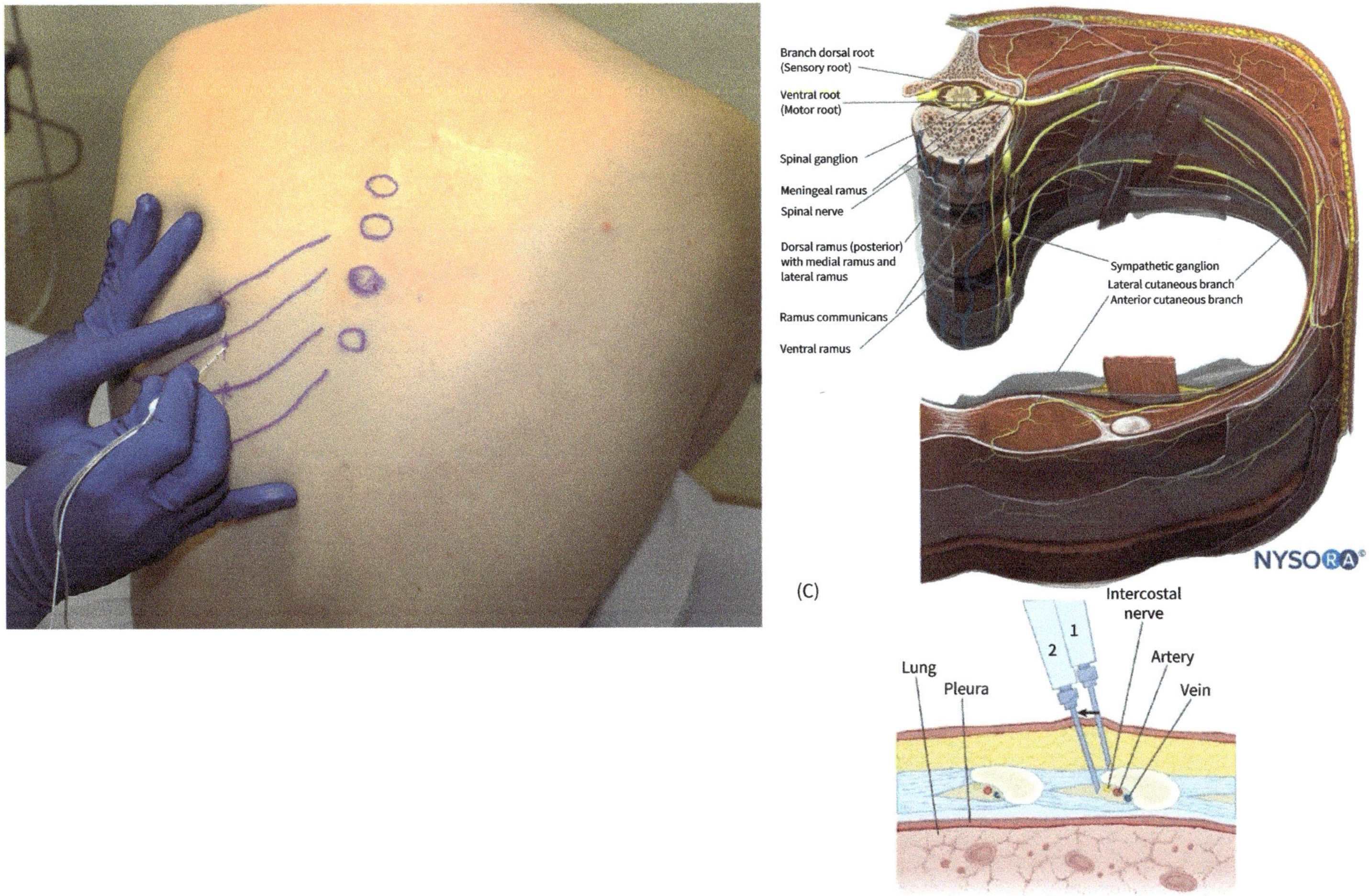

Figure 20.4 (A) Needle positioning for the intercostal nerve block. Upward traction is applied with index finger of the nondominant hand. Spinous processes and ribs are marked, with the angle of the rib denoted by an "X". (B) Anatomy of the intercostal nerve. (C) With the release of skin traction, the needle is walked off the inferior margin of the rib. The needle is advanced in close proximity to the neurovascular bundle.

(B) Reprinted with permission from NYSORA.

(C) Reprinted with permission from Morgan GE, Mikhail MS, Murray MJ. *Clinical Anesthesiology.* 4th ed. New York, NY: McGraw-Hill Medical, 2012: Figure 17-33.

Complications

- Intercostal nerve injury
- Intravascular injection via intercostal artery or vein
- Local anesthetic toxicity
- Pneumothorax

Serratus Anterior Plane Block

Introduction

The serratus anterior plane (SAP) block was introduced in 2013 by Blanco et al. as a progression of the Pecs I and II blocks to allow a more targeted approach in providing analgesia to the lateral thorax. Through local anesthetic spread superficially to the serratus anterior, broad craniocaudal coverage of the lateral cutaneous branches of the intercostal nerves has been demonstrated, reaching as far as T2 to T9 with a single injection.[18]

The SAP block has shown significant benefit in lowering perioperative pain scores and opioid consumption for patients undergoing surgery of the breast or thorax and may be preferable to neuraxial techniques in the setting of coagulopathy, platelet dysfunction, and/or thrombocytopenia.[19–21]

Indications

Indications include breast surgery including axillary dissection and chest wall and thoracic wall surgery.

Anatomy

The SAP block provides multilevel analgesia to the axilla and anterolateral thorax through local anesthetic distribution to the lateral cutaneous branches of the intercostal nerves as they exit the serratus anterior.[22] The serratus anterior is a fan-shaped muscle comprising serrated projections that function to pull the scapula forward. It originates from the lateral surfaces of ribs 1 through 8 or 9 and inserts on the medial border of the scapula. As a relatively broad muscle sheet, the serratus anterior serves as a plane for the local anesthetic to distribute along several thoracic levels.[23]

The major nerve targets of the SAP block are the lateral cutaneous branches of the intercostal nerves.[18] Beginning in the posterolateral thorax as branches of the intercostal nerves, the lateral cutaneous branches travel anterolaterally through the intercostal muscles and serratus anterior to the axilla, where they terminate as the anterior and posterior branches (Figure 20.5C). Here, they provide sensory innervation to the skin of the axilla and anterolateral thorax.[22,23] The lateral cutaneous branch of T2 is unique in that it does not divide into anterior and posterior branches but provides sensory innervation to the arm as the

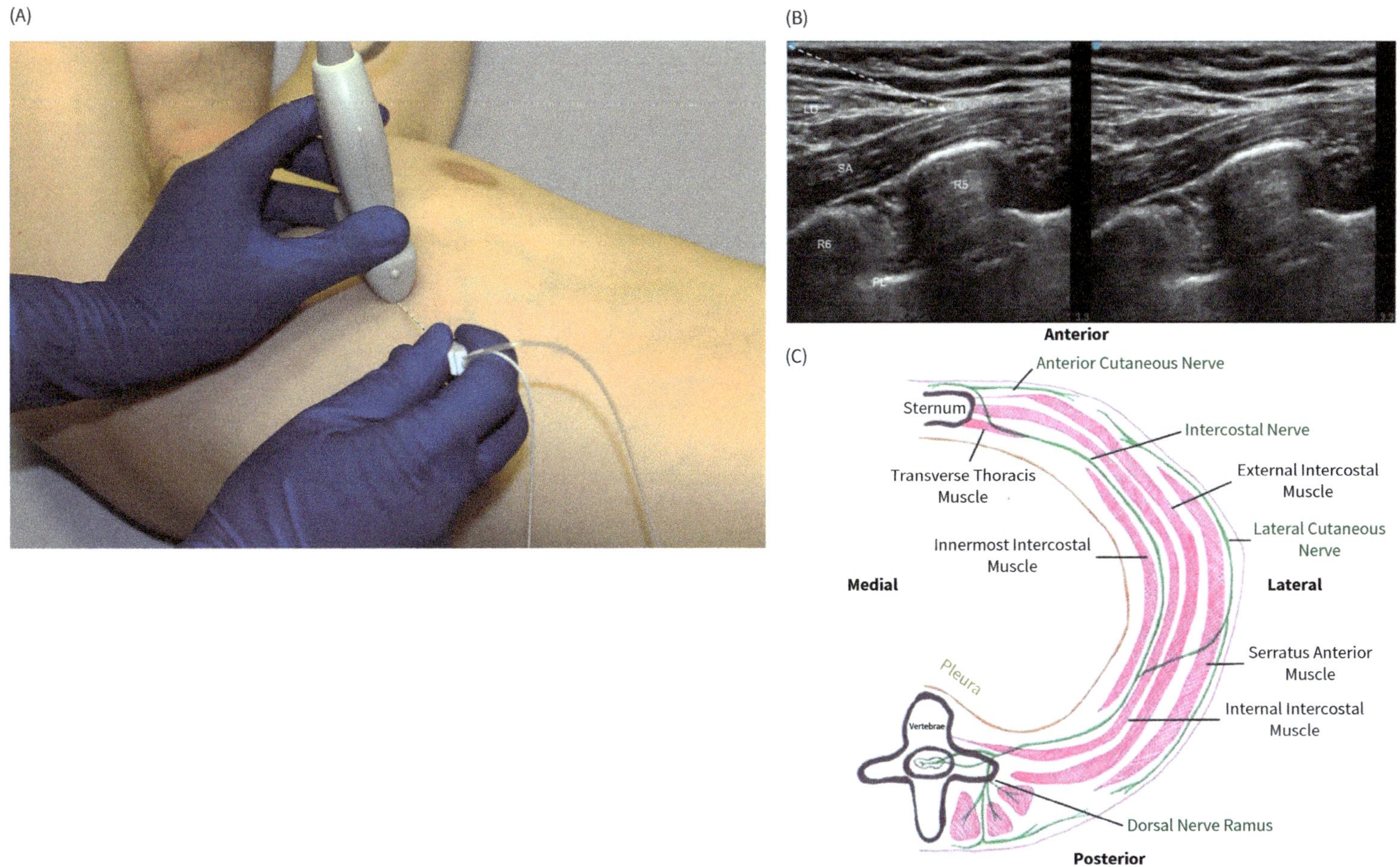

Figure 20.5 (A) Ultrasound transducer and needle positioning for the serratus anterior plane block. (B) Ultrasound anatomy and needle trajectory of the serratus anterior plane block. (C) Anatomy of the intercostal nerve and branches. The lateral cutaneous branch is shown overlying the serratus anterior muscle.

(C) Reprinted with permission from Mayes J, Davison E, Panahi P, et al. An anatomical evaluation of the serratus anterior plane block. *Anaesthesia*. 2016;71:1064–1069, Figure 4.

Abbreviations: LD, latissimus dorsi muscle; PL, pleura; R5, rib 5; R6, rib 6; SA, serratus anterior muscle.

intercostobrachial nerve.[17] The long thoracic nerve, which innervates the serratus anterior, is also anesthetized in the SAP block. Its course begins posterior to the brachial plexus, traveling inferolaterally along the midaxillary line and terminating within the outer surface of the serratus anterior.[22]

Local Anesthetic

Long-acting local anesthetics, such as bupivacaine or ropivacaine, are most commonly used: 0.25% bupivacaine or 0.375% ropivacaine can be given as a single 30-mL injection.

Equipment

- 22-gauge regional block needle
- Linear, high-frequency ultrasound transducer
- Sterile draping
- Syringe and needle for cutaneous local infiltration
- Syringe with extension tubing for block injection

Procedural Technique

>> Tip on Technique

The latissimus dorsi muscle lies just superficial to the serratus anterior and may be seen along the posterior aspect of the image, serving as a useful anatomic landmark.

Position the patient in the lateral decubitus position, with the arm abducted and resting above the head. Prepare and drape the midaxillary region at the level of the fifth rib, approximately at the level of the nipple. Place a linear, high-frequency ultrasound transducer in the transverse plane of the midaxillary line at the level of the fifth rib. Identify the rib, pleura, and intercostal muscles. The serratus anterior muscle lies just superficial to the ribs and intercostal muscles (Figure 20.5B).

Infiltrate a local anesthetic (most commonly, 1% lidocaine) to create a skin wheal just posterior to the ultrasound probe. With an in-plane approach, advance a 22-gauge needle to the fascial layer superficial to the serratus anterior muscle (Figure 20.5A). With negative aspiration, inject 1 to 2 mL of local anesthetic and confirm a slight downward displacement of the serratus anterior muscle and hydrodissection of the fascial plane. Avoid intramuscular injection, which will fail to open the fascial plane. Continue to inject a total volume of 30 mL of local anesthetic under direct visualization of needle tip.

Complications

- Intercostal nerve injury
- Intravascular injection via intercostal artery or vein
- Local anesthetic toxicity
- Pneumothorax

Pecs I and II Blocks

Introduction

The Pecs I and II blocks are ultrasound-guided regional techniques of the anterolateral thorax that rely on two fascial planes: the plane between the pectoralis major and minor and the plane between the pectoralis minor and serratus anterior. The Pecs I block, first described in 2011, includes a single injection between the pectoralis major and minor. This technique provides analgesic coverage of the medial and lateral pectoral nerves and is most frequently used for breast surgeries such as expander or prosthesis placement.[24] Although the Pecs I block is effective for surgical pain involving the pectoral muscles, it has not been shown to provide analgesic coverage of the overlying skin or axilla.[25] The Pecs II block was first described in 2012 and includes both the Pecs I and an additional injection in the fascial plane between the pectoralis minor and serratus anterior. Allowing local anesthetic to distribute along the serratus anterior provides additional coverage of the long thoracic and thoracodorsal nerves, as well as the lateral cutaneous branches of the T2 to T6 intercostal nerves. The Pecs II block is therefore able to provide analgesia to the axilla, latissimus dorsi, pectoral muscles, serratus anterior, and overlying skin.[26,27]

Indications

Indications are breast surgery including axillary dissection and chest wall and thoracic wall surgery.

Anatomy

The Pecs II block provides analgesia to the anterolateral chest wall and axilla through local anesthetic spread in two fascial planes: between the pectoralis major and minor (Pecs I block) and between the pectoralis minor and serratus anterior. The first fascial plane, between the pectoral muscles, provides anesthetic coverage of two major nerve targets: the medial pectoral nerve and the lateral pectoral nerve (Figure 20.6C).[24] Both nerves have been described as purely motor in function yet may provide nociceptive input from pectoral muscle spasm or stretching following surgery of the chest wall or breast.[25,28] The lateral pectoral nerve runs

(A)

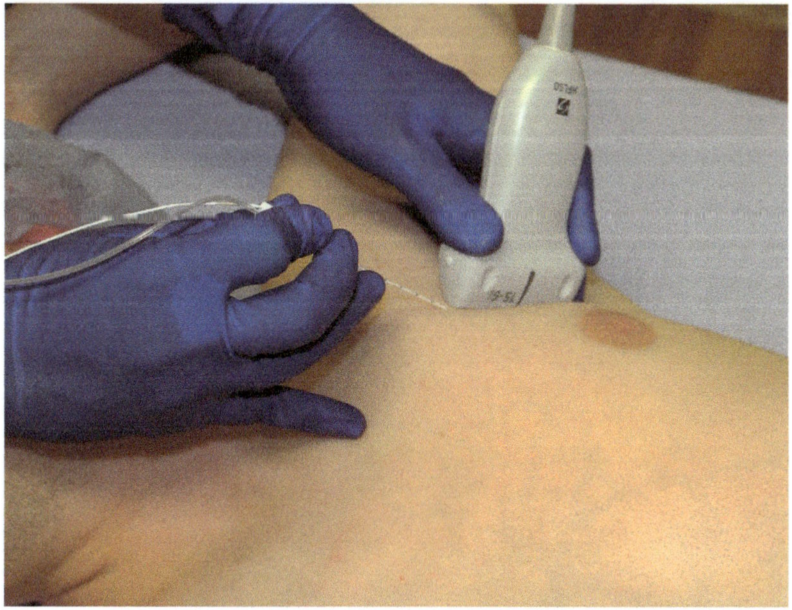

(B)

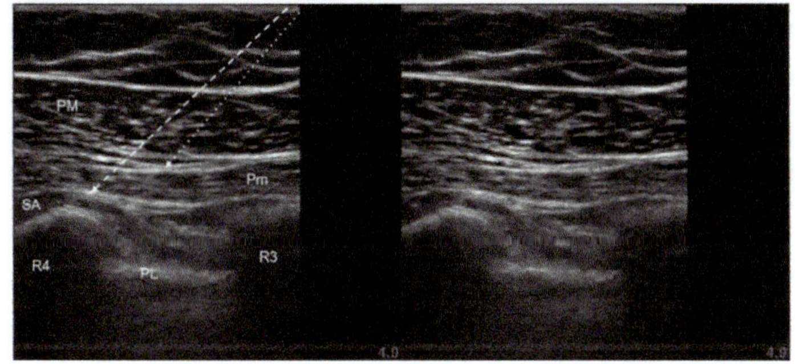

(C)

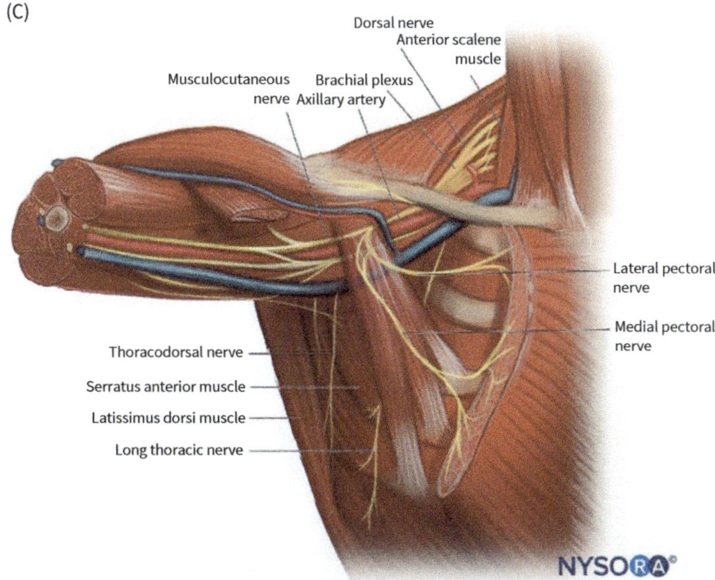

Figure 20.6 (A) Ultrasound transducer and needle positioning for the Pecs 1 and 2 blocks. (B) Ultrasound anatomy and needle trajectory of the Pecs 1 and 2 blocks. Dotted line = needle trajectory for Pecs 1 block; segmented line = needle trajectory to complete Pecs 2 block. (C) Pectoral anatomy.

(C) Reprinted with permission from NYSORA.

Abbreviations: PL, pleura; PM, pectoralis major muscle; Pm, pectoralis minor muscle; R3, rib 3; R4, rib 4; SA, serratus anterior muscle.

between the pectoralis major and minor near the pectoral branch of the thoracoacromial artery and terminates within the pectoralis major. The medial pectoral nerve runs beneath the pectoralis minor and moves anteriorly, penetrating the pectoralis minor and terminating within the pectoralis major.[24,26]

The second fascial plane, between the pectoralis minor and serratus anterior, provides anesthetic coverage to several nerves, including the long thoracic nerve, thoracodorsal nerve, and lateral cutaneous branches of the T2 to T6 intercostal nerves.[26,28] The long thoracic nerve provides innervation to the serratus anterior through a relatively protracted course within the axilla. It begins posterior to the brachial plexus and travels inferolaterally, running deep to the clavicle and traveling along the midaxillary line just superficial to the serratus anterior. The thoracodorsal nerve similarly travels within the axilla just superficial to the serratus anterior but is found more posteriorly and provides innervation to the latissimus dorsi. The lateral cutaneous branches of T3 to T6 provide sensory innervation to the skin of the axilla and anterolateral thorax. They begin as branches of the intercostal nerves, traveling anterolaterally through the intercostal muscles and serratus anterior to the axilla, where they terminate as the anterior and posterior branches. The lateral cutaneous branch of T2 is unique in that it does not divide into anterior and posterior branches but provides sensory innervation to the arm as the intercostobrachial nerve.[17,26]

Local Anesthetic

Long-acting local anesthetics, such as 0.25% bupivacaine, are most frequently used. The Pecs I injection (between pectoralis major and minor) should include 10 mL of local anesthetic followed by 20 mL of local anesthetic for the deeper plane (between the pectoralis minor and serratus anterior) to complete the Pecs II block.

Equipment

- 22-gauge regional block needle
- Linear, high-frequency ultrasound transducer
- Sterile draping
- Syringe and needle for cutaneous local infiltration
- Syringe with extension tubing for block injection

Procedural Technique

Position the patient supine, with the arm abducted 90°. Prepare and drape the superolateral chest and axilla. Place a linear, high-frequency ultrasound transducer in the midclavicular parasagittal plane and move caudally until the third rib is identified.

>>Tip on Technique

The second rib will be the first visualized rib with a caudal motion of the ultrasound probe.

> **>> Tip on Technique**
>
> The pectoral branch of the thoracoacromial artery resides between the pectoralis major and the pectoralis minor.
>
> The caudal end of the transducer is rotated laterally and moved toward the axilla at the lateral aspect of the pectoralis minor. Identify the rib, serratus anterior, pectoralis minor, and pectoralis major (Figure 20.6B).
>
> Infiltrate a local anesthetic (most commonly, 1% lidocaine) to create a skin wheal at the superomedial end of the ultrasound probe. With an in-plane approach, advance a 22-gauge needle to the fascial plane between the pectoralis major and minor (Figure 20.6A). With negative aspiration, inject 10 mL of local anesthetic and confirm hydrodissection of the fascial plane.
>
> Next, advance the needle to the fascial plane between the pectoralis minor and serratus anterior muscles. With negative aspiration, inject 20 mL of local anesthetic and confirm hydrodissection of the fascial plane.

Complications

- Intravascular injection via pectoral branch of the thoracoacromial artery
- Local anesthetic toxicity
- Neuraxial spread
- Pneumothorax

Erector Spinae Plane Block

Introduction

The erector spinae plane (ESP) block was first described by Forero et al. in 2016 as a new regional technique for treating thoracic neuropathic pain.[29] Current evidence suggests that the ESP block may provide analgesia via local anesthetic spread to the epidural space, neuroforamina, and dorsal and ventral rami of the thoracic spinal nerves. Cadaveric studies combined with computed tomography and magnetic resonance imaging have demonstrated multilevel craniocaudal spread of injectate with penetration to the epidural space and intercostal nerves.[29,30]

The ESP block has most notably been used to provide analgesia to thoracic nerve distributions with coverage of the posterior, lateral, and anterolateral thorax, yet its use in surgeries of the abdomen and upper and lower extremities has been well documented.[31] This fascial plane block offers the advantage of broad analgesic coverage similar to neuraxial techniques and may be preferred in the setting of coagulopathy, platelet dysfunction, and/or thrombocytopenia.

Indications

Indications are breast, chest wall, and thoracic wall surgery.

Anatomy

The ESP block provides broad analgesic coverage through local anesthetic spread along the fascial plane between the erector spinae muscles and vertebral transverse processes. The erector spinae muscles consist of a group of three paraspinal muscles extending from the base of the skull to the sacrum. They include the spinalis, longissimus thoracis, and iliocostalis (Figure 20.7C). Collectively, the erector spinae muscles create a deep tissue plane for local anesthetic spread in a craniocaudal fashion.[29]

The dorsal rami of the thoracic spinal nerves are one of the primary targets for the ESP block. They travel posteriorly through the costotransverse foramen into the erector spinae muscles, providing motor and sensory innervation to the erector spinae muscles and overlying skin. The costotransverse foramen (bordered laterally by the superior costotransverse ligament, medially by the lamina, superiorly by the transverse process, and inferiorly by the rib below) may have a critical role in permitting local anesthetic spread anteriorly from the ESP and allowing a broad mediolateral coverage, ranging from the intercostal nerves and ventral rami laterally to the neuroforamina and epidural space medially.[29,31]

Local Anesthetic

Long-acting local anesthetics, such as bupivacaine or ropivacaine, are most commonly used: 0.25% bupivacaine or 0.375% ropivacaine can be given as a single 20- to 30-mL injection.

Equipment

- 22-gauge regional block needle
- Linear, high-frequency ultrasound transducer
- Sterile draping
- Syringe and needle for cutaneous local infiltration
- Syringe with extension tubing for block injection

Procedural Technique

Position the patient seated with the head resting in the forward position. Identify the target vertebral level for injection by palpation and surface anatomic landmarks or with ultrasound. Identify the level most closely representing the craniocaudal midpoint of the target analgesic region.

Prepare and drape the thoracic paraspinal area. With a linear, high-frequency ultrasound transducer oriented in the paramedian sagittal plane, identify the transverse process at the selected vertebral level. The transverse process can be visualized approximately 2 to 3 cm lateral to the spinous process (Figure 20.7B). Move the ultrasound probe laterally and medially to identify the ribs and transverse processes.

(A) (B) (C)

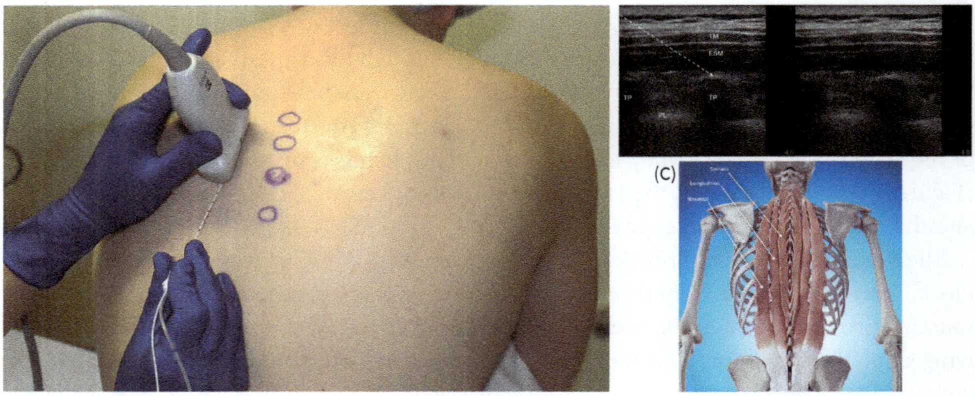

Figure 20.7 (A) Ultrasound transducer and needle positioning for the erector spinae plane block. Purple markings indicate spinous processes. (B) Ultrasound anatomy and needle trajectory of the erector spinae plane block. (C) Anatomy of the erector spinae muscles.

Abbreviations: ESM, erector spinae muscles; PL, pleura; TM, trapezius muscle; TP, transverse process.

Infiltrate a local anesthetic (most commonly, 1% lidocaine) to create a skin wheal at the inferior end of the ultrasound probe. With an in-plane approach, advance a 22-gauge needle in a caudad to cephalad direction to contact the transverse process (Figure 20.7A). The needle tip should be positioned between the transverse process and overlying erector spinae muscles. With negative aspiration, inject 20 to 30 mL of local anesthetic and confirm a hydrodissection of the fascial plane.

Complications

- Local anesthetic toxicity
- Pneumothorax

Transversus Thoracis Muscle Plane Block

Introduction

The transversus thoracis muscle plane (TTP) block is a relatively novel regional anesthesia technique first described in 2015 by Ueshima and Kitamura. It provides analgesia to the anterior chest wall by targeting the anterior cutaneous branches of the intercostal nerves.[32,33] Cadaveric studies have shown that a single-shot injection of local anesthetic deposited in the fascial plane between the internal intercostal muscle and transversus thoracis can cover the T2 to T6 intercostal nerves.[34]

The TTP block was originally applied to surgeries of the breast as an adjunct to the Pecs II block; however, recent data have suggested a benefit in cardiac surgery involving median sternotomy, implantable cardioverter defibrillator placement, and pericardial drainage.[35]

Indications

Indications include anterior thoracic wall and breast surgery and implantable cardioverter defibrillator placement.

Anatomy

The TTP block provides analgesia to the internal mammary region by targeting the anterior cutaneous branches of the intercostal nerves.[32,33] Intercostal nerves, originating from the ventral rami of the thoracic spinal nerves, give rise to the lateral cutaneous branches and the anterior cutaneous branches. The anterior branches of T2 to T6 are terminal intercostal nerves that penetrate the overlying external intercostal muscles and pectoralis major to provide skin innervation of the anterior thoracic wall.[17]

The transversus thoracis muscle is located in the anterior chest wall, on the inner surface of the body of the sternum and ribs (Figure 20.8C). It has insertion sites on the costal cartilages of ribs 2 through 6 and lies between the internal intercostal muscle and parietal pleura. The internal thoracic artery may also be identified approximately 2 cm lateral to the sternal border, traveling between the internal intercostal muscle and transversus thoracis.[36]

Local Anesthetic

For patients <75 kg, 10 to 20 mL of 0.3% ropivacaine may be used. For patients ≥75 kg, 10 to 20 mL of 0.5% ropivacaine may be used. Due to limited data, local anesthetic type and dosing have not yet been standardized.

Equipment

- 22-gauge regional block needle
- Linear, high-frequency ultrasound transducer
- Sterile draping
- Syringe and needle for cutaneous local infiltration
- Syringe with extension tubing for block injection

Procedural Technique

Position the patient supine with arms resting at the side. Prepare and drape the parasternal chest wall. Place a linear, high-frequency ultrasound transducer in the parasagittal plane

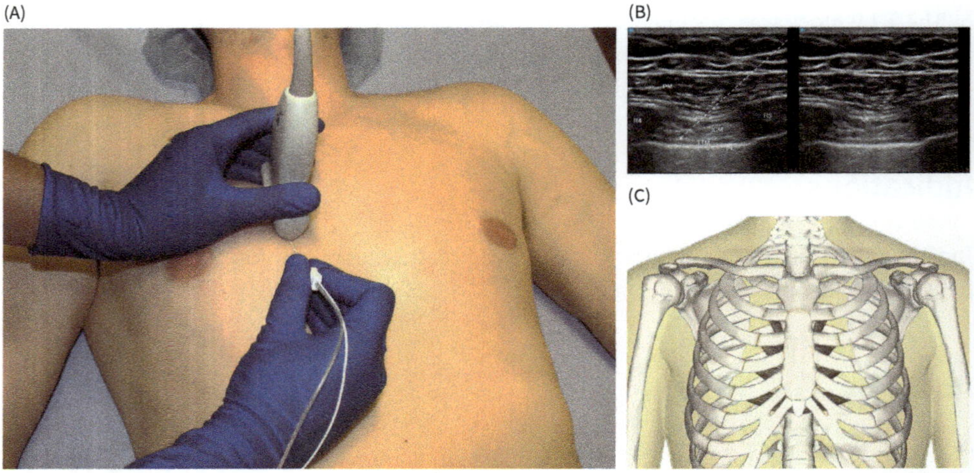

Figure 20.8 (A) Ultrasound transducer and needle positioning for the transversus thoracis muscle plane block. (B) Ultrasound anatomy and needle trajectory of the transversus thoracis muscle plane block. (C) Transversus thoracis muscle.

(C) Modified from Andrewmeyerson, CC BY-SA 3.0 https://creativecommons.org/licenses/by-sa/3.0 via Wikimedia Commons

Abbreviations: ICM, intercostal muscles; PL, pleura; PM, pectoralis major muscle; R4, rib 4; R5, rib 5; TTM, transversus thoracis muscle.

1 cm lateral to the sternal border. Identify the T4 to T5 intercostal space, intercostal muscles, transversus thoracis muscle, and pleura (Figure 20.8B).

Infiltrate a local anesthetic (most commonly, 1% lidocaine) to create a skin wheal at the caudal end of the ultrasound probe. With an in-plane approach, advance a 22-gauge needle to the fascial plane between the internal intercostal and transversus thoracis muscles (Figure 20.8A).

With negative aspiration, inject 10 to 20 mL of local anesthetic and confirm a hydrodissection of the fascial plane.

Complications

- Intravascular injection via internal thoracic artery or vein
- Local anesthetic toxicity
- Pericardial puncture
- Pneumothorax

Further Reading

New York School of Regional Anesthesia. [Home page]. http://www.nysora.com.

Rosenblatt MA, Lai Y. Thoracic nerve block techniques. *UpToDate*. https://www.uptodate.com/contents/thoracic-nerve-block-techniques. Published 2019. Accessed November 25, 2019.

References

1. Franco A, Diz JC. The history of the epidural block. *Curr Anaesth Crit Care*. 2000;11:274–276.
2. Block BM, Liu SS, Rowlingson AJ, Cowan AR, Cowan JA Jr, Wu CL. Efficacy of postoperative epidural analgesia: a meta-analysis. *JAMA*. 2003;290:2455–2463.
3. GA McLeod, C Cumming. Thoracic epidural anaesthesia and analgesia. *Cont Ed Anaesth Crit Care Pain*. 2004;4:16–19.
4. Bromage PR. Mechanism of action of extradural analgesia. *Br J Anaesth*. 1975;47(Suppl):199–211.
5. Richardson J, Groen GJ. Applied epidural anatomy. *Cont Education in Anaesthesia Critical Care & Pain*. 2005;5:98–100.
6. Reina MA, Franco CD, López A, Dé Andrés JA, van Zundert A. Clinical implications of epidural fat in the spinal canal: a scanning electron microscopic study. *Acta Anaesthesiol Belg*. 2009;60:7–17.
7. Wiltse LL. Anatomy of the extradural compartments of the lumbar spinal canal. Peridural membrane and circumneural sheath. *Radiol Clin North Am*. 2000;38:1177–1206.
8. Karmakar MK. Thoracic paravertebral block. *Anesthesiology*. 2001;95:771–780.
9. Naja ZM, El-Rajab M, Al-Tannir MA, et al. Thoracic paravertebral block: influence of the number of injections. *Reg Anesth Pain Med*. 2006;31:196–201.
10. Davies RG, Myles PS, Graham JM. A comparison of the analgesic efficacy and side-effects of paravertebral vs epidural blockade for thoracotomy: a systematic review and meta-analysis of randomized trials. *Br J Anaesth*. 2006;96:418–426; erratum in *Br J Anaesth*. 2007;99:768.
11. Richardson J, Lönnqvist PA. Thoracic paravertebral block. *Br J Anaesth*. 1998;81:230–238.
12. Helm EJ, Rahman NM, Talakoub O, Fox DL, Gleeson FV. Course and variation of the intercostal artery by CT scan. *Chest*. 2013;143:634–639.
13. Bennett HA, Dodson HC, Bamforth BJ. Intercostal nerve block in upper abdominal and chest surgery. *Curr Res Anesth Analg*. 1956;35:123–130.
14. Baxter CS, Fitzgerald BM. Intercostal nerve block. *StatPearls*. https://www.ncbi.nlm.nih.gov/books/NBK482273/. Published 2019. Accessed November 25, 2019.
15. Sabanathan S, Mearns AJ, Bickford Smith PJ, et al. Efficacy of continuous extrapleural intercostal nerve block on post-thoracotomy pain and pulmonary mechanics. *Br J Surg*. 1990;77:221–225.
16. Wurnig PN, Lackner H, Teiner C, et al. Is intercostal block for pain management in thoracic surgery more successful than epidural anaesthesia? *Eur J Cardiothorac Surg*. 2002;21:1115–1119.
17. Glenesk NL, Lopez PP. Anatomy, thorax, intercostal nerves. *StatPearls*. https://www.ncbi.nlm.nih.gov/books/NBK538238/. Published 2019. Accessed November 25, 2019.
18. Blanco R, Parras T, McDonnell JG, Prats-Galino A. Serratus plane block: a novel ultrasound-guided thoracic wall nerve block. *Anaesthesia*. 2013;681107–681113.
19. Khalil AE, Abdallah NM, Bashandy GM, Kaddah TA. Ultrasound-guided serratus anterior plane block versus thoracic epidural analgesia for thoracotomy pain. *J Cardiothorac Vasc Anesth*. 2017;31:152–158.
20. Park MH, Kim JA, Ahn HJ, Yang MK, Son HJ, Seong BG. A randomised trial of serratus anterior plane block for analgesia after thoracoscopic surgery. *Anaesthesia*. 2018;73:1260–1264.
21. Rahimzadeh P, Imani F, Faiz SHR, Boroujeni BV. Impact of the ultrasound-guided serratus anterior plane block on post-mastectomy pain: a randomised clinical study. *Turk J Anaesthesiol Reanim*. 2018;46:388–392.
22. Mayes J, Davison E, Panahi P, et al. An anatomical evaluation of the serratus anterior plane block. *Anaesthesia*. 2016;71:1064–1069.
23. Southgate SJ, Herbst MK. Ultrasound guided serratus anterior blocks. *StatPearls*. https://www.ncbi.nlm.nih.gov/books/NBK538476/. Published 2019. Accessed November 25, 2019.
24. Blanco R. The "pecs block": a novel technique for providing analgesia after breast surgery. *Anaesthesia*. 2011;66:847–848.
25. Desroches J, Belliveau M, Bilodeau C, Landry M, Roy M, Beaulieu P. Pectoral nerves I block is associated with a significant motor blockade with no dermatomal sensory changes: a prospective volunteer randomized-controlled double-blind study. *Can J Anaesth*. 2018;65:806–812.
26. Blanco R, Fajardo M, Parras Maldonado T. Ultrasound description of Pecs II (modified Pecs I): a novel approach to breast surgery. *Rev Esp Anestesiol Reanim*. 2012;59:470–475.

27. Goswami S, Kundra P, Bhattacharyya J. Pectoral nerve block1 versus modified pectoral nerve block2 for postoperative pain relief in patients undergoing modified radical mastectomy: a randomized clinical trial. *Br J Anaesth.* 2017;119:830–835.
28. Versyck B, Groen G, van Geffen GJ, Van Houwe P, Bleys RL. The pecs anesthetic blockade: A correlation between magnetic resonance imaging, ultrasound imaging, reconstructed cross-sectional anatomy and cross-sectional histology. *Clin Anat.* 2019;32:421–429.
29. Forero M, Adhikary SD, Lopez H, Tsui C, Chin KJ. The erector spinae plane block: a novel analgesic technique in thoracic neuropathic pain. *Reg Anesth Pain Med.* 2016;41:621–627.
30. Adhikary SD, Bernard S, Lopez H, Chin KJ. Erector spinae plane block versus retrolaminar block: a magnetic resonance imaging and anatomical study. *Reg Anesth Pain Med.* 2018;43:756–762.
31. Kot P, Rodriguez P, Granell M, et al. The erector spinae plane block: a narrative review. *Korean J Anesthesiol.* 2019;72:209–220.
32. Ueshima H, Kitamura A. Blocking of multiple anterior branches of intercostal nerves (Th2-6) using a transversus thoracic muscle plane block. *Reg Anesth Pain Med.* 2015;40:388.
33. Ueshima H, Kitamura A. Clinical experiences of ultrasound-guided transversus thoracic muscle plane block: a clinical experience. *J Clin Anesth.* 2015;27:428–429.
34. Ueshima H, Takeda Y, Ishikawa S, Otake H. Ultrasound-guided transversus thoracic muscle plane block: a cadaveric study of the spread of injectate. *J Clin Anesth.* 2015;27:696.
35. Fujii S, Bairagi R, Roche M, Zhou JR. Transversus thoracis muscle plane block. *Biomed Res Int.* 2019;2019:1716365.
36. Tang A, Bordoni B. Anatomy, thorax, muscles. *StatPearls.* http://www.ncbi.nlm.nih.gov/books/NBK538321/. Published 2019. Accessed December 13, 2019.

21
Minimally Invasive Thoracic Surgery

Joseph Capone and Antony Tharian

Introduction

Traditionally, thoracic surgery has involved large incisions to gain access to the lungs and other intrathoracic structures. As techniques in other surgical specialties began to trend toward less and less invasive, thoracic surgery has followed suit. The first thoracoscopy was performed in 1910; however, it was not until 1991 when the first video-assisted thoracoscopic surgery (VATS) lobectomy was performed, forever revolutionizing the approach to diagnosis and treatment of conditions in the chest. The goals for minimally invasive thoracic surgery are no different than other minimally invasive surgical approaches and can be found listed in Box 21.1.

The focus of this chapter is primarily on the anesthetic implications of minimally invasive thoracic surgeries (MITS) or thoracic surgeries performed through incisions other than sternotomy or thoracotomy, with a specific focus on novel approaches including single port and robotic-assisted thoracic surgery (RATS). The common incisions used for these approaches can be seen in Figure 21.1 and include the original three-port VATS as well as modified three-port, two-port, and single-port VATS. This chapter focuses primarily on novel minimally invasive approaches to surgery on the lung, esophagus, thymus, and other noncardiac mediastinal structures.

Box 21.1 Goals of Minimally Invasive Thoracic Surgery

- Improved postoperative pain
- Reduced length of hospitalization
- Accelerated recovery
- Decreased complication rates
- Improved cosmesis
- Optimize quality of life post-operatively
- All while achieving similar or better outcome when compared to conventional approaches.

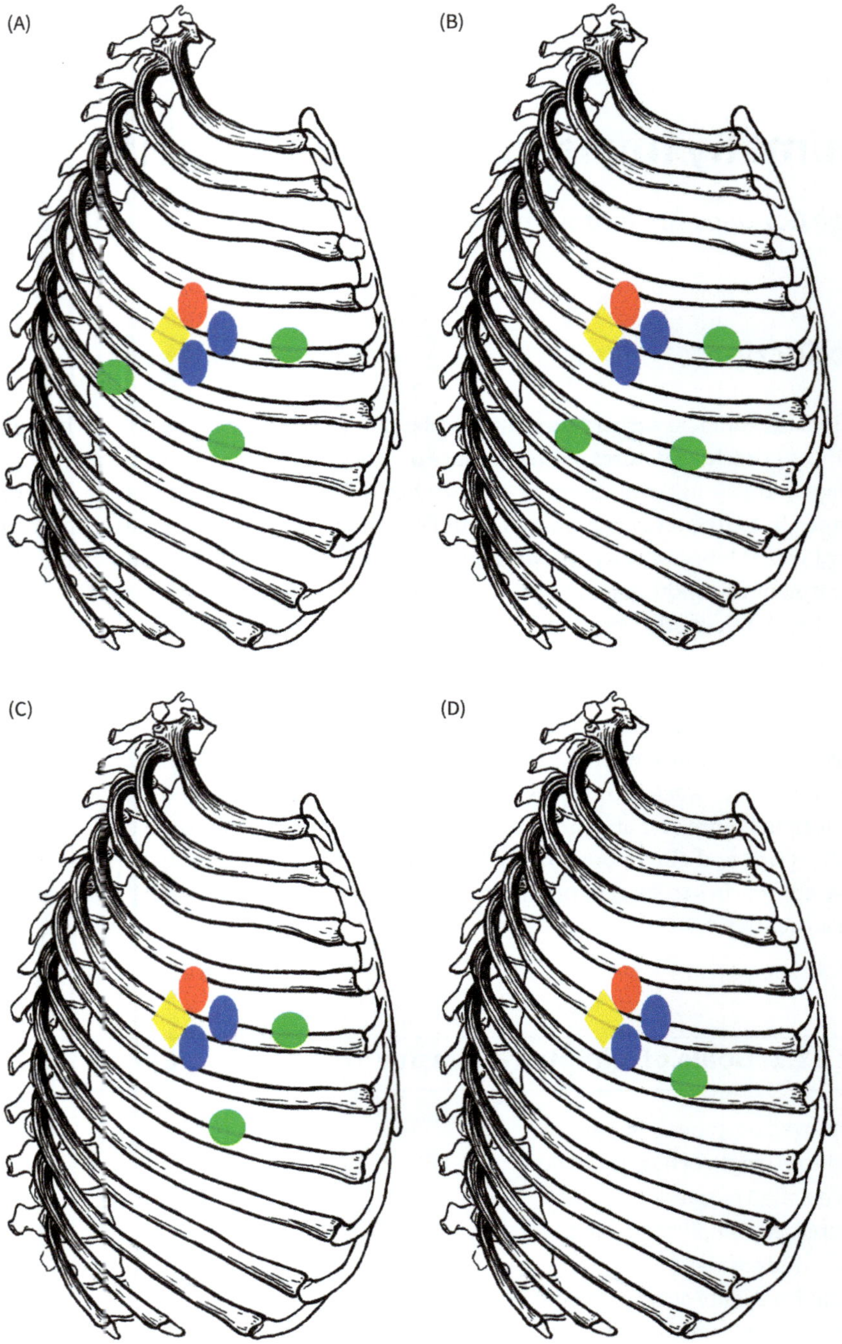

Figure 21.1 (A) Three-port video-assisted thoracoscopic surgery (VATS). (B) Modified 3-port VATS. (C) Two-port VATS. (D) Single-port VATS.

Yellow = bronchi; red = pulmonary artery; blue = pulmonary veins; green = port site.

Minimally Invasive Approaches to Thoracic Surgery

Overview

To perform surgery in the thorax, surgeons need the ability to operate with a left and a right hand as well as adequate visualization of the surgical field. The early days of thoracic surgery involved either large intercostal incisions with rib spreading or a median sternotomy to accomplish this. Progression from open thoracic surgery to VATS is one of the greatest achievements in thoracic surgery in a generation. The original VATS required placement of two or three 10-mm ports in addition to a 3 to 6 cm utility port for specimen removal (1,2). Over time it was realized that the additional retraction and manipulation provided by the third port provided little benefit in certain surgical scenarios leading to the progression from three-port to two-port VATS.

Single-Port Video-Assisted Thoracoscopic Surgery

From two-port VATS, the next logical progression was to remove the second port all together and place the video thoracoscope through the utility port along with the other instruments (3). This single port approach allows for achievement of the same goals of standard VATS techniques including decreased postoperative pain, faster recovery, and improved cosmesis while maintaining adequate surgical exposure (4–7) and remaining even more minimally invasive (8). Preoperative evaluation of imaging studies for surgical planning and port placement are essential when employing a single port technique. For operative single-port VATS, a 2 to 3 cm incision is typically adequate, with even smaller incisions, 1 to 1.5 cm, being adequate for relatively minor diagnostic procedures such as pleurodesis or sympathectomies (9).

To achieve adequate thoracoscopic visualization for single-port VATS, the target lesion is approached in a craniocaudal fashion. This falls in contrast to the laterolateral "baseball diamond" approach typically employed for conventional VATS. By rotating the complement of instruments 90 degrees, optimal visualization is maintained. To avoid interference with one another, while still maintaining 360-degree maneuverability, special articulating instruments are required (9).

Selecting the appropriate incision site is of crucial importance when employing a single-port technique. Inadequate distance between the port site and the target lesion can cause interference between instruments resulting in additional incisions or conversion to an open technique, negating many of the benefits of a single-port VATS (9,10).

Since the advent of single-port VATS, progress in minimally invasive thoracic surgery has only accelerated. In just a few short years, surgeons have gone from performing simple procedures such as wedge resections and sympathectomies to surgeries with increasing complexity including tracheal resection and reconstruction, esophagectomy, bronchoplastic procedures and resections for advanced lung cancer (3,11–14). Although most VATS still take place under general anesthesia, utilization of single-port techniques has allowed for the utilization of nonintubated anesthetic techniques in select patients.

Robotic-Assisted Thoracic Surgery

Around the turn of the century, the next evolution in thoracic surgery was beginning. The use of robotic surgical platforms (Figure 21.2) was no longer limited to simple intra-abdominal or pelvic procedures. The hopes of improved surgical precision and decreased morbidity piqued the interest of thoracic surgeons as well. Although data have shown improved outcomes when compared with open thoracotomy (15–17), no trial has demonstrated superiority over VATS for lung resections (18–28). Similar results have been seen with robotic-assisted esophageal surgery. Although it is widely regarded as a technically superior operation, there are no high-quality data demonstrating superiority of robotic-assisted esophagectomy over conventional approaches regarding patient-centered outcomes (29–34). Common minimally invasive approaches to lung resection and esophagectomy are outlined in Figure 21.3.

For several years progress in RATS stagnated. Many centers resisted the trend given the considerable upfront cost of the robotic surgical system as well as the ongoing cost of its consumable components. RATS for lung surgery required the same number of incisions as conventional VATS, often even requiring a fourth. The robotic surgical system's claims of 3D vision and improved dexterity showed promise; however, these benefits failed to make up for the loss of haptic feedback to the surgeon (35). Prolonged set-up time eating up valuable operating room time further detracted from its use. Examples of robotic approaches to the thymus and posterior mediastinal masses are noted in Figure 21.4.

The robotic surgical system did show some promise in the thoracic landscape. Utilization of RATS for anterior mediastinal procedures—namely, thymectomies—has been demonstrated to increase remission rates in myasthenia gravis as well as decreased morbidity and shorter hospitalizations when compared with VATS (31–41). Although no prospective randomized controlled trials have been done comparing RATS versus open thoracic surgery or RATS versus VATS for posterior mediastinal procedures, the available data suggest

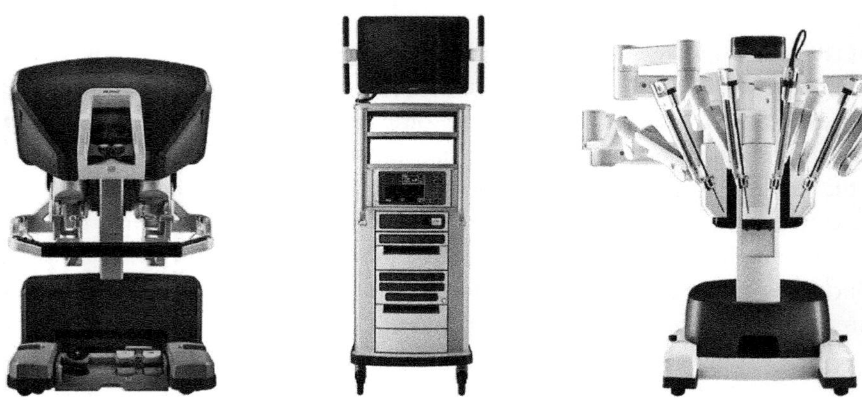

Figure 21.2 The Da Vinci Xi Robotic Surgical System (Intuitive Surgical, Mountain View, CA, US). From left to right: surgeon console, vision cart, patient cart.

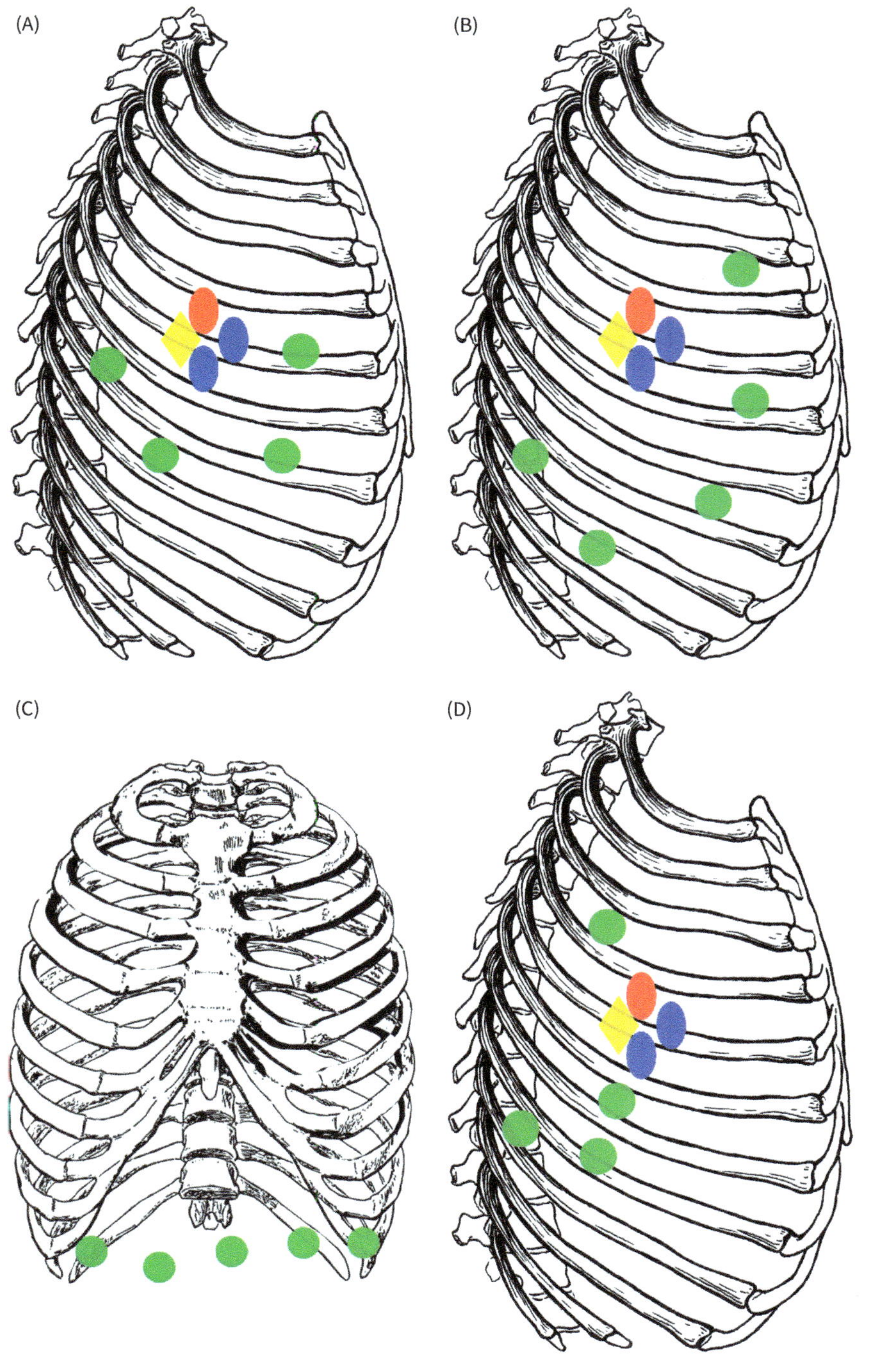

Figure 21.3 (A) Lateral decubitus robot-assisted lung resection. (B) Lateral decubitus robot-assisted esophagectomy. (C) Supine transhiatal robot-assisted esophagectomy. (D) Prone robot-assisted esophagectomy.

Yellow = bronchi; red = pulmonary artery; blue = pulmonary veins; green = port site.

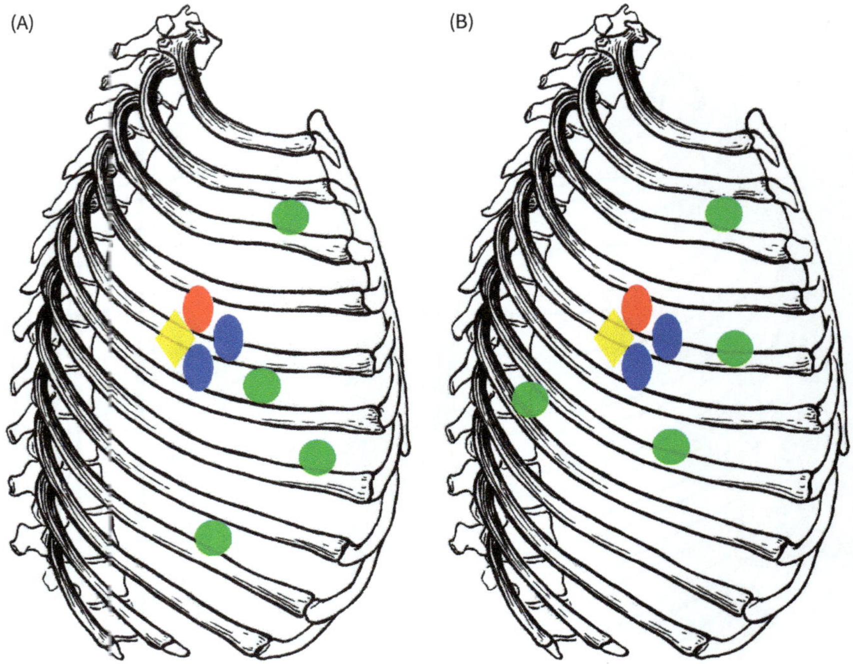

Figure 21.4 (A) Lateral decubitus robot-assisted thymectomy. (B) Lateral decubitus robot-assisted approach to posterior mediastinum.
Yellow = bronchi; red = pulmonary artery; blue = pulmonary veins; green = port site.

utilization of the robotic surgical system appears to confer some benefit with shorter hospital stays, less tissue trauma and fewer complications (42–45).

Single-Port Robotic-Assisted Thoracic Surgery

Nearly a decade after the first RATS, a further refinement was made with release of the first single-port site robotic surgical platform pictured in Figure 21.5. This system employs a single 25 mm trocar with an articulating endoscopic camera and three articulating 5 mm instruments. Although initially utilized for cholecystectomy (46), its use was quickly expanded to include gynecologic (47) and complex urologic surgeries (48,49). Although not yet approved by the US Food and Drug Administration for this purpose, some providers have already begun to explore its use in thoracic surgeries (50). Similar to single-port VATS, utilization of single-port RATS provides the opportunity to utilize nonintubated anesthetic techniques in selected patients.

No compelling outcome driven data exist comparing single-port robotic with single-port or conventional VATS. However, use of this system does provide some benefit. For traditional single-port VATS, the surgeon stands beside the patient; however, the axis of operation is

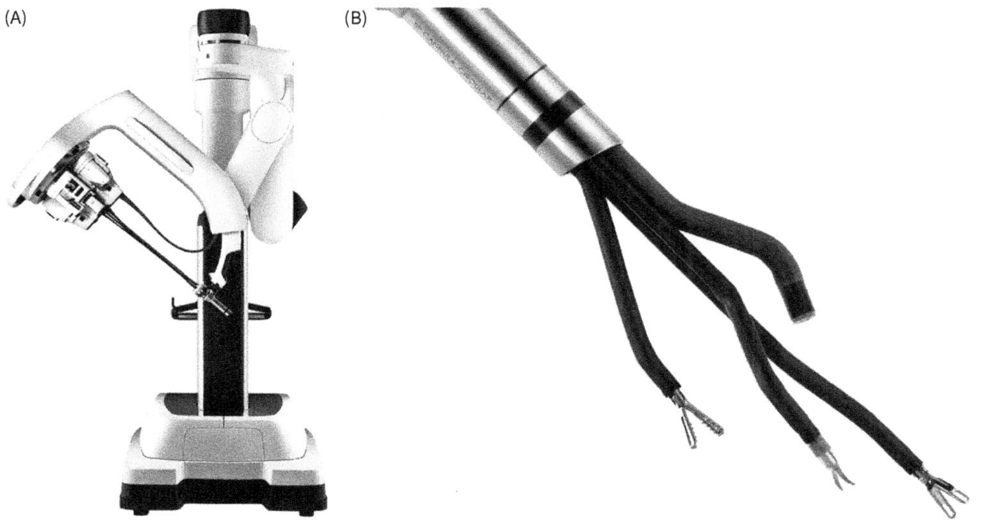

Figure 21.5 The Da Vinci SP (Intuitive Surgical, Mountain View, CA, US).

typically craniocaudal, making for awkward and uncomfortable positioning for the surgeon, especially for long operative times (9). The single-site robotic surgical system significantly improves ergonomics, with the surgeon seated at the robotic console, making for a much more comfortable and user-friendly experience for the surgeon. In addition, the option of a physiologic tremor filter improves surgical dexterity. These factors potentially facilitate faster operative times and the ability to perform more complex operations (50). Utilization of this system also eliminates the interference between instruments that contributes to both the steep learning curve and unpopularity of single-port VATS for many users.

Despite clear advances made with the single-site surgical platform, it is still not without its limitations. The trocar through which the instruments emerge is nonarticulating, reducing overall degrees of freedom, thus limiting its operative maneuverability and, in some cases, its ability to perform complex tasks. Due to the intrinsic shape and length of the semirigid instruments, the surgical target must be between 8 and 24 cm away from the port to be operated on. Meticulous preoperative evaluation of imaging studies for optimal port placement is essential. Further, not all instruments traditionally employed for thoracic surgery are yet available for this relatively new surgical system. In some situations, this may require the addition of a second port or wider initial incision to facilitate entry of otherwise unavailable but necessary instruments (50).

Thoracic surgeons continue to push the envelope by attempting new approaches and techniques in their efforts to improve patient outcomes. One such example has demonstrated feasibility of utilizing the single-port robotic platform in a subxiphoid or subcostal approach to lung surgery in cadavers as seen in Figure 21.6 (51). This approach eliminates mechanical compression of the intercostal neurovascular bundle, a major source of postoperative pain. It also addresses the problem of where to place the bulky 2.5 cm trocar in smaller patients whose intercostal space may not accommodate it.

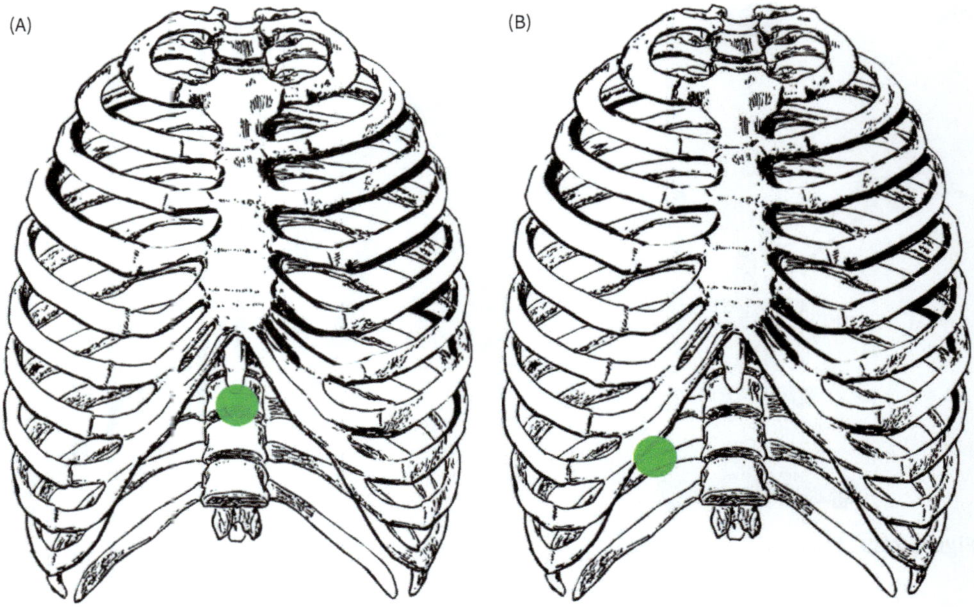

Figure 21.6 (A) Subxiphoid single port robot-assisted approach. (B) Right subcostal single port robot-assisted approach.
Yellow = bronchi; red = pulmonary artery; blue = pulmonary veins; green = port site.

Anesthetic Considerations

Patient Positioning

Patient positioning is procedurally dependent and is the responsibility of both the anesthesia and surgical team as well as the operating room staff. For most MITS involving the lung, patients are placed in the lateral decubitus position with the operative side up. Surgeries involving the thymus can be done in lateral decubitus from the left or right. As noted in Figure 21.2, esophageal surgeries can be approached with the patient in lateral decubitus, supine and even prone positioning has been described (52). For patients in lateral decubitus position, care should be taken to ensure pressure points are appropriately padded. The operative side arm should be fully supported with either an arm rest, separate freestanding table, or pillows stacked on top of the dependent arm. The patient's waist should be aligned with the break in the bed and a kidney rest utilized to allow for lateral flexion toward the dependent side if needed to improve surgical exposure. Conforming bean bags, peg boards or other similar devices are frequently employed to maintain lateral positioning. Once the patient has been positioned endotracheal tube and lung isolation device placement should again be confirmed via both visual and fiberoptic examination.

Temperature Management

As is the case with most surgeries, for minimally invasive thoracic procedures, normothermia should be maintained, with close monitoring of temperature throughout. Special care should be taken to avoid hypothermia as this can contribute to increased blood loss and transfusion requirements, cardiac arrythmias, and hypertension, as well as an increased risk of infection (53–55). Strategies to mitigate drops in temperature include utilizing water or forced air warmers and using warmed intravenous (IV) fluids as well as increasing the ambient temperature of the room. Warming the patient prior to undergoing a general anesthetic has also been shown to attenuate drops in temperature intraoperatively (56).

Monitoring

Monitors utilized for MITS should include at a minimum electrocardiogram, noninvasive blood pressure cuff, pulse oximetry (SpO_2), end tidal carbon dioxide ($ETCO_2$) monitoring, and some form of temperature monitor. Invasive beat-by-beat blood pressure monitoring with an intraarterial catheter should be utilized whenever there is risk for hemodynamic instability. This can be due to patient factors (e.g., significant cardiovascular comorbidities) or surgical factors (e.g., hilar involvement or adhesions contributing to significant bleeding).

Additional invasive monitoring devices such as central venous catheters and pulmonary artery catheters are rarely employed in the absence of patient specific indications (e.g., shock states requiring vasoactive medications or severe pulmonary hypertension). In the event of unexpected hemodynamic instability, transesophageal echocardiography can be utilized as a rescue device to diagnose underlying causes; however, its routine use is not typically employed.

Anesthetic Management

General Endotracheal Anesthesia

The most common technique employed for MITS is general endotracheal anesthesia. Induction agent and technique varies greatly and should be tailored to patient comorbidities. Surgeries taking place within the pleural space typically utilize a lung isolation technique with the most common being placement of a left-sided double-lumen tube. Other approaches exist including bronchial blockers; however, lung isolation techniques are covered elsewhere in this textbook. To provide favorable operating conditions, patients should be kept anesthetized and paralyzed. Patients should be mechanically ventilated utilizing some form of lung protective ventilation strategy to mitigate acute lung injury, especially during one-lung ventilation (57). Management of mechanical ventilation and one-lung ventilation are covered in depth elsewhere in this textbook. In the absence of significant blood loss, crystalloid administration should be limited to no more than 6 to 8 mL/kg/hour as volumes greater than this have been associated with increased pulmonary complications (58–62).

Nonintubated Thoracic Surgery

Ever since the advent of the double-lumen tube in the 1950s, general endotracheal anesthesia with lung isolation has been considered the standard of care for anesthesia for thoracic surgery. Although this remains the most common approach to MITS, since the advent of single-port VATS and RATS, it has become increasingly feasible to perform selected procedures without lung isolation in nonintubated, spontaneously breathing patients (63). Patients who stand to benefit most from this approach include those with comorbidities for which undergoing general anesthesia or one-lung ventilation would pose undue risk or those who might have increased difficulty weaning from mechanical ventilation at the conclusion of surgery. Utilizing a nonintubated technique has been shown to be safe and feasible for the management of pleural and pericardial effusions, lung and pleural biopsies, pneumothorax, empyema, thymectomy, and even lung cancer resections (64–75).

Utilization of regional and local anesthesia forms the cornerstone of anesthetic management for nonintubated thoracic surgery. Commonly employed regional techniques include placement of a thoracic epidural catheter or performing paravertebral blocks. In addition to providing appropriate surgical anesthesia, both these techniques also provide excellent postoperative analgesia (67,76,77). There has been no well-documented difference in analgesic effects between thoracic epidural and paravertebral blocks for this purpose. As such, the choice of analgesic technique is based primarily on provider preference and local practice patterns. A number of additional regional techniques have been described and are listed in Box 21.2 (63,73,78,79).

Supplemental sedation is typically employed but is by no means required for nonintubated thoracic surgery. Short-acting, easily titratable medications such as propofol and remifentanil are the ideal agents (68,69,79–84). These medications should be used judiciously and titrated carefully to avoid over sedation and airway loss, especially with patients in the lateral decubitus position. Dexmedetomidine, another suitable agent, has the added benefit of providing anxiolysis and sedation while maintaining spontaneous ventilation (85,86). Conversion to general anesthesia can be challenging, especially for patients in the lateral decubitus position. Should the need arise, whether due to airway loss, hemorrhage, or hemodynamic instability, a well-established protocol should be in place to facilitate optimal resuscitation and conversion to general anesthesia (63).

Box 21.2 Regional Techniques for Nonintubated Thoracic Surgery and Postoperative Pain Management

- Thoracic epidural catheter
- Paravertebral block with or without catheter placement
- Intercostal nerve block with or without catheter placement
- Serratus anterior plane block
- Intrapleural local anesthetic administration
- Intrathoracic vagal nerve block

Postoperative Pain Management

One of the primary benefits of performing MITS is the significant reduction in postoperative pain when compared to open techniques (4,5,87,88). Despite this advantage, mild to moderate pain may still be present and should be addressed. Common causes of postoperative pain include incisional pain, nerve compression from manipulation of instruments through ports, rib trauma, pleural pain, or visceral pain from injury to lung parenchyma or mediastinal structures. A significant proportion of patients will develop ipsilateral shoulder pain (ISP) following MITS. Some sources estimate the incidence of ISP being as high as 53% (6,7). In the presence of good-quality regional anesthesia, especially when single-port techniques are utilized, ISP may be the patient's only pain-related complaint.

The exact etiology of ISP is not known and is thought to be multifactorial. Myofascial pain related to positioning and transection of major bronchi have been suggested as contributory (89). One popular theory suggests it results from irritation of pleural surfaces receiving sensory innervation from the phrenic nerve causing referred pain to the similarly innervated skin overlying the shoulder. Infiltration of the phrenic nerve has been shown to delay onset as well as significantly reduce the occurrence of ISP following thoracic surgery (90–92).

No consensus currently exists regarding the best practice for pain management following MITS. Most practitioners advocate for a multimodal approach using a combination of locoregional anesthesia and IV medications including opioids, nonsteroidal anti-inflammatory drugs, gabapentinoids, and *N*-methyl-D-aspartate antagonists. Thoracic epidurals or paravertebral blocks have historically been viewed as the gold standard for postoperative pain control following thoracic surgery. Good pain control has also been achieved using IV opioids in combinations with intercostal nerve blocks, serratus anterior plane blocks, and erector spinae plane blocks (93–98). However, as the invasiveness of surgical techniques has decreased, so too has the need for invasive measures for pain control. For VATS, good pain control can even be achieved with local infiltration at incision sites (96,97). If there is a high risk of conversion to an open procedure or if a patient comorbidity precludes the use of IV pain medications (e.g., nonsteroidal anti-inflammatory drugs in chronic kidney disease, opioid allergy, etc.), thoracic epidural or paravertebral block can be utilized. If a patient has undergone nonintubated thoracic surgery, the regional technique utilized as the primary anesthetic will contribute significantly to postoperative pain control (59,63,73).

References

1. Ghee CD, Fortes DL, Liu C, Khandar SJ. A randomized controlled trial of continuous subpleural bupivacaine after thoracoscopic surgery. *Sem Thorac Cardiovasc Surg*. 2017;30(2): 240–249.
2. Sihoe AD, Yim AP. Video-assisted pulmonary resections. In: Patterson FG, Cooper JD, Deslauriers J., eds. *Thoracic Surgery*. 3rd ed. Philadelphia, pA: Elsevier; 2008: 970–988.
3. Sihoe AD, Yim AP. VATS as a diagnostic tool. In: Shields TW, LoCicero J, Reed CE, et al. eds. *General Thoracic Surgery*. 7th ed. Philadelphia, PA: Lippincott Williams & Wilkins; 2009: 313–332.
4. Kneuertz PJ, Kamel MK, Stiles BM, et al. Robotic thymectomy is feasible for large thymomas: a propensity-matched comparison. *Anna Thorac Surg*. 2017;104:1673–1678.
5. Cerfolio RJ, Bryant AS, Minnich DJ. Operative techniques in robotic thoracic surgery for inferior or posterior mediastinal pathology. *J Thorac Cardiovasc Surg*. 2012;143:1138–1143.

6. Zirafa CC, Melfi F. Robot-assisted surgery for posterior mediastinal mass. *J Thorac Dis.* 2017;9:4929–4931.
7. Ruurda JP, Hanlo PW, Hennipman A, Broeders IA. Robot assisted thoracoscopic resection of a benign mediastinal neurogenic tumor: technical note. *Neurosurgery.* 2003;52:462–464.
8. Gonzalez D, Paradela M, Garcia J, Dela Torre M. Single-port video-assisted thoracoscopic lobectomy. *Interact Cardiovasc Thorac Surg.* 2011;12(3):514–515.
9. Rocco G, Martin-Ucar A, Passera E. Uniportal VATS wedge pulmonary resections. *Anna Thorac Surg.* 2004;77(2):726–728.
10. Rocco G. Single-port video-assisted thoracic surgery (uniportal) in the routine general thoracic surgical practice. *Op Tech Thorac Cardiovasc Surg.* 2009;14(4):326–335.
11. Bertolaccini L, Terzi A, Viti A. Why should we prefer the single port access thoracic surgery?. *J Visual Surg.* 2016;2:43.
12. Liu Z, Yang R, Shao F. Uniportal video-assisted thoracoscopic tracheal resection. *Anna Thorac Oncol Res.* 2017;1(1):1004–1006.
13. Gonzalez-Rivas D, Fieira E, Delgado M, de la Torre M, Mendez L, Fernandez R. Uniportal video-assisted thoracoscopic sleeve lobectomy and other complex resections. *J Thorac Dis.* 2014;6(Suppl 6):S674–S681
14. Dmitrii S, Pavel K. Uniportal video-assisted thoracic surgery esophagectomy. *Thorac Surg Clin.* 2017;27(4):407–515.
15. Gonzalez-Rivas D, Fernandez R, Fieira E, Mendez L. Single-incision thoracoscopic right upper lobectomy with chest wall resection by posterior approach. *Innovations.* 2013;8(1):70–72.
16. Cerfolio RJ, Bryant AS, Skylizard L, Minnich DJ. Initial consecutive experience of completely portal robotic pulmonary resection with 4 arms. J Thorac Cardiovasc Surg. 2011;142:740–746.
17. Farivar AS, Cerfolio RJ, Vallieres E, et al. Comparing robotic lung resection with thoracotomy and video-assisted thoracoscopic surgery cases entered into the Society of Thoracic Surgeons database. *Innovations.* 2014;9(1):10–15.
18. Paul S, Jalbert J, Isaacs AJ, Altorki NK, Isom OW, Sedrakyan A. Comparative effectiveness of robotic-assisted vs. thoracoscopic lobectomy. *Chest.* 2014;146(6):1505–1512.
19. Jang HJ, Lee HS, Park SY, Zo JI. Comparison of the early robot-assisted lobectomy experience to video assisted thoracic surgery lobectomy for lung cancer: a single-institution case series matching study. *Innovations.* 2011;6:305–310.
20. Louie BE, Farivar AS, Aye RW, Vallières E. Early experience with robotic lung resection results in similar operative outcomes and morbidity when compared with matched video-assisted thoracoscopic surgery cases. Anna Thorac Surg. 2012;93:1598–1604.
21. Augustin F, Bodner J, Maier H, et al. Robotic-assisted minimally invasive vs. thoracoscopic lung lobectomy: Comparison of perioperative results in a learning curve setting. *Langenbecks Arch Surg.* 2013;398:895–901.
22. Kent M, Wang T, Whyte R, Curran T, Flores R, Gangadharan S. Open, video-assisted thoracic surgery, and robotic lobectomy: review of a national database. *Anna Thorac Surg.* 2014;97(1):236–242.
23. Swanson SJ, Miller DL, McKenna RJ Jr, et al. Comparing robot-assisted thoracic surgical lobectomy with conventional video-assisted thoracic surgical lobectomy and wedge resection: Results from a multihospital database. *J Thorac Cardiovasc Surg.* 2014;147(3):929–937.
24. Nakamura H. Systematic review of published studies on safety and efficacy of thoracoscopic and robot-assisted lobectomy for lung cancer. *Anna Thorac Cardiovasc Surg.* 2014;20(2):93–98.
25. Cao C, Manganas C, Ang SC, Yan TD. A systematic review and meta-analysis on pulmonary resections by robotic video-assisted thoracic surgery. *Anna Cardiothorac Surg.* 2012;1(1):3–10.
26. Adams RD, Bolton WD, Stephenson JE, Henry G, Robbins ET, Sommers E. Initial multicenter community robotic lobectomy experience: comparisons to a national database. *Anna Thorac Surg.* 2014;97(6):1893–1898.
27. Paul S, Jalbert J, Isaacs AJ, Altorki NK, Isom OW, Sedrakyan A. Comparative effectiveness of robotic-assisted vs thoracoscopic lobectomy. *Chest.* 2014;146(6):1505–1512.
28. Park BJ, Melfi F, Mussi A, et al. Robotic lobectomy for non-small cell lung cancer (NSCLC): long-term oncologic results. *J Thorac Cardiovasc Surg.* 2012;143(2):383–389.

29. Demir A, Ayalp K, Ozkan B, Kabe E, Toker A. Robotic and video-assisted thoracic surgery lung segmentectomy for malignant and benign lesions. *Interact Cardiovasc Thorac Surg.* 2015;20(3):304–309.
30. Seto Y, Mori K, Aikou S. Robotic surgery for esophageal cancer: merits and demerits. *Anna Gastroenterol Surg.* 2017;1(3):193–198.
31. Suda K, Nakauchi M, Inaba K, Ishida Y, Uyama I. Robotic surgery for upper gastrointestinal cancer: current status and future perspectives. *Digest Endosc.* 2016;28(7):701–713.
32. Weksler B, Sharma P, Moudgill N, Chojnacki KA, Rosato EL. Robot-assisted minimally invasive esophagectomy is equivalent to thoracoscopic minimally invasive esophagectomy. *Dis Esophagus.* 2012;25(5):403–409.
33. Clark J, Sodergren MH, Purkayastha S, et al. The role of robotic assisted laparoscopy for oesophagogastric oncological resection: an appraisal of the literature. *Dis Esophagus.* 2011;24(4):240–250.
34. Ruurda JP, van der Sluis PC, van der Horst S, van Hilllegersberg R. Robot-assisted minimally invasive esophagectomy for esophageal cancer: a systematic review. *J Surg Oncol.* 2015;112:257–265.
35. Qureshi YA, Dawas KI, Mughal M, Mohammadi B. Minimally invasive and robotic esophagectomy: evolution and evidence. *J Surg Oncol.* 2016;114:731–735.
36. D'Amico TA. Robotics in thoracic surgery: applications and outcomes. *J Thorac Cardiovasc Surg.* 2006;131:19–20.
37. Ruckert JC, Swierzy M, Ismail M. Comparison of robotic and nonrobotic thoracoscopic thymectomy: a cohort study. J Thorac Cardiovasc Surg. 2011;141:673–277.
38. Rueckert J, Swierzy M, Badakhshi H, Meisel A, Ismail M. Robotic-assisted thymectomy: surgical procedure and results. *Thorac Cardiovasc Surg.* 2015;63:194–200.
39. Ricciardi R, Melfi F, Maestri M, et al. Endoscopic thymectomy: a neurologist's perspective. *Anna Cardiothorac Surg.* 2016;5(1):38–44.
40. Keijzers M, Dingemans AM, Blaauwgeers H, et al. 8 years' experience with robotic thymectomy for thymomas. *Surg Endoscop.* 2014;28:1202–1208.
41. Marulli G, Maessen J, Melfi F, et al. Multi-institutional European experience of robotic thymectomy for thymoma. *Anna Cardiothorac Surg.* 2016;5:18–25.
42. Kajiwara N, Kakihana M, Usuda J, Ohira T, Kawate N, Ikeda N. Extended indications for robotic surgery for posterior mediastinal tumors. *Asian Cardiovasc Thorac Anna.* 2012;20:308–313.
43. Kroh M, El-Hayek K, Rosenblatt S, et al. First human surgery with a novel single-port robotic system: cholecystectomy using the da Vinci single-site platform. *Surg Endosc.* 2011;25(11):3566–3573.
44. Scheib SA, Fader AN. Gynecologic robotic laparoendoscopic single-site surgery: prospective analysis of feasibility, safety, and technique. *Am J Obstet Gynecol.* 2015;212(2):179e1–8.
45. Ramirez D, Maurice MJ, Kaouk JH. Robotic perineal radical prostatectomy and pelvic lymph node dissection using a purpose-built single-port robotic platform. *BJU Int.* 2016;118:829–833.
46. Maurice MJ, Ramirez D, Kaouk JH. Robotic laparoendoscopic single-site retroperitioneal renal surgery: Initial investigation of a purpose-built single-port surgical system. *Eur Urol.* 2017;71:643–647.
47. Park SY, Kim HK, Jang DS, Han KN, Kim DJ. Initial experiences with robotic single-site thoracic surgery for mediastinal masses. *Anna Thorac Surg.* 2019;107(1):242–247.
48. Gonzalez-Rivas D, Ismail M. Subxiphoid or subcostal uniportal robotic-assisted surgery: early experimental experience. *J Thorac Dis.* 2019;11(1):231–239.
49. Kim DJ, Hyung WJ, Lee CY, et al. Thoracoscopic esophagectomy for esophageal cancer: feasibility and safety of robotic assistance in the prone position. *J Thorac Cardiovasc Surg.* 2010;139:53–59.
50. Schmied H, Kurz A, Sessler DI, Kozek S, Reiter A. Mild hypothermia increases blood loss and transfusion requirements during total hip arthroplasty. *Lancet.* 1996;347:289–292.
51. Frank SM, Fleisher LA, Breslow MJ, at al. Perioperative maintenance of normothermia reduces the incidence of morbid cardiac events: a randomized clinical trial. *JAMA.* 1997;277(14): 1127–1134.
52. Kurz A, Sessler DI, Lenhardt R. Perioperative normothermia to reduce the incidence of surgical-wound infection and shorten hospitalization: study of wound infection and temperature group. *N Engl J Med.* 1996;334:1209–1215.

53. Hynson JM, Sessler DI, Moayeri A, McGuire J, Schroeder M. The effects of preinduction warming on temperature and blood pressure during propofol/nitrous oxide anesthesia. Anesthesiology. 1993;79(2):219–228.
54. Lohser J, Slinger P. Lung injury after one-lung ventilation: a review of the pathophysiologic mechanisms affecting the ventilated and the collapsed lung. *Anesth Analg.* 2015;121(2):302–318.
55. Arslantas MK, Kara HV, Tuncer BB, et al. Effect of the amount of intraoperative fluid administration on postoperative pulmonary complications following anatomic lung resections. *J Thorac Cardiovasc Surg.* 2015;149(1):314–321.
56. Zeldin RA, Normandin D, Landtwing D, Peters RM. Postpneumonectomy pulmonary edema. *J Thorac Cardiovasc Surg.* 1984;87:359–365.
57. Alam N, Park BJ, Wilton A, et al. Incidence and risk factors for lung injury after lung cancer resection. *Anna Thorac Surg.* 2007;84:1085–1091.
58. Brandstrup B, Tønnesen H, Beier-Holgersen R, et al. Effects of intravenous fluid restriction on postoperative complications: comparison of two perioperative fluid regimens: a randomized assessor-blinded multicenter trial. *Anna Surg.* 2003;238:641–648.
59. Licker M, de Perrot M, Spiliopoulos A, et al. Risk factors for acute lung injury after thoracic surgery for lung cancer. *Anesth Analg.* 2003;97:1558–1565.
60. Sunaga H, Blasberg JD, Heerdt PM. Anesthesia for nonintubated video-assisted thoracic surgery. *Curr Opin Anaesthesiol.* 2017;30(1):1–6.
61. Katlic MR. Five hundred seventy-six cases of video-assisted thoracic surgery using local anesthesia and sedation: lessons learned. *J Am Coll Surg.* 2018;226(1):58–63.
62. Pompeo E, Tacconi F, Mineo D, Mineo T. The role of awake video-assisted thoracoscopic surgery in spontaneous pneumothorax. *J Thorac Cardiovasc Surg.* 2007;133:786–790.
63. Noda M, Okada Y, Maeda S, et al. Is there a benefit of awake thoracoscopic surgery in patients with secondary spontaneous pneumothorax? *J Thorac Cardiovasc Surg.* 2012;143:613–616.
64. Pompeo E, Dauri M. Is there any benefit in using awake anesthesia with thoracic epidural in thoracoscopic talc pleurodesis? *J Thorac Cardiovasc Surg.* 2013;146:495–497.
65. Hung MH, Chan KC, Liu YJ, et al. Nonintubated thoracoscopic lobectomy for lung cancer using epidural anesthesia and intercostal blockade. *Anna Surg.* 2011;254:1038–1043.
66. Wu CY, Chen JS, Lin YS, et al. Feasibility and safety of nonintubated thoracoscopic lobectomy for geriatric lung cancer patients. *Anna Thorac Surg.* 2013;95:405–411.
67. Mineo TC, Sellitri F, Tacconi F, Ambrogi V. Quality of life and outcomes after nonintubated versus intubated video-thoracoscopic pleurodesis for malignant pleural effusion: comparison by a case-matched study. *J Pall Med.* 2014;17:761–768.
68. Liu J, Cui F, Li S, et al. Nonintubated video-assisted thoracoscopic surgery under epidural anesthesia compared with conventional anesthetic option: a randomized control study. *Surg Innov.* 2015;22:123–130.
69. Vanni G, Tacconi F, Sellitri F, Ambrogi V, Mineo TC, Pompeo E. Impact of awake videothoracoscopic surgery on postoperative lymphocyte responses. *Anna Thorac Surg.* 2010;90:973–978.
70. Katlic MR, Facktor MA. Video-assisted thoracic surgery utilizing local anesthesia and sedation: 384 consecutive cases. *Anna Thorac Surg.* 2010;90:240–245.
71. Pompeo E, Rogliani P, Cristino B, Schillaci O, Novelli G, Saltini C. Awake thoracoscopic biopsy of interstitial lung disease. *Anna Thorac Surg.* 2013;95:445–452.
72. Ambrogi V, Mineo TC. VATS biopsy for undetermined interstitial lung disease under non-general anesthesia: comparison between uniportal approach under intercostal block vs. three-ports in epidural anesthesia. *J Thoracd Dis.* 2014;6:888–895.
73. Kiss G, Claret A, Desbordes J, Porte H. Thoracic epidural anaesthesia for awake thoracic surgery in severely dyspnoeic patients excluded from general anaesthesia. *Interact Cardiovasc Thorac Surg.* 2014;19(5):816–823.
74. Piccioni F, Langer M, Fumagalli L, Haeusler E, Conti B, Previtali P. Thoracic paravertebral anaesthesia for awake video-assisted thoracoscopic surgery daily. *Anaesthesia.* 2010;65(12):1221–1224.
75. Kiss G, Castillo M. Non-intubated anesthesia in thoracic surgery-technical issues. *Anna Transl Med.* 2015;3(8):109.

76. Chen KC, Cheng YJ, Hung MH, Tseng YD, Chen JS. Nonintubated thoracoscopic surgery using regional anesthesia and vagal block and targeted sedation. *J Thorac Dis*. 2014;6(1):31–36.
77. Tseng YD, Cheng YJ, Hung MH, Chen KC, Chen JS. Nonintubated needlescopic video-assisted thoracic surgery for management of peripheral lung nodules. *Anna Thorac Surg*. 2012;93:1049–1054.
78. Guo Z, Shao W, Yin W, et al. Analysis of feasibility and safety of complete video-assisted thoracoscopic resection of anatomic pulmonary segments under non-intubated anesthesia. *J Thorac Dis*. 2014;6(1):37–44.
79. Chen KC, Cheng YJ, Hung MH, Tseng YD, Chen JS. Nonintubated thoracoscopic lung resection: a 3-year experience with 285 cases in a single institution. *J Thorac Dis*. 2012;4:347–351.
80. Gonzalez-Rivas D, Fernandez R, de la Torre M, Benome C. Uniportal video-assisted thoracoscopic left upper lobectomy under spontaneous ventilation. *J Thorac Dis*. 2015;7:494–495.
81. Dong Q, Liang L, Li Y, et al. Anesthesia with nontracheal intubation in thoracic surgery. *J Thorac Dis*. 2012;4:126–130.
82. Iwata Y, Hamai Y, Koyama T. Anesthetic management of nonintubated video-assisted thoracoscopic surgery using epidural anesthesia and dexmedetomidine in three patients with severe respiratory dysfunction. *J Anesth*. 2016;30(2):324–327.
83. Gallego-Ligorit L, Vives M, Vallés-Torres J, Sanjuán-Villarreal TA, Pajares A, Iglesias M. Use of dexmedetomidine in cardiothoracic and vascular anesthesia. *J Cardiothorac Vasc Anesth*. 2018(3);32:1426–1438.
84. Salati M, Brunelli A. Uniportal VATS for pneumothorax and interstitial lung disease. *J Thorac Dis*. 2013;5(Suppl 3):S217–S220.
85. Gonzalez-Rivas D. Uniportal thoracoscopic surgery: from medical thoracoscopy to non-intubated uniportal video-assisted major pulmonary resections. *Anna Cardiothorac Surg*. 2016;5:85–91.
86. Halezeroğlu S. Advantages and disadvantages of single incision VATS in major anatomical resection for lung cancer. *J Visual Surg*. 2017;3:115.
87. Harris CG, James RS, Tian DH, et al. Systematic review and meta-analysis of uniportal versus multiportal video-assisted thoracoscopic lobectomy for lung cancer. *Anna Cardiothorac Surg*. 2016;5:76–84.
88. Bunchungmongkol N, Pipanmekaporn T, Paiboonworachat S, Saeteng S, Tantraworasin A. Incidence and risk factors associated with ipsilateral shoulder pain after thoracic surgery. *J Cardiothorac Vasc Anesth*. 2014;28(4):979–982.
89. Ohmori A, Iranami H, Fujii K, Yamazaki A, Doko Y. Myofascial involvement of supra- and infraspinatus muscles contributes to ipsilateral shoulder pain after muscle-sparing thoracotomy and video-assisted thoracic surgery. *J Cardiothorac Vasc Anesth*. 2013;27:1310–1314.
90. Yousefshahi F, Predescu O, Colizza M, Asenjo JF. Postthoracotomy ipsilateral shoulder pain: a literature review on characteristics and treatment. *Pain Res Manage*. 2016;2016:3652726.
91. Scawn ND, Pennefather SH, Soorae A, Wang JY, Russell GN. Ipsilateral shoulder pain after thoracotomy with epidural analgesia: the influence of phrenic nerve infiltration with lidocaine. *Anesth Analg*. 2001;93(2):260–264.
92. Danelli G, Berti M, Casati A, et al. Ipsilateral shoulder pain after thoracotomy surgery: a prospective, randomized, double-blind, placebo-controlled evaluation of the efficacy of infiltrating the phrenic nerve with 0.2%wt/vol ropivacaine. *Eur J Anaesthesiol*. 2007;24(7):596–601.
93. Martinez-Barenys C, Busquets J, de Castro PE, et al. Randomized double-blind comparison of phrenic nerve infiltration and suprascapular nerve block for ipsilateral shoulder pain after thoracic surgery. *Eur J Cardiothorac Surg*. 2011;40(1):106–112.
94. Umari M, Falini S, Segat M, et al. Anesthesia and fast-track in video-assisted thoracic surgery (VATS): from evidence to practice. *J Thorac Dis*. 2018;10(Suppl 4):S542–S544.
95. Park MH, Kim JA, Ahn HJ, Yang MK, Son HJ, Seong BG. A randomised trial of serratus anterior plane block for analgesia after thoracoscopic surgery. *Anaesthesia*. 2018;73(10):1260–1264.
96. Hu B, Zhou H, Zou X. The erector spinae plane block (ESPB) for non-intubated video-assisted thoracoscopic surgery. *J Clin Anesth*. 2019;54:50–51.
97. Parascandola SA, Ibañez J, Keir G, Anderson J, Plankey M, Flynn D, et al. Liposomal bupivacaine versus bupivacaine/epinephrine after video-assisted thoracoscopic wedge resection. *Interact Cardiovasc Thorac Surg*. 2017;24(6):925–930.

22
Enhanced Recovery in Thoracic Surgery

Manxu Zhao, Zhongyuan Xia, and Henry Liu

Introduction

Implementation of enhanced recovery after surgery (ERAS) protocols is achieved through multiple evidence-based perioperative measures [1,2]. ERAS has been shown to improve the patient's perioperative outcomes, facilitate recovery, decrease the incidence of postoperative complications with shorter hospital length of stay (LOS) and overall cost savings [2,3]. Multiple small-element improvements in patient care from referral to discharge have been developed to cover various aspects related to preadmission, admission, intraoperative care, and postoperative care [3,4]. ERAS protocols for thoracic surgery include elements such as regional anesthesia, euvolemic fluid management, early chest tube removal, deep vein thrombosis (DVT), and atrial fibrillation prevention to reduce pulmonary and cardiac complications [2,5,6].

Preadmission Counseling and Education

Comprehensive preoperative counseling helps to set realistic expectations and provides better understanding about surgical and anesthetic procedures and may reduce anxiety, pain, and fatigue and enhance recovery and early discharge. Patients should receive written and verbal instructions and multimedia information containing explanations of the procedure and anesthesia (Table 22.1).

Preoperative Care

With patient education and counseling in the preoperative units, anesthesia care providers can focus on preventing dehydration, DVT, postoperative nausea and vomiting (PONV) and decreasing postoperative pain [Table 22.2].

Intraoperative Period

Antibiotic Prophylaxis

With postoperative pulmonary infection rate as high as 7% to 14% after thoracic surgery [15], it is important to ensure adequate antibiotic concentration in the serum and tissue during

Table 22.1 ERAS in Thoracic Surgery: Pre-admission Preparations

	Evidence-Based Recommendations
Nutrition assessment and supplement	Oral supplement 5–7 days prior to surgery to patient: • Weight lost >10%, • BMI <18.5 kg/m^2, • Albumin <30g/L [7]. Improve quality of life and muscle function and decreased complication rate and chest tube removal time [4,8]
Smoking cessation	Stop 4 weeks before surgery • Behavioral therapy • Pharmacotherapy • Nicotine replacement • Immersing E-cigarettes [9]
Alcohol abuse management	Stop 4–8 weeks before surgery [10]
Management of anemia	• Treat with iron supplement as indicated • Avoid erythropoietin and blood transfusion in cancer patients (poorer outcomes) [11] • Lowering triggering level of hemoglobin for transfusion
Pulmonary rehabilitation	Indication: • Poor exercise tolerance • Borderline Pulmonary function test Goal: • Improve peak oxygen consumption or functional capacity (measured with the 6-minute walk test) aerobic training (lower and/or upper limbs) • Strength training • Respiratory exercises • Relaxation techniques • Exercise intensity, frequency (1–10 weeks), duration (2–14 weeks) [12]

Abbreviation: BMI, body mass index; ERAS, enhanced recovery after surgery.

incision. Antibiotics should cover bacteria colonized in the airway and skin. Usually the first antibiotic choice is cephalosporins with amoxicillin–clavulanic acid as an alternative, especially with targeted prophylactic antibiotics for the prevention of postoperative pneumonia [16]. Vancomycin or teicoplanin may be used in penicillin-allergic patients. Antibiotics should be given no more than 60 minutes prior to skin incision with repeated doses for prolonged operations or with more than 1500 ml blood loss.

Skin Preparation

Patients should take a shower or bath the night before or in the morning of the operative day using plain soap [17]. Chlorhexidine–alcohol is preferred over povidone-iodine solutions, showing a 40% reduction in surgical site infection. Deep or subcutaneous tissues irrigation with aqueous iodophor solution also helps. It is not recommended to remove hair, apply plastic adhesive drapes, soak prosthetic devices in antiseptic solutions before implantation, or lavage the pleural cavity with aqueous iodophor solution [17].

Table 22.2 ERAS in Thoracic Surgery: Preoperative Care

	Evidence-based Recommendation
Preoperative fasting	• Allows clear liquid 2 hours prior to surgery • Allows solid 6 hours prior to surgery • Except patient with delayed gastric emptying [13]
Preoperative carbohydrate	To be given 2 hours prior to surgery
Pre-anesthetic medications	• Avoid sedatives • Opioid-sparing medication • Patient education • Relaxation techniques • Music interventions [14]
Venous thromboembolic prophylaxis	Pharmacological: • Low molecular weight heparin • Unfractionated heparin Mechanical: • Compression stockings • Intermittent pneumatic compression devices • Foot impulse devices • Cancer patient should have 4 weeks prophylactic treatment
PONV prevention	Nonpharmacologic approach for all patients • Avoidance of prolonged fasting and dehydration • Preoperative carbohydrate loading • Peripheral nerve blocks or neuraxial anesthesia • P6 acupoint stimulation Multimodal pharmacological control for mod-high risk patients • 1st line: ondansetron, corticosteroids to all patients • 2nd line: scopolamine, compazine, metoclopramide, aprepitant to moderate to high risk patient • 3nd line: promethazine as rescue

Abbreviations: ERAS, enhanced recovery after surgery; PONV, postoperative nausea and vomiting.

Preventing Intraoperative Hypothermia

Perioperative hypothermia is present when the patient's temperature is less than 36°C. It increases bleeding, wound infections, and cardiovascular complications, including myocardial and bowel ischemia, and prolongs hospital LOS. Hypothermia prevention should start in the preoperative area and continue to the operating room until the postoperative period with a forced air and fluid warming system to maintain normothermia [3,18].

Management of One-Lung Ventilation

Two main concerns of one-lung ventilation (OLV) are hypoxemia and postoperative acute lung injury (ALI). Ventilation/perfusion mismatch and malposition of double-lumen tube contribute to hypoxemia. ALI occurs in 4% to 15% of patients during lung resections and affects both lungs. Lung-protective ventilation strategies may reduce inflammation response [19,20], and result in fewer postoperative pulmonary complications [21,22].

- FiO_2: lowest to maintain SpO_2 >90%
- TV: 4 to 6 ml/kg based on ideal bodyweight
- PEEP: 5 to 10 cmH_2O to dependent lung
- CPAP: 2 to 5 cmH_2O (disrupt when visibility impaired) to nondependent lung
- $PaCO_2$: <60 to 70 mmHg

Recruitment maneuvers improve gas exchange and ventilation efficiency during OLV with improved oxygenation, better compliance, and decreased dead space and may reduce inflammatory cytokines release [23]. The peak airway pressure for recruitment in the healthy lung should be less than 40 cmH_2O, with a PEEP slowly increasing up to 20 cmH_2O. It should be lower in a diseased lung. The final recruitment maneuvers with TLV should be performed at lower pressure levels to prevent disrupting surgical staples.

Nonintubated Anesthesia

The nonintubated video-assisted thoracoscopic surgical procedures (VATS) have a lower risk of postoperative complications and a shorter mean LOS [24] for procedures including lobectomy, pneumonectomy, excision of bullae, and lung volume reduction. While maintaining spontaneous ventilation, anesthesia management involves regional anesthesia, intravenous sedation, and well-planned airway management to convert to general anesthesia and lung separation when needed. Although the technique shows potential, the routine use of nonintubated anesthesia cannot be recommended [24].

Postoperative Period

Multimodal Pain Relief

Effective analgesia is essential so the patient can cough with minimal pain, breathe deeply, and ambulate early. Multimodal analgesia with regional analgesia or local anesthetic techniques may avoid or minimize opioids and their side effects. The additive or synergistic effects of different types of analgesics minimize the side effects of individual drugs while potentiating the desired effects.

Regional Analgesia

Thoracic epidural analgesia (TEA) is commonly used in thoracic surgery. There are several side effects including the possibility of urinary retention, hypotension, muscular weakness, and epidural hematoma or abscess. It is placed at level of T3–T4 or T4–T5 with achievable dermatome of T1 to T10 with continuous infusion of a local anesthetic agent with or without opioids.

Intercostal catheter is as effective as TEA in terms of postoperative analgesia. It is potentially more cost-effective, requires less time, can be placed by the surgeon at the end of the operation, and may be associated with fewer complications.

Paravertebral block (PVB) provides a unilateral block of somatic and sympathetic nerves. Local anesthetic agent is injected into the paravertebral space that is lateral to the epidural space where the spinal nerves travel (Figure 22.1). Two or more PVBs are injected to ensure

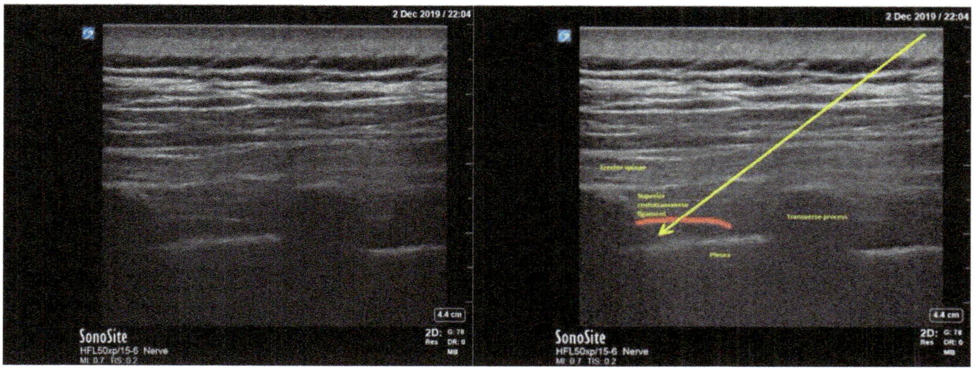

Figure 22.1 Paravertebral block under ultrasound guidance in parasagittal approach. Yellow line indicates the needle trajectory with arrow showing local anesthetic deposition.

the distribution of several dermatomes. PVB can be achieved through a loss of resistance technique, under thoracoscopic or ultrasound guidance, or under direct vision during thoracotomy. PVB has similar analgesic efficacy but fewer side effects of PONV, pruritus, hypotension and urinary retention, respiratory complications, and hemodynamic instability when compared to TEA [5].

The serratus anterior plane block provides adequate analgesia for the first 24 hours after thoracotomy [25]. Under ultrasound guidance, the patient is placed in the lateral position with the probe overlying the fifth rib at the midclavicular region. Three muscles are identified: the latissimus dorsi (superficial and posterior), teres major (superior), and serratus anterior muscle (deep and inferior). The needle is advanced from posterior to anterocaudal direction to reach the plane superficial to serratus anterior muscle (Figure 22.2).

Erector spinae plane block (ESPB) is a novel technique providing analgesia after VATS. ESPB is not inferior to that of PVB 24 hours postoperatively [26]. The ESPB is a fascial plane

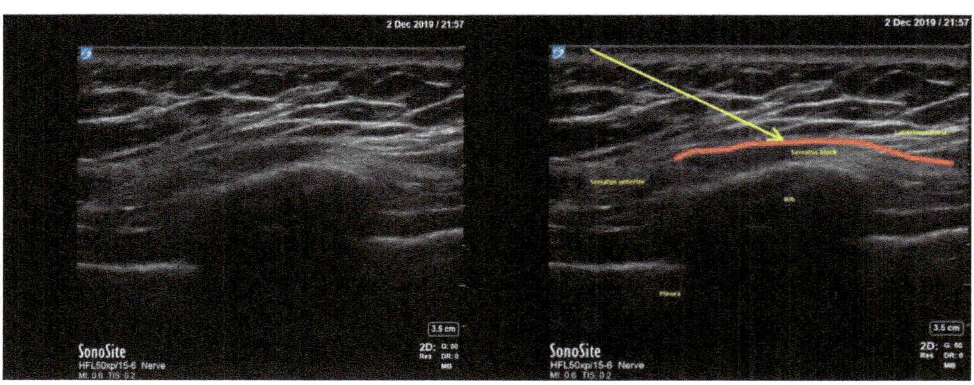

Figure 22.2 Serratus anterior plane block. Yellow line presents the needle trajectory and arrow presents the needle end point for local anesthetic medication deposition.

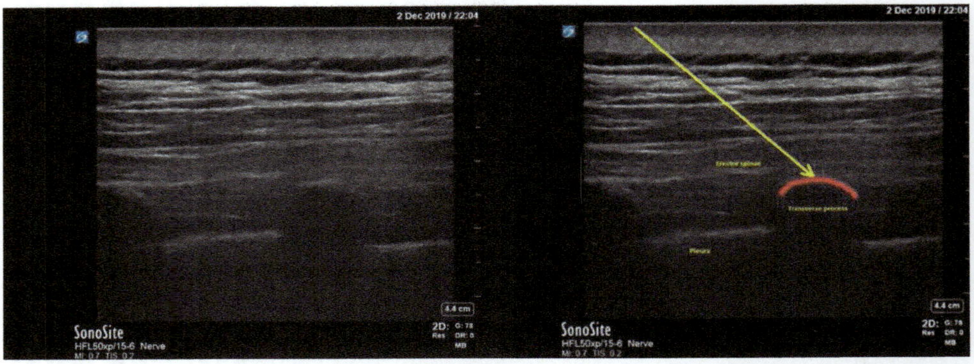

Figure 22.3 Erector spinae plane block. Yellow line indicates the needle trajectory with arrow showing the needle tip above transverse process and below erector spinae muscle.

block with local anesthetic injected beneath erector spinae muscle (Figure 22.3). Under ultrasound guidance, the needle is placed between the transverse process and erector spinae muscle. Clinical effects of the ESPB depend on the spread of the local anesthetic volume. ESPB may potentially block both dorsal ramus and ventral ramus of the spinal nerve through the intercostal space and paravertebral space [27,28].

Opioids

Opioids should be used as part of multimodal regimens for major thoracic surgery. However, opioid-related adverse drug events are common and have been associated with increased inpatient mortality, prolonged LOS, high cost of hospitalization, and higher rate of 30-day readmission; opioid-sparing interventions should be employed, whenever possible [33] (Table 22.3).

Fluid Management

Fluid management is challenging during thoracic surgery as patients are prone to developing pulmonary and interstitial edema. Pre-existing lung disease, chemoradiotherapy, direct surgical lung manipulation, one-lung ventilation, and reperfusion injury predispose patients to lung injury [34] Perioperative fluid management is restricted to 1 to 3 ml/kg/h with positive fluid balance of <1500 ml (or 20 ml/kg/24 h) to minimize the hydrostatic pressure in the pulmonary capillaries [35]. Additional fluid is given to replenish blood or exudative loss. Oral fluids and diet should resume as soon as the patient is lucid and able to swallow (Table 22.4).

Arrythmia Prevention

Postoperative atrial fibrillation and flutter (POAF) is one of the most common cardiac complications following thoracic surgery. It is associated with an increased LOS, higher rates of readmission and stroke, and increased morbidity and mortality [36]. Recommendations in the 2014 American Association for Thoracic Surgery guidelines to prevent and manage POAF include continuation of β-blockers perioperatively, supplementation of magnesium in

Table 22.3 ERAS in Thoracic Surgery: Opioid-sparing medications

Group	Medication	Benefit
Acetaminophen	Acetaminophen	Decreases ipsilateral shoulder pain after thoracotomy
NSAIDs	Ketorolac	Decreases ipsilateral post-thoracotomy shoulder tip pain [29]
		Prolong survival in cancer patients [30]
NMDA Antagonists	Ketamine, magnesium	Improve early postoperative lung function [31]
Gabapentinoids	Gabapentin, pregabalin	Treat neuropathic pain
Glucocorticoids	Dexamethasone, methylprednisolone	Prevent PONV, prolongs the duration of peripheral nerve block [32]

Abbreviations: ERAS, enhanced recovery after surgery; NSAID, nonsteroidal anti-inflammatory drugs; NMDA, *N*-methyl-D-aspartate; PONV, postoperative nausea and vomiting.

magnesium-depleted patients, and administration of diltiazem preoperatively or amiodarone postoperatively in high-risk patients [37].

Chest Drain Management

The chest tube provides important monitoring and recovery means post-thoracic surgery. A retained chest tube is painful, decreases respiratory function, and delays ambulation. The routine application of external suction offers no advantages and should be avoided. No suction reduces the duration of air leak but increases the risk of pneumonia and arrhythmia due to air accumulation [38]. The amount of pleural fluid output observed daily influences the timing of chest tube removal. Pleural effusion of 450 mL/day is the highest volume threshold for the removal of a chest tube after pulmonary resection [39]. Digital chest drainage devices

Table 22.4 ERAS in Thoracic Surgery: Postoperative Management

	Evidence-Based Recommendation
Fluid management	Restricted to 1–3 mL/kg/h with positive fluid balance of <1500 mL
Arrhythmia prevention and management	• Beta-blocker continuation • Magnesium supplement • Diltiazem preoperatively or amiodarone postoperatively in high risk patients
Chest drain management	• D/C chest tube if 450 mL/day of fluid drainage or less • Single chest tube to be placed • Digital drainage system
Urinary drain	Unnecessary except patient with TEA or urinary retention
Early mobilization	Within 24 hours postoperative

Abbreviations: ERAS, enhanced recovery after surgery; TEA, thoracic epidural analgesia.

provide more reliable and objective airflow measurements to guide chest tube management. A single chest drain instead of two after a routine anatomical lung resection is safe and effective to adequately manage air leak and pleural effusion and is less painful (Table 22.4).

Urinary Drainage

Urinary drainage is used to prevent urinary retention (incidence of 11.6%) and monitor urine output during and after thoracic surgery. The causes of urinary retention may include increasing age, being male, diabetes mellitus, pain, and TEA [40]. It is associated with increased LOS and an increased risk of urinary tract infection and impedes postoperative mobilization. A Foley catheter is unnecessary for the sole purpose of monitoring urine output. Urinary output is an ineffective indicator of fluid status and does not influence the occurrence of renal dysfunction perioperatively with fluid management [41].

Early Mobilization

Postoperative immobility is associated with increased morbidity and LOS due to diminished muscle mass, increased risk of pulmonary complications, and VTE. Early ambulation within 24 hours is beneficial in terms of early discharge of patients and low morbidity [2].

Outcomes: ERAS in Thoracic Surgery

Multiple studies have shown different clinical outcomes after ERAS protocol implementation in thoracic surgery [2,3,18,42]. Brunelli et al. compared ERAS pathway versus standard care in patients undergoing video-assisted thoracoscopic lobectomy and found no benefit conferred by the ERAS program on outcomes such as cardiopulmonary complications, 30- and 90-day mortality, LOS, and readmissions [18]. While Rogers et al. conducted a prospective cohort study on 422 consecutive patients undergoing lung resection for primary lung cancer and followed a standardized, 15-element ERAS protocol in all patients. They concluded that increased compliance with an ERAS pathway is associated with improved clinical outcomes after resection for primary lung cancer, and they emphasized that several elements, including early mobilization, appeared to be more influential than other measures [2]. A report from the United Kingdom by Scarci et al. found that patients on the ERAS program had a significantly reduced postoperative LOS in thoracic surgery. Patient satisfaction was also higher in the ERAS group, and ERAS implementation resulted in a significant financial benefit. Thus they believe that the ERAS pathway is a safe perioperative management strategy to improve patient satisfaction and reduce LOS and cost after major thoracic surgery without increasing morbidity or mortality [43].

Summary

Accumulating evidence suggests that ERAS protocols show efficacy and benefits in thoracic surgery. ERAS implementation will take some time and initial investment from the hospital. It will take a multidisciplinary approach and involve continuous education and training of pertinent personnel. The ERAS program demands streamlining the preoperative, intraoperative, and postoperative care of surgical patients. Continuously monitoring the compliance of individual patients and surgeons are also important to gain all the benefits of an ERAS program [2].

References

1. Kehlet H, Wilmore DW. Evidence-based surgical care and the evolution of fast-track surgery. *Ann Surg.* 2008;248:189–198.
2. Rogers LJ, Bleetman D, Messenger DE, et al. The impact of enhanced recovery after surgery (ERAS) protocol compliance on morbidity from resection for primary lung cancer. *J Thorac Cardiovasc Surg.* 2018;155:1843–1852.
3. Coleman SR, Chen M, Patel S, Yan H, Kaye AD, Zebrower M, et al. Enhance Recovery Pathways for Cardiac Surgery. *Curr Pain Headache Rep.* 2019;23(4):28. doi:10.1007/s11916-019-0764-2. PMID: 30868281
4. Collins PF, Elia M, Stratton RJ. Nutritional support and functional capacity in chronic obstructive pulmonary disease: a systematic review and meta-analysis. *Respirology.* 2013;18:616–629.
5. Liu H, Emelife PI, Moll V, et al. Regional anesthesia for cardiac surgery. *Best Pract Res Clin Anaesthesiol.* 2019;33(4):387–406. doi:10.1016/j.bpa.2019.07.008
6. Van Haren RM, Mehran RJ, Correa AM, et al. Enhanced recovery decreases pulmonary and cardiac complications following thoracotomy for lung cancer. *Ann Thorac Surg.* 2018;106:272–279.
7. Weimann A, Braga M, Carli F, et al. ESPEN guideline: clinical nutrition in surgery. *Clin Nutr.* 2017;36:623–650.
8. Matzi V, Lindenmann J, Muench A, et al. The impact of preoperative micronutrient supplementation in lung surgery: a prospective randomized trial of oral supplementation of combined alpha-ketoglutaric acid and 5-hydroxymethylfurfural. *Eur J Cardiothorac Surg.* 2007;32:776–782.
9. Lee SM, Tenney R, Wallace AW, Arjomandi M. E-cigarettes versus nicotine patches for perioperative smoking cessation: a pilot randomized trial. *Peer J.* 2018:28;6.
10. Egholm JW, Pedersen B, Møller AM, Adami J, Juhl CB, Tønnesen H. Perioperative alcohol cessation intervention for postoperative complications. *Cochrane Database Syst Rev.* 2018;11:CD008343.
11. Tonia T, Mettler A, Robert N, et al. Erythropoietin or darbepoetin for patients with cancer. *Cochrane Database Syst Rev* 2012;12:CD003407.
12. Kadiri SB, Kerr AP, Oswald NK, et al. Fit 4 surgery, a bespoke app with biofeedback delivers rehabilitation at home before and after elective lung resection. *J Cardiothorac Surg.* 2019;14(1):132. doi:10.1186/s13019-019-0951-6.
13. Fawcett WJ, Thomas M. Pre-operative fasting in adults and children: clinical practice and guidelines. *Anesthesia.* 2019;74:83–88.
14. Stamenkovic DM, Rancic NK, Latas MB, et al. Preoperative anxiety and implications on postoperative recovery: what can we do to change our history? *Minerva Anesth.* 2018;84:1307–1317.
15. Oxman DA, Issa NC, Marty FM, et al. Postoperative antibacterial prophylaxis for the prevention of infectious complications associated with tube thoracostomy in patients undergoing elective general thoracic surgery: a double-blind, placebo-controlled, randomized trial. *JAMA Surg.* 2013;148:440–446.
16. Villeneuve PJ. Interventions to avoid pulmonary complications after lung cancer resection. J Thorac Dis 2018;10(Suppl. 32): S3781–S3788.
17. Berrios-Torres SI, Umscheid CA, Bratzler DW, et al. Centers for Disease Control and Prevention guideline for the prevention of surgical site infection, 2017. *JAMA Surg.* 2017;152:784–791.
18. Brunelli A, Thomas C, Dinesh P, Lumb A. Enhanced recovery pathway versus standard care in patients undergoing video-assisted thoracoscopic lobectomy. *J Thorac Cardiovasc Surg.* 2017;154:2084–2090.

19. Schilling T, Kozian A, Huth C, Kretzschmar M, Welte T, Hachenberg T. The pulmonary immune effects of mechanical ventilation in patients undergoing thoracic surgery. *Anesth Analg.* 2005;101:957–965.
20. Michelet P, D'Journo X-B, Roch A, et al. Protective ventilation influences systemic inflammation after esophagectomy: a randomized controlled study. *Anesthesiology.* 2006;105:911–919.
21. Licker M, Diaper J, Villiger Y, et al. Impact of intraoperative lung-protective interventions in patients undergoing lung cancer surgery. *Crit Care.* 2009;13:R41.
22. Fernández-Pérez ER, Keegan MT, Brown DR, et al. Intraoperative tidal volume as a risk factor for respiratory failure after pneumonectomy. *Anesthesiology.* 2006;105:14–18.
23. Blank RS, Colquhoun DA, Durieux ME, et al. Management of one-lung ventilation: impact of tidal volume on complications after thoracic surgery. *Anesthesiology*. 2016;124:1286–1295.
24. Deng HY, Zhu ZJ, Wang YC, Wang WP, Ni PZ, Chen LQ. Non-intubated video-assisted thoracoscopic surgery under loco-regional anaesthesia for thoracic surgery: a meta-analysis. *Interact Cardiovasc Thorac Surg.* 2016;23:31–40.
25. Saad FS, El Baradie SY, Abdel Aliem MAW, Ali MM, Kotb TAM. Ultrasound-guided serratus anterior plane block versus thoracic paravertebral block for perioperative analgesia in thoracotomy. *Saudi J Anaesth.* 2018;12:565–570.
26. Taketa Y, Irisawa Y, Fujitani T. Comparison of ultrasound-guided erector spinae plane block and thoracic paravertebral block for postoperative analgesia after video-assisted thoracic surgery: a randomized controlled non-inferiority clinical trial. *Reg Anesth Pain Med.* 2019; Nov 8:rapm-2019-100827. doi:10.1136/rapm-2019-100827 [Online ahead of print]
27. Bang S, Chung K, Chung J, Yoo S, Baek S, Lee SM. The erector spinae plane block for effective analgesia after lung lobectomy: Three cases report. *Medicine (Baltimore).* 2019;98(29):e16262.
28. Forero M, Adhikary SD, Lopez H, Tsui C, Chin KJ. The erector spinae plane block: a novel analgesic technique in thoracic neuropathic pain. *Reg Anesth Pain Med.* 2016;41:621–627.
29. Pipanmekaporn T, Punjasawadwong Y, Charuluxananan S, et al. The effectiveness of intravenous parecoxib on the incidence of ipsilateral shoulder pain after thoracotomy: a randomized, double-blind, placebo-controlled trial. *J Cardiothorac Vasc Anesth.* 2018;32:302–308.
30. Jiang WS, Wang LG, Zhang JG, et al. Effects of postoperative non-steroidal anti-inflammatory drugs on long-term survival and recurrence of patients with non-small cell lung cancer. *Medicine (Baltimore).* 2018;97(39):e12442. doi: 10.1097/MD.0000000000012442.
31. De Oliveira GS Jr, Castro-Alves LJ, Khan JH, McCarthy RJ. Perioperative systemic magnesium to minimize postoperative pain: a meta-analysis of randomized controlled trials. *Anesthesiology.* 2013;119:178–190.
32. Pehora C, Pearson AM, Kaushal A, Crawford MW, Johnston B. Dexamethasone as an adjuvant to peripheral nerve block. Cochrane Database Syst Rev 2017;11:CD011770.
33. Shafi S, Collinsworth AW, Copeland LA, et al. Association of opioid-related adverse drug events with clinical and cost outcomes among surgical patients in a large integrated health care delivery system. *JAMA Surg.* 2018;153:757–763.
34. Ware LB, Fremont RD, Bastarache JA, Calfee CS, Matthay MA. Determining the etiology of pulmonary edema by the edema fluid-to-plasma protein ratio. *Eur Respir J.* 2010;35:331–337.
35. Evans RG, Naidu B. Does a conservative fluid management strategy in the perioperative management of lung resection patients reduce the risk of acute lung injury. *Interact Cardiovasc Thorac Surg.* 2012;15:498–504
36. Onaitis M, D'Amico T, Zhao Y, O'Brien S, Harpole D. Risk factors for atrial fibrillation after lung cancer surgery: analysis of the Society of Thoracic Surgeons general thoracic surgery database. *Ann Thorac Surg.* 2010;90:368–374.
37. Frendl G, Sodickson AC, Chung MK, et al. 2014 AATS guidelines for the prevention and management of perioperative atrial fibrillation and flutter for thoracic surgical procedures. *J Thorac Cardiovasc Surg.* 2014;148:e153–193.
38. Gocyk W, Kużdzał J, Włodarczyk J, et al. Comparison of suction versus nonsuction drainage after lung resections: a prospective randomized trial. *Ann Thorac Surg.* 2016;102:1119–1124.

39. Motono N, Iwai S, Funasaki A, Sekimura A, Usuda K, Uramoto H. What is the allowed volume threshold for chest tube removal after lobectomy: a randomized controlled trial. *Ann Med Surg (Lond)*. 2019;43:29–32.
40. Kim KW, Lee JI, Kim JS, et al. Risk factors for urinary retention following minor thoracic surgery. *Interact Cardiovasc Thorac Surg*. 2015;20:486–492.
41. Egal M, de Geus HR, van Bommel J, Groeneveld AB. Targeting oliguria reversal in perioperative restrictive fluid management does not influence the occurrence of renal dysfunction: a systematic review and meta-analysis. *Eur J Anesthesiol*. 2016;33:425–435.
42. Li M, Zhang J, Gan TJ, et al. Enhanced recovery after surgery pathway for patients undergoing cardiac surgery: a randomized clinical trial. *Eur J Cardiothorac Surg*. 2018;54(3):491–497. doi:10.1093/ejcts/ezy100.
43. Scarci M, Solli P, Bedetti B. Enhanced recovery pathway for thoracic surgery in the UK. *J Thorac Dis*. 2016 Feb;8(Suppl 1):S78–S83. doi:10.3978/j.issn.2072-1439.2015.11.07

Index

Tables, figures, and boxes are indicated by *t*, *f*, and *b* following the page number.